Quick Reference to
Critical Care Nursing

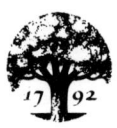

J.B. Lippincott Company Philadelphia

London   Mexico City   New York   St. Louis   São Paulo   Sydney

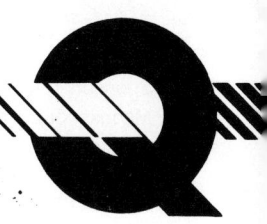

Quick Reference to

Critical Care Nursing

Betsy Jones Fletcher, R.N., B.A., M.Ed.

Artwork by Mary S. Jones

Sponsoring Editor: Jeanne H. Wallace
Manuscript Editor: Shirley Kuhn
Indexer: Julie Schwager
Art Director: Tracy Baldwin
Designer: William Boehm

Production Supervisor: N. Carol Kerr
Production Assistant: J. Corey Gray
Compositor: Hampton Graphics
Printer/Binder: R. R. Donnelly & Sons Company

6

Library of Congress Cataloging in Publication Data

Fletcher, Betsy Jones.
    Quick reference to critical care nursing.

    (Lippincott's quick references)
    Bibliography
    Includes index.
    1. Intensive care nursing. I. Title.
    RT120.I5F53   610.73'61   82-262
    ISBN 0-397-54367-0   AACR2

The author and publisher have exerted every effort to ensure that drug selection and dosage set forth in this text are in accord with current recommendations and practice at the time of publication. However, in view of ongoing research, changes in government regulations, and the constant flow of information relating to drug therapy and drug reactions, the reader is urged to check the package insert for each drug for any change in indications and dosage and for added warnings and precautions. This is particularly important when the recommended agent is a new or infrequently employed drug.

This information does not preclude the reader from administering medications under the supervision of the attending physician.

Nursing procedures outlined in the text should serve as guidelines only and do not preclude the reader from performing procedures according to individual institution's policies or from performing them under the supervision of the attending physician.

To the ones in my life who make the world just a bit better and brighter by being there—my mother and father, Mary and Carl Jones; my sister, Elinor Jones; my husband, Kent; my little ones, Brian and Kimberly; and the One who made it all possible

And in loving memory of my grandmothers, Lettie C. Smith and Annie P. Jones.

Contents

Preface

The fields of medicine and nursing are changing constantly, and an ever-increasing amount of new facts and technology is continually being added to the current body of knowledge. This is especially true in the area of critical care. It is imperative that the health professional keep abreast of these changes. *Quick Reference to Critical Care Nursing* was written with this objective in mind—to provide the most current information available in a readily accessible and easily understandable form.

The conditions and the procedures commonly associated with the care of the critically ill are covered in this text in an outline format designed for easy reference and quick comprehension. Different age groups are considered throughout where applicable. Conditions encountered frequently in the critical care setting are presented in depth, proceeding from the description, cause, and clinical manifestations of the condition to the appropriate diagnostic tests, treatment, and nursing actions. The detailed information on procedures includes equipment lists, complications, actions for assisting with the procedure, and general nursing care. Procedural problem solving is emphasized in discussions of specific problems and appropriate nursing actions. Pertinent "helpful hints" and items of crucial interest are found throughout and are specially designed for emphasis. Diagrams are included when needed for clarification.

Heavy emphasis is placed on the cardiac arrhythmias. Detailed descriptions and ECG patterns are presented in Chapter 4, which is devoted to commonly seen arrhythmias. One feature of this chapter is an innovative table for determining arrhythmias from description.

A number of useful features are provided. Frequently used emergency drugs are presented alphabetically for ready reference. Dosages and methods for obtaining the desired concentration of drugs, as well as special requirements for adults, children, and maternity patients, are covered. A review of normal and abnormal vital signs for all age groups includes sophisticated criteria required in critical care nursing in addition to the significance of abnormal findings. Conversion tables, several methods for calculating the heart rate, and laboratory values most commonly used in critical care are provided in an appendix.

My desire in writing this book was to fill a felt need for an up-to-date, compact reference that would present complicated information clearly and concisely—one that would be a valuable tool for nurses in many health-care settings, and also for students engaged in the study of critical care nursing.

Care of the critically ill patient is both an art and a science. Even as we master the sophisticated technology associated with critical care, it is imperative that the entire health-care team remember that a human being, a very vulnerable one at that, is the object of all the attention and is literally dependent on us for life in many situations.

We owe them all, even the most "hopeless," the best that we have to give—our love, compassion, and dedication.

Betsy Jones Fletcher, R.N., B.A., M.Ed.

Acknowledgments

I would like to extend my deepest appreciation to the following people for their help in making *Quick Reference to Critical Care Nursing* possible:

James LeFevre, Sales Representative for J. B. Lippincott, expressed an interest in my ideas for a book for my students and thus started it all.

Diana Intenzo, Executive Editor for J. B. Lippincott, gave me the opportunity to write this book. She also provided expert guidance, supervision, a personal interest in my endeavors, and a delightful working relationship.

Jeanne Wallace, Associate Editor for J. B. Lippincott, offered her expert and very helpful editorial skills, graciously worked around my schedule without complaint, and offered a personal interest in *Quick Reference to Critical Care Nursing.*

Shirley Kuhn, Manuscript Editor for J. B. Lippincott, cheerfully worked closely with me on all the fine details of *Quick Reference to Critical Care Nursing.*

Marie Robeson, R.N., B.N.Ed., M.A., Director of Nursing, Durham County General Hospital, Durham, North Carolina, provided a friendly interest and helped facilitate my use of the clinical facilities at Durham County General Hospital.

Beverly Smith, R.N., B.S.N., M.Ed., Director of Nursing Education, Watts School of Nursing, Durham County General Hospital, gave me permission to use the school library and offered her interest and encouragement throughout my tenure as a faculty member.

Priscilla Hoover, B.A., M.L.S., Librarian, Watts School of Nursing, Durham County General Hospital, allowed me very liberal use of the library facilities and encouraged me to write this book.

Betty Faulkner, R.N., B.S.N., M.S.N., Instructor in Nursing, Watts School of Nursing, cheerfully offered me constant encouragement and suggestions, and was always available to answer my questions and share her reference books.

Ginnie (Virginia) Ingram, R.N., B.S.N., formerly Instructor in Nursing, Watts School of Nursing, offered her encouragement and suggestions, and shared her clinical expertise.

Gail Rigsbee, R.N., Head Nurse, Coronary Intensive Care Unit, Durham County General Hospital, always took the time to answer my questions and shared her reference material.

J. Kenneth Powell, Jr., R.R.T., Director of Respiratory Therapy, Durham County General Hospital, provided information concerning current practices in an ever-changing field.

Greta Brooks, R.N., B.S.N., Assistant to the Director of Nursing Education, Watts School of Nursing, offered pertinent suggestions and information.

The nursing supervisors of the various clinical areas at Durham County General Hospital, especially Doris Baldwin, Marguerite Hilliard, and Kyle Howard, allowed me to do clinical research in their areas as my schedule allowed.

The nurses at Durham County General Hospital, especially Kay Parker and Clara Sharpe, took the time to fill out a questionnaire or to discuss with me their thoughts concerning the contents that they would like to see in a book of this nature.

Elinor Jones, B.S., M.Ed., not only worked diligently to type the majority of the manuscript but offered her editorial skills as well.

Polly Haugland cheerfully offered her expert typing skills at a most propitious time.

Mary S. Jones, professional artist, worked long and hard to prepare the artwork.

And most especially I thank my family, who offered their love, support, and encouragement, and gave their time freely to help in any way—my husband, Kent; my parents, Carl and Mary Jones; my sister, Elinor Jones; my mother-in-law and father-in-law, Margaret and J. D. Fletcher; and last but certainly not least, my little ones, Brian and Kimberly, who were extraordinarily patient while Mommie worked on the book.

Cardiovascular Nursing

1

Myocardial Infarction

The most common condition seen in the intensive coronary unit is presented in this chapter. Nursing considerations are discussed in detail.

Description

Myocardial infarction (MI) is defined as acute local necrosis (tissue death) of the myocardium, resulting from insufficient blood supply through the coronary arteries and associated oxygen deficiency.

Synonyms

• Heart attack
• Coronary
• Coronary thrombosis
• Coronary occlusion

Causes

Obstruction (occlusion) of a coronary artery due to the following:
• Atherosclerosis
• Embolism
• Collagen diseases

Decrease in coronary blood flow due to causes other than obstruction of a coronary vessel, for example:
• Myocardial hypertrophy seen in congestive heart failure and hypertension
• Shock
• Hypotension
• Hemorrhage
• Sudden, extreme physical activity
• Severe dehydration

Clinical Manifestations

"Classical" Myocardial Infarction

Chest pain
• Severe quality

- Usually located in the substernal region
- May radiate across the chest, involve either arm and shoulder, throat, jaw, or teeth
- Usually occurs suddenly but may build over a period of hours
- Continuous
- Not necessarily associated with physical activity
- Described as crushing, viselike, heavy weight, ache, knot in chest, or feeling of bursting
- Unaffected by rest or by administration of nitroglycerin tablets or over-the-counter medications such as antacids

Profuse sweating

Nausea and vomiting

Dyspnea

Apprehension

Weakness

Atypical Situations

Serious complications that overshadow the situation immediately following infarction include life-threatening arrhythmias, sudden collapse or death of the patient, and cardiogenic shock.

Referred pain as the presenting complaint may be located in the lower jaw, one or both arms, or both sides of chest or neck. (Classical symptoms may not be present.)

Silent infarction is said to occur when none of the symptoms are present, or when the patient denies any knowledge of same. Evidence of "old" infarction is detected sometime later on a routine ECG.

Diagnostic Tests

Characteristic ECG Changes

ECG changes specific to infarction comprise a triad of electrical events—ST-segment elevation, T-wave inversion, and significant Q wave. Characteristics of the triad and the order in which they occur are as follows.

ST-Segment Elevation

Significance: Recent, acute injury

Time Sequence: Minutes to hours after infarction

Accuracy: Changes are generally due to MI but not specifically. A diagnosis of MI may be made if characteristic pattern develops and enzyme abnormalities occur over a period of days. This test returns to normal days to weeks later.

T-Wave Inversion

Significance: Myocardial ischemia

Time sequence: Hours to days after infarction

Accuracy: This is not very specific for MI. This change is seen in many other conditions. A diagnosis of MI should not be made if this is the only change detected. This test returns to normal weeks to months later.

Significant (Pathologic) Q Wave

"Significant" is described as over 0.04 seconds wide or greater in depth than 1/3 the height of the QRS complex.

Significance: Necrosis (infarction) has occurred

Time sequence: Hours to days after infarction

Accuracy: This is more specific than the other two changes. Since necrosis is indicated, a diagnosis of MI may be made even without enzyme changes. Age of infarction is not indicated. This characteristic may or may not return to normal.

NOTE. Initially, the ECG may not indicate the presence of an infarction. To establish documentation of an MI, additional ECGs (serial) will be taken over a period of several days. Characteristic ECG changes may never be documented in patients whose hearts are in abnormal positions or those with abnormally shaped chests. Small infarctions may not be detected on the ECG. ECG changes may be so transient that they will not be documented on routine tracings. The patient's history, physical exam, and signs and symptoms must be relied upon in these cases. Specifically, the infarction site corresponds to the particular coronary artery or arteries affected. The location is indicated by the ECG changes specific for the area. The left ventricle is most often affected because of its heavier workload.

Serum Enzymes in Myocardial Infarction

Enzymes are proteins that function as cellular regulators of the cell's metabolism and chemical activity. When the cell membrane is destroyed, as in infarction, these enzymes are released into the blood, resulting in increased serum enzyme levels. Particular enzymes are specific for different types of cells. The cardiac enzymes are creatine phosphokinase (CPK), serum glutamic-oxaloacetic transaminase (SGOT), lactic dehydrogenase (LDH), and hydroxybutyric dehydrogenase (HBD).

Creatine Phosphokinase (CPK)

Normal value: Female—2–49 IU/L
  Male—2–83 IU/L

Elevation in MI: CPK level increases within 4 to 9 hours after infarction. Peak value occurs during first 24 hours. This returns to normal by the fourth or fifth day.

Other factors that cause elevation: CPK level is elevated in patients with brain damage and musculoskeletal diseases or injuries (including IM injections).

Serum Glutamic Oxaloacetic Transaminase (SGOT)

Normal value: 7–26 IU/L

Elevation in MI: SGOT level increases within 8 to 12 hours after infarction.

It reaches a peak in 24 hours and usually returns to normal after 4 to 5 days.

Other factors that cause elevation: Elevation occurs in patients with acute pericarditis, congestive heart failure, coronary insufficiency, and hepato-cellular disease.

Serum Lactic Dehydrogenase (LDH)
Normal value: 52–149 IU/L

Elevation in MI: The level increases within 12 to 24 hours postinfarction. It reaches a peak in 72 hours. It usually returns to normal 10 days later.

Other factors that cause elevation: Elevation occurs in a variety of muscular, renal, neoplastic, hepatic, and hemolytic disases, as well as in a number of pulmonary conditions simulating MI.

Hydroxybutyric Dehydrogenase (HBD)
Normal value: 50–250 IU/L

Elevation in MI: Elevation increases within 12 to 24 hours after infarction. Peak value occurs within 72 hours. It usually returns to normal 10 days later.

Other factors that cause elevation: HBD is also elevated in patients with liver disease, neoplasms, muscular dystrophy, and musculoskeletal injury.

Isoenzymes in Myocardial Infarction

Lactic dehydrogenase (LDH) isoenzymes and creatine phosphokinase (CPK) isoenzymes obtained by electrophoresis that prove to be even more specific for infarction have also been identified. (Isoenzymes are separate molecular structures of an enzyme.)

LDH_1 and LDH_2
Normal value: LDH_1 is less than LDH_2. (LDH_1 = 17%–32%, LDH_2 = 23%–36%)

Elevation in MI: LDH_1 is greater than LDH_2 or LDH_1 almost equals LDH_2, with both isoenzymes significantly elevated in 12 to 24 hours. Although variable, it usually returns to normal in less than 7 days.

Other factors that cause elevation: Rarely, other conditions which are easy to differentiate from an MI may cause this type of elevation (*e.g.*, renal infarction).

CPK–MB (CPK_2)
Normal value: 0

Elevation in MI: Elevation increases within 4 to 8 hours after infarction. It reaches a peak within 24 hours and usually returns to normal within 3 days.

Other factors that cause elevation: CPK–MB is specific for the myocardium, especially MI.

NOTE. Normal values may vary with different laboratory determinations.

White Blood Cell Count (WBC)

This is generally elevated the first day following infarction and remains elevated for 5 to 7 days. The extent of the elevation indicates the severity of infarction. Levels over 15,000 leukocytes per cubic millimeter suggest other complications.

Erythrocyte Sedimentation Rate (ESR)

This becomes elevated, but on a slower scale than the WBC, and remains elevated for several weeks following infarction.

Nuclear Imaging

Isotopes technetium pyrophosphate or diphosphonate are injected intravenously. The isotope accumulates in the cells of new infarctions or ischemic myocardium. "Hot spot" scanning is done to pick up MI. Because this test is still under development, its specificity is still undetermined.

Treatment and Nursing Actions

Monitor the Heart

1. Explain what you are doing and describe function of equipment to the patient.
2. Attach patient to monitor.
3. Run a rhythm strip to establish a baseline, and use for comparison.
4. Watch closely to detect arrhythmias, recording and documenting any abnormality.
5. Treat arrhythmias according to physician's orders or standing orders (see Arrhythmias).

Monitor and Record Vital Signs

1. Check apical and radial pulses, respirations, temperature, and blood pressure per unit routine, physician's order, or as indicated.
   - If unstable, vital signs may be monitored every 15 minutes or less.
   - If stable and patient appears to be in no distress or is not exhibiting signs of complications, may be monitored every 2 to 4 hours.
2. Once again, explain what you are doing. Fear and apprehension can adversely affect vital signs (*i.e.,* may cause significant rise in vital signs).
3. Be alert for abnormal vital signs and treat accordingly.
   Temperature
   - Temperature is usually elevated after first 24 hours.
   - Generally, elevation is around 37.8°C to 38.3°C (100–101°F) or more and lasts for 2 to 3 days, returning to normal by the fifth day.
   - Abnormally high temperatures suggest other complications (*i.e.,* systemic infection, pulmonary infarction, pneumonia, thrombophlebitis).

- Avoid taking temperatures rectally because slowing of the heart and arrhythmias may occur in response to vagal stimulation.

Pulse
- Count pulse for a full minute to check for presence of abnormality.
- An irregular pulse may precede a life-threatening arrhythmia.
- A ventricular gallop (S_3 gallop—heard after the second heart sound) or gallop rhythm may indicate acute left ventricular failure.
- An elevated pulse may suggest cardiogenic shock.

Respirations
- Rales heard in bases of the lungs may indicate acute left ventricular failure.
- Frothy sputum that may be blood-tinged and gurgling respirations are indicative of acute pulmonary edema.

Blood pressure
- A drop in blood pressure and narrowed pulse pressure may indicate cardiogenic shock.

Hemodynamic Monitoring (central venous pressure [CVP], Swan–Ganz catheter, arterial line)

This type of monitoring may be indicated, especially in the presence of complications (*i.e.,* acute left ventricular failure and cardiogenic shock).
1. Prepare for and assist physician with insertion of devices.
2. Follow hospital routine for taking readings, changing tubing, changing the dressing, and cleaning the site.

Provide Comfort Measures
1. Administer pain medication as prescribed, usually morphine sulfate or meperidine hydrochloride (Demerol). Analgesics may affect vital signs adversely.
2. Administer oxygen to relieve pain due to hypoxia.

NOTE. Keep in mind that severe pain may precede arrhythmias and shock.

3. Administer hypnotics, sedatives, or tranquilizers as ordered to promote rest and lessen fear and apprehension.
4. Remove tight clothing and dress patient in patient gown.
5. Assist with finding position of comfort.
6. Provide basic patient care as the condition permits.
   - A complete bed bath may tire the patient. Postpone bathing until condition stabilizes, or sponge bathe if it is warranted or requested.
   - Basic care should be done at patient's convenience. Most people are accustomed to bathing at a certain time and feel more comfortable with this regimen.
   - Frequent mouth care is essential for all patients.

Promote Cardiac Rest

1. Encourage rest to reduce the work of the myocardium. The method of rest is generally one of the following or a combination of the two:
   - Complete bed rest is the most popular method prescribed during the acute stage. Placing the patient in semi-Fowler's position is recommended because it aids ventilation and increases expansion of the lungs by naturally lowering the diaphragm. If the patient is stable, chair rest may be permitted after 3 or 4 days.
   - Chair rest is another method that may be prescribed starting the day after infarction. A chair with a straight backrest should be placed beside the bed and the patient assisted into it. The amount of time sitting in the chair is increased gradually and is gauged by the patient's tolerance or fatigue. This method is thought to be less strenuous on the heart than complete bed rest. Some contraindications are severe hypotension, presence of shock, and administration of narcotics for severe pain which may cause a slow heart rate.

2. Take precautions to prevent thromboembolism—a complication of bed rest.

3. Keep in mind that the critically ill patient should not be expected to perform the strenuous activity of moving from stretcher to bed.

4. When changing the patient's position in bed, remind him to breathe normally rather than hold his breath. Breath holding induces the Valsalva maneuver, which may cause death due to reflex bradycardia.

   NOTE. Valsalva maneuver may also occur during vomiting, gagging, straining at stool or urination, and during bouts of severe coughing.

5. Assist the patient in using the bedside commode.
   - This method is generally considered less strenuous than using the bedpan.
   - Male patients may be allowed to stand or sit on the side of the bed with assistance to use the urinal.
   - Method used (*i.e.*, bedside commode or bedpan) depends on doctor's order and patient's condition.

6. The patient may be allowed to perform some routine activities, depending on his condition and the physician's orders.
   - Brush teeth
   - Comb hair
   - Wash face, hands, and genital area
   - Feed himself

7. Passive exercises, especially of the lower extremities, should be encouraged and performed by the nurse, if necessary.

   NOTE. If the patient complains of chest pain or dyspnea on exertion, or if any undesirable ECG changes occur during these periods of activity, the activity should be curtailed, documented, and reported to the physician.

Promote Proper Elimination

1. Administer stool softeners as ordered to encourage bowel movements.
2. Caution patient not to strain at stool or urination. (See note listed under Promote Cardiac Rest.)
3. Avoid enemas which may cause vagal stimulation. (See Temperature listed under Monitor and Record Vital Signs.)
4. Monitor patient's output, both feces and urine (may be on hourly urine measurements and specific gravity checks).
5. Be alert for abnormal signs.
   • Oliguria or anuria may be indicative of cardiogenic shock.
   • High specific gravity or concentrated urine may indicate dehydration.
6. Administer diuretics as ordered to maintain urine output of over 30 ml/hr.

Promote Proper Nutrition

1. A liquid diet is usually ordered initially, until the nausea and vomiting have subsided. It is easier to digest and also lessens the danger of aspiration should cardiac arrest occur.
2. Avoid beverages containing caffeine (*i.e.*, tea, coffee, and some carbonated drinks), and hot or cold beverages, which may affect the heart rate and rhythm.
3. The type of diet ordered following full liquids will depend on the patient's condition and the physician's preference.
4. A lower intake of salt is recommended.

NOTE. Not all patients can use the salt substitutes because of the large amount of potassium involved. Check with the physician before administering.

5. Intravenous solutions are administered to the patient who is critically ill and unable to eat.
6. Monitor the fluid intake closely, whether oral or intravenous, to detect or prevent overload of the circulatory system and subsequent complications (*i.e.*, congestive heart failure.)

Provide Emotional Support

1. The post MI patient is very apprehensive. Reassure him that he has passed the most dangerous stage and that he is being closely watched to prevent or control any complications that may occur.
2. Explain nursing care and procedures and encourage other health team members to do the same.
3. Encourage patient to vent feelings.
4. Be optimistic, avoiding both overly positive or negative remarks.
5. Encourage family participation in patient care. Remember that the family's emotional needs may be just as great as the patient's. (This would depend on patient's approval and condition.)

6. Avoid sensory overload or deprivation.
   - Sensory overload—avoid excess noise; organize nursing care to prevent constant interruptions of rest.
   - Sensory deprivation—talk to patient regarding everyday happenings, his interests, and his family; encourage family participation in care; provide diversion, such as books, magazines, radio, or TV (if not contraindicated).
7. Contact pastor, rabbi, priest, or chaplain as requested.

Administer Oxygen Therapy as Ordered

1. Use oxygen therapy with extreme caution in patients whose history is unknown. High concentrations of oxygen administered to a patient with chronic respiratory insufficiency will result in the patient "pinking up" initially, followed by hypoventilation, stupor, coma, apnea, and death (*i.e.*, CO_2 narcosis).
2. Check frequently to see if oxygen therapy is effective.
   - Oxygen helps relieve cardiac pain, cyanosis, and dyspnea.
3. Enforce safety precautions.
4. Monitor arterial blood gases closely and report as indicated.
   - Maintain satisfactory pO_2 to prevent complications (*i.e.*, CO_2 narcosis or oxygen toxicity).

Obtain a Thorough History

1. Obtain history from patient, family or significant other. This is vital information and may be as important and possibly as life-saving as the treatment for the MI.
2. Secure the old chart if at all possible.
3. Determine medications or treatments used prior to admission and check to see if patient has any of the following problems:
   - Is patient diabetic and taking insulin,
   - Is patient epileptic and taking Dilantin,
   - Is patient an alcoholic,
   - Is patient a drug abuser,
   - Does patient have any allergies (Chart and medication sheets should be flagged appropriately.),
   - Does patient have glaucoma,
   - Does patient have symptoms of urinary obstruction,
   - Does patient have a chronic respiratory disease and use any special treatment for it (*e.g.* nebulizer)?

Obtain an Emergency Drug Route

1. Start an IV to provide a direct line to venous circulation for emergency administration of drugs. Heparin locks or wells are also being used.
2. Use special precautions in preventing phlebitis (aseptic insertion technique and dressing change).
   - Use upper extremity veins.
   - If the patient is paralyzed, start the IV on the unaffected side if possible.

- Follow hospital routine for changing tubing, adaptor, and dressing, and cleaning the site (usually every 24 hrs).

Have Emergency Equipment and Drugs Available to Treat Complications
1. Keep "crash cart" nearby and well stocked.
2. Have easy access to a defibrillator and suction apparatus.

Prepare for Transfer from the Coronary Care Unit (CCU)
at Appropriate Time
1. After the acute stage, and if there are no serious complications, the patient may be transferred to another critical care area generally referred to as a progressive care unit where his progress in rehabilitation and ambulation will be closely monitored.
   - Explain to the patient that he will be closely monitored by telemetry.
   - A nurse from the progressive care unit should visit the patient and family prior to the move.
   - Stress to the patient that this area is an extension of the CCU and that the staff is well trained.
   - To prevent or lessen feelings of fear and abandonment, nurses from the CCU should periodically visit the patient and check on his progress.
2. Hemodynamic monitoring is discontinued prior to transfer.
3. Although most of the patient's needs remain unchanged after the transfer to the progressive care unit, some significant changes include the following:
   - Patient will be monitored by telemetry.
   - A highly individualized progressive program of rehabilitation is instituted according to the patient's condition and physician's orders (*e.g.*, over a period of several days the patient may gradually progress to bathing or perhaps showering himself). The heart should be closely monitored during periods of activity to see how the patient tolerates the activity. Any abnormality should be recorded, documented, and reported if necessary.
   - The patient is out of the confines of the CCU and placed in a regular hospital room, which may lift the spirits of some patients, depress some patients who fear they will not be closely watched, or provide false security for others (*i.e.*, the patient tends to overdo.)
   - The IV is usually converted to a heparin lock for an emergency drug route.

Be Prepared for Possible Complications
Keep in mind that complications may occur at any time—during the acute, subacute, or convalescent stages.
- Emergency equipment and drugs should be easily accessible.
- Listen closely to the patient's complaints. Many times the patient will "sense" impending danger and convey these feelings to family or staff.

2
Complications Related to Myocardial Infarction

It should be noted that many of the cardiac conditions discussed in this chapter can and do occur independently of myocardial infarction, although they are discussed here chiefly as complications of MI. Arrhythmias, a major complication, are described in detail in Chapter 4. Congestive heart failure, thromboembolic events, ventricular aneurysm, ventricular rupture, pericarditis, recurrent MI, papillary muscle rupture, Dressler's syndrome, and shoulder–hand syndrome are considered in this chapter.

CONGESTIVE HEART FAILURE

Description

Congestive heart failure (CHF) is an inability of the heart, for any reason, to maintain an adequate cardiac output to meet metabolic demands which can occur when the cardiac output is normal, decreased, or increased. This causes congestion in the systemic circulation (referred to as right-sided heart failure) or pulmonary circulation (referred to as left-sided heart failure), or both.

Congestive Heart Failure Terminology

Other terms used to describe CHF include
- *Backward failure*—excessive buildup of pressure in the venous system and heart
- *Forward failure*—poor cardiac output
- *High-output failure*—when peripheral demands exceed the heart's capacity to perfuse the tissues
- *Low-output failure*—when the heart muscle is unable to pump adequately to perfuse the tissues, even when the tissue demands are normal

Causes

Diseases of the myocardium (*e.g.*, MI)

Infections (*i.e.* subacute bacterial endocarditis)

Hypertension

Pregnancy

Hemorrhage and anemia

Transfusions

Infusions

Arrhythmias (bradycardia or tachycardia)

Hyperthyroidism

Excessive intake of sodium

Ruptured chordae tendineae causing acute mitral valve regurgitation

Congenital heart anomalies

Surgery and anesthesia

Clinical Manifestations

Symptoms will depend on the side of the heart affected. Generally, there is a combination of symptoms (*i.e.*, symptoms showing right-sided and left-sided heart failure).

Left-sided heart failure is more common because myocardial infarction usually affects the left ventricle.

Right-sided heart failure generally occurs as a sequel to left-sided heart failure.

Left-sided Heart Failure

This is related to pulmonary circulation and generally means left ventricular failure. The following are symptoms of left-sided heart failure:

- Dyspnea—the most common clinical manifestation and the earliest to appear as a consequence of left ventricular failure and resulting pulmonary engorgement; initially, may be apparent only on exertion but eventually progresses to dyspnea at rest
- Paroxysmal nocturnal dyspnea (cardiac asthma)—sudden onset of dyspnea and general respiratory distress, occurring 1 to 2 hours after patient goes to sleep
- Orthopnea
- Cough which may be unproductive
- Fatigue
- Restlessness—seen more commonly in elderly patients
- Acute pulmonary edema—most advanced stage of acute left heart failure
- Rales—A classical sign initially found at the bases of the lungs but progress upward as left heart failure continues
- Gallop rhythm a classical sign, ventricular gallop or S_3 gallop. (Atrial gallop or S_4 gallop may sometimes occur in the absence of ventricular failure.)
- Tachycardia
- Hypotension
- Sweating

Right-sided Heart Failure

This generally means right ventricular failure. The following are symptoms of right-sided heart failure:

- Peripheral edema—Generalized peripheral edema (anasarca) is rare; edema found in feet and legs (ambulatory patient); edema found on back, especially the sacral area (patients on bed rest)
- Enlarged liver and upper abdominal pain due to congested liver
- Positive hepatojugular reflux—elicited by exerting pressure over the right upper quadrant of the abdomen; pressure increases amount of blood re-

turning to the heart, venous pressure rises, and neck veins become distended because the failing right heart is unable to handle this excess blood flow

- Weight gain—caused by peripheral edema, whether mild (1+) or severe (4+).
- Nausea and loss of appetite—caused by enlarged liver and edema of the bowel
- Distended neck veins in a semi-upright position (45° angle)—indicate increase in venous pressure in superior vena cava; one of the earliest signs of right heart failure
- Pleural effusion due to edema fluid in pleural cavity—detected by diminished or absent breath sounds or lung auscultation
- Nocturia
- General weakness
- Sweating
- Ascites

Treatment and Nursing Actions

1. Administer prescribed drugs.
   Digitalis preparations
   - One of the digitalis preparations is used to support left ventricular function.
   - The drug is usually administered intravenously.
   - May be given orally in right-sided heart failure because this is not usually an emergency
   Rapid-acting diuretics
   - Lasix or Edecrin is used to aid in reducing blood volume.
   - The drug is usually administered intravenously (may be given orally in right-sided heart failure).
   - Closely monitor intake and output.
   - Watch closely for signs of bladder distention.
   - Indwelling catheter should be inserted after administration of these drugs.
2. Institute rotating tourniquets.
   Rotating tourniquets further reduce the amount of blood returning to the heart.

NOTE. Phlebotomy (removal of blood) is sometimes instituted.

3. Administer oxygen therapy.
   A face mask is a most desirable method because it delivers a high concentration of oxygen.
   Oxygen administered by positive pressure devices is necessary for the critically ill patient.
   Closely monitor arterial blood gases.
   - Report to physician if results are above or below set rate.
4. Monitor vital signs closely.
   - Report to physician if readings are above or below set rate.
   - Neurologic checks should also be performed.

- Check pulses.
- Check heart and breath sounds.

5. Monitor ECG continuously.
   - Observe closely for arrhythmias.
   - Notify physician of occurrence of arrhythmias.
   - Treat condition accordingly.
6. Monitor arterial, central, venous, and pulmonary artery pressures.
   - Report to physician if readings are above or below set rate.
7. Start an IV or ensure the patency of IV in place
   - Most drug therapy is administered intravenously.
   - An emergency venous access route is necessary.
8. Encourage rest to lessen cardiac demands.
   - As condition improves, activity will be gradually increased, with patient response closely monitored.
9. Promote comfort.
   Assist patient to comfortable position.
   - Semi-Fowler's position is usually most comfortable because it aids in lessening blood flow to the heart and in preventing pulmonary congestion.
10. Provide support for emotional needs.
    - Answer patient's questions.
    - Explain activities (*i.e.*, vital sign checks, administration of medications).
11. Assist patient to bedside commode for bowel movements.
    - Using the bedside commode is not as strenuous as using the bedpan.
    - Caution not to strain at stool.
12. Promote adequate nutrition.
    - Diet is usually low sodium.
    - Fluids are generally restricted, but any fluid intake should be monitored closely.
    - Weigh patient daily.
13. Provide special care when needed.
    - Intra-aortic balloon pump may be used to support the left ventricle in the acutely ill patient.
    - Monitor closely.

THROMBOEMBOLIC EVENTS

There are three forms of thromboembolic events commonly associated with MI—pulmonary, peripheral, and cerebral. Pulmonary embolism occurs most frequently and is described in detail in Chapter 10. Peripheral thromboembolism and cerebral thromboembolism are discussed in this chapter.

PERIPHERAL THROMBOEMBOLIC EVENTS

Cause

- Peripheral emboli generally occur as a result of clots (*i.e.*, mural thrombi) within the left side of the heart, usually with involvement of the iliac or femoral arteries.

Clinical Manifestations

Sudden onset of numbness, pallor, and coldness in the affected extremity

Pain in the affected extremity

No arterial pulses in the extremity

Involvement of both extremities if the embolus is located at the bifurcation of the aorta

Treatment

Possible embolectomy

Anticoagulant therapy

Prevention

- Encourage passive or active exercises and movement of feet and legs as the condition warrants and as ordered. A footboard would be valuable.
- Avoid placing any pressure behind the knee, from improperly fitted elastic hose or bandages, gatching the foot of the bed too severely, or placing pillows under the knee.
- Patient should use properly fitted anti-embolic hose that extend well above the knee.
- Proper hydration is needed to prevent increased viscosity of blood.
- Administer anticoagulant therapy prophylactically.
- Caution patient not to strain at stool.
- Increase level of activity gradually and monitor effects closely.

CEREBRAL THROMBOEMBOLIC EVENTS

Cause

- Cerebral emboli generally occur as a result of mural thrombi.

Clinical Manifestations

Sudden cerebrovascular accident (CVA)
- Patient may present with symptoms of CVA, of which the underlying cause is an MI that is possibly going undetected.
- Patient presents with symptoms of an MI, and suddenly shows symptoms of a CVA.

Speech disturbances

Motor weakness

Paralysis

Loss of consciousness

NOTE. Clinical manifestations depend on the area affected.

Treatment

- Possible embolectomy
- Anticoagulant therapy

Prevention

See Prevention of Peripheral Thromboembolic Events, p 17.

VENTRICULAR ANEURYSM

Description

Ventricular aneurysm may occur following myocardial infarction when a full thickness of the ventricular wall is affected by infarction. Congestive heart failure and cardiac enlargement are frequently present. These aneurysms rarely rupture. They occur in fewer than 25% of patients.

Clinical Manifestations

Third and fourth heart sounds are present.

ECG shows old MI; large Q waves and ST-segment elevation (more pronounced with exercise) in affected leads may be present.

Systolic expansion is visible and palpable in anterior chest wall.

Double apical pulse may be auscultated due to paradoxical movement.

Emboli occur systemically.

Cardiac failure and arrhythmias do not respond to treatment but persist.

Diagnostic Tests

Chest x-ray film—the rounded bulge of the aneurysm may be visible

Cineventriculography—the paradoxical movement of the aneurysm is detected

Treatment

• May be removed surgically if symptoms demand

VENTRICULAR RUPTURE

Description

Ventricular rupture is a rupture or perforation of the myocardium, generally within 10 days following MI. It is usually the result of an extensive transmural infarction. Rupture may occur in the interventricular septum or outer wall of the ventricles. Of the major complications, it is the least common and one of the most deadly.

Causes

The exact cause of ventricular rupture is uncertain; however, there are some unproven theories (*i.e.*, physical activity, anticoagulant therapy). It has been found to occur more frequently in women than in men.

Clinical Manifestations

Rupture of outer wall of the ventricle
• Usually sudden death, although patient may survive for an hour; death appears to be caused by an arrhythmia.
• Recurrent chest pain prior to rupture
• Sudden hypotension
• Sudden unexplained slowing of heart rate

NOTE. Electrical activity of the heart may be noted on the monitor for several minutes or longer, following ventricular rupture (Inherent electrical activity continues for a short time even though the ventricules do not respond by contracting.)

Rupture of the interventricular septum
• Sudden right heart failure (caused by communication between right and left ventricles)
• Sudden development of loud systolic murmur
• Does not always result in immediate death, but prognosis is poor

Diagnostic Tests

ECG—may show electrical activity (sinus rhythm), although no pulse or blood pressure is detected

Insertion of Swan-Ganz catheter into the right side of the heart—shows increased oxygen saturation in the right heart.

Pericardiocentesis—diagnosis by needle aspiration of blood

Treatment and Nursing Actions

1. If sudden death occurs, begin cardiopulmonary resuscitation (CPR) immediately. Rule out other causes of sudden death (*i.e.*, ventricular fibrillation or standstill).

   ALERT. Notify the physician immediately, as surgical repair may be possible with an interventricular rupture.

2. Prepare equipment for Swan–Ganz catheter insertion.
3. Prepare equipment for pericardiocentesis.
4. Prepare for surgery. If the patient is too acutely ill to undergo surgery, the intra-aortic balloon may be used to temporarily maintain the patient until surgical repair is possible.
5. Prepare for insertion of intra–aortic balloon.
6. Monitor vital signs, ECG, and arterial blood gases.
7. Start intravenous therapy—to establish a line for emergency drugs and blood transfusions (patient should be typed and cross-matched.)
8. Treat symptoms of cardiogenic shock.

Prevention

• Encourage bed rest during the acute phase of an MI.
• Caution patient not to strain at stool; administer laxatives or stool softeners; allow patient to use bedside commode for defecation.
• If hypertension is present, treat and control with antihypertensive medications.

PERICARDITIS

Description

Pericarditis is an inflammation of the pericardium. Pericarditis associated with MI generally occurs a day or two after MI and is seen in fewer than 25% of these patients.

Causes

Nonspecific causes

Trauma (including surgical trauma)

Neoplastic processes

Myocardial infarction

Collagen diseases and allergies

Infections (viral, bacterial [*e.g.*, TB], fungal)

Drugs

Clinical Manifestations

Chest pain increases with swallowing, deep breathing, or lying flat.

Transient pericardial rub may be detected (generally lasts minutes–hours only).

Chest pain is usually relieved by leaning forward.

NOTE. ECG changes—ST-segment elevation

Treatment

Relieve pain.
• Provide bed rest.
• Place patient in comfortable position (usually with head elevated).
• Administer medication as prescribed for pain.

Discontinue anticoagulants unless contraindicated.
• Tamponade is a potential problem with hemorrhagic pericarditis.

RECURRENT MI

Clinical Manifestations

(See pp 3–4.)

Treatment

(See pp 7–12.)

Prevention

Proper diet

Prescribed exercise, especially brisk walking (the best exercise for improving collateral circulation)

Control of underlying cardiac conditions (*i.e.*, hypertension)

Prevention of physical and emotional stress

NOTE. The use of anticoagulants (warfarin or Coumadin) is thought to aid in the prevention of recurrent MI; however, this is controversial.

RUPTURE OF PAPILLARY MUSCLE

Description

Papillary muscle rupture occurs as a complication of MI in a small number of patients.

NOTE. Papillary muscle malfunction during the first few days following **MI** is common; it causes transient mitral systolic murmurs.

Clinical Manifestations

Severe cardiac failure

Loud systolic murmur with thrill located internal to the apex of the heart

Treatment

Surgical repair (mitral valve repair) may be necessary.

Prognosis is poor, death ensuing within hours or days following rupture.

The intra-aortic balloon may temporarily maintain the patient until surgery is performed.

DRESSLER'S SYNDROME (POSTMYOCARDIAL INFARCTION SYNDROME)

Dressler's syndrome occurs in a small percentage of patients following MI, generally in 1 to 6 weeks.

Cause

Cause is linked to autoimmune reaction to myocardial damage.

Clinical Manifestations

Pericardial or pleural pain

Malaise

Pyrexia

Treatment

Anticoagulants are contraindicated because they may cause hemopericardium

In severe cases, indomethacin or corticosteroids are indicated.

In minor cases, the syndrome resolves quickly.

SHOULDER–HAND SYNDROME

Description

This residual effect occurs in a small number of patients; the specific cause is unknown.

Clinical Manifestations

Shoulder joint, generally the left one, has limited movement.

Arm is stiff and painful.

Hand may be swollen with skin shiny and tense.

Treatment

1. Physical therapy
2. May possibly be prevented by passive exercises

3
Electrocardiography

Cardiac monitoring is obtained by attaching electrodes to the skin to detect the electrical stimulus transmitted from the heart that causes the heart to beat. This electrical stimulus is amplified in the cardiac monitor and displayed on a screen (oscilloscope).

Monitoring systems vary according to manufacturer and hospital need. There are basically three types of systems—monitor with lead selection; monitor without lead selection; and telemetry, a battery operated system. In the first two systems the patient is attached to the monitor by a cable; no cable is used in telemetry.

LEAD PLACEMENT SYSTEMS
LEAD PLACEMENT WHEN LEAD SELECTION IS NOT PART OF MONITOR
LEAD II
- One of most commonly used methods
- Utilizes 3 leads
- Placement of electrodes is as follows:
  - *Negative*—first intercostal space, right side of sternal border
  - *Positive*—fourth intercostal space, left side, midclavicular line
  - *Ground*—fourth intercostal space, right side of sternal border

MODIFIED CHEST LEAD I (MCL₁)
- One of most commonly used methods
- Utilizes 3 leads
- Placement of electrodes is as follows:
  - *Negative*—left shoulder, just below clavicle, midclavicular line
  - *Positive*—fourth intercostal space, right side of sternal border
  - *Ground*—right shoulder, just below clavicle, midclavicular line

LEAD PLACEMENT WHEN LEAD CAN BE SELECTED ON MONITOR
4-LEAD SYSTEM
- Leads I, II, or III may be selected.

- Placement of electrodes is as follows:
  - *Negative*—just below the clavicle, right side, midclavicular line
  - *Inactive*—just below the clavicle, left side, midclavicular line
  - *Ground*—lower rib cage, right side, in line with shoulder or midaxilla
  - *Positive*—lower rib cage, left side, in line with shoulder or midaxilla

5-LEAD SYSTEM

- Leads I, II, or III may be selected.
- Chest lead is added, permitting a 12-lead ECG to be obtained by moving the position of this lead.
- Placement of electrodes is as follows:
  - (See 4-lead system for limb leads.)
  - Chest V1—fourth intercostal space, right of sternal border
  - Chest V2—fourth intercostal space, left of sternal border
  - Chest V3—midway between V2 and V4
  - Chest V4—fifth intercostal space, left side, midclavicular line
  - Chest V5—midway between V4 and V6
  - Chest V6—fifth intercostal space, left side, midaxillary line

TELEMETRY
LEAD II

- Placement of electrodes is as follows:
  - *Negative*—first intercostal space, right side of sternal border
  - *Positive*—fourth intercostal space, left side, midclavicular line

MODIFIED CHEST LEAD I (MCL₁)

- Placement of electrodes is as follows:
  - *Negative*—just below the clavicle, left side, midclavicular line
  - *Positive*—fourth intercostal space, right side of sternal border

NOTE. No ground electrode is necessary for telemetry monitoring.

PREPARATION OF THE SKIN FOR ELECTRODE PLACEMENT

Proper skin preparation is necessary for the success of cardiac monitoring. The following steps should be taken when preparing for electrode placement.
1. Skin must be dry. Remove lotion or oil with alcohol. Allow to dry thoroughly.
2. If the selected area has excessive body hair, shave just enough for electrode application. Be very careful not to cause skin irritation.
3. Using a dry washcloth or 4 × 4, rub each site briskly for a few seconds.
4. Apply electrodes. Do not apply to joints, bony protuberances, skin folds, or areas that may have excessive motion.

NOTE. Excessive perspiration will prevent adequate adherence of electrodes. To keep the area dry, apply a thin coat of tincture of benzoin where the electrode will come in contact with the skin or apply an antiperspirant spray.

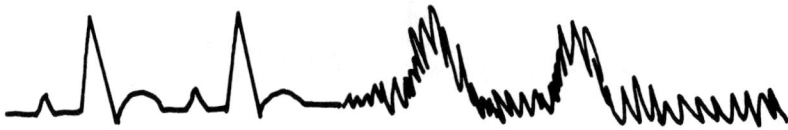

FIG. 3-1. *Artifact.*

NURSING CARE OF THE ELECTRODE SITE

Daily inspection and care of the electrode site is necessary to ensure accurate and continuous service and to prevent or detect possible complications.

Disposable electrodes—change as necessary (electrode not adhering to skin, skin irritation, excessive perspiration, drying of electrode gel, poor quality tracing); may be left in place for several days if no complications.

Nondisposable electrodes—change daily or more often if necessary, as with disposable electrodes.

NOTE. Some patients may be sensitive to the electrode gel or tape.

COMMON MONITORING PROBLEMS
EXCESSIVE ARTIFACT (Fig. 3-1)

Causes

Patient movement

Electrical interference

Poor electrode contact

Nursing Action

Always check patient to be sure that the problem is artifact.

Check all electrodes for proper contact.

Prevent tension on lead wires during movement because it could cause poor electrode contact.

SIXTY CYCLE INTERFERENCE

This is an interference, of mechanical or electrical origin, that causes distortions in the tracing (Fig. 3-2).

Causes

Electrical interference

Poor electrode contact

X-ray equipment

Diathermy

Damaged lead wires and connections

Loose connections

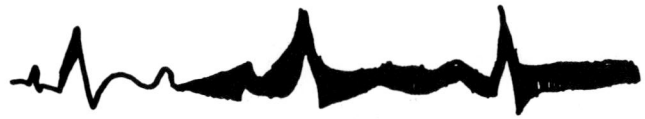

FIG. 3-2. *Electrical interference.*

Nursing Action

Check area to ascertain if any equipment is responsible.

Check lead wires and connections for damage. Replace.

Tighten loose connections.

Check all electrodes for proper contact.

LEAD REVERSAL

With lead reversal, signal on scope is opposite of what it should be.

Cause

Incorrect placement of leads

Nursing Action

Correct lead placement.

BASELINE APPEARS, BUT NO ECG

Causes

Low gain setting on monitor

Loose connections

Damage to cable or lead wires

Disconnected lead wires or cables

Nursing Action

Increase gain setting.

Check all connections and tighten if necessary.

Replace damaged equipment.

Reconnect lead wires or cable as indicated.

Make sure monitor has "warmed up" thoroughly before attaching.

EXCESSIVE TRIGGERING OF ALARMS (HIGH OR LOW)

Causes

Damage to cable or lead wires

Alarms set too close to patient's normal rate

Poor electrode contact

Patient movement

Excessive cable or lead wire movement

Improper site selection, resulting in low amplitude

Wandering baseline

Loose connections

Nursing Action

Replace damaged equipment.

Set alarms appropriately.

Check all electrodes for proper contact.

Secure cable and lead wires to patient's clothing.

Reapply electrode as indicated.

Tighten all loose connections.

WANDERING BASELINE (Fig. 3-3)

Causes

Poor electrode contact

Patient movement

Excessive movement of cable

Excessive tension of electrode and lead wires

Electrodes applied at improper site

Nursing Action

Check all electrodes for proper contact.

Attach cable to patient's clothing to prevent excessive movement.

Prevent tension on lead wires during movement.

Reapply electrodes as necessary.

WEAK SIGNAL

Causes

Low gain setting on monitor

Poor electrode contact

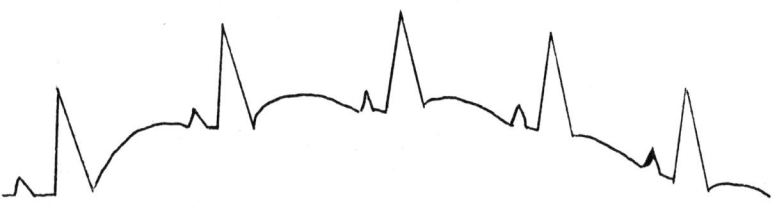

FIG. 3-3. *Wandering baseline.*

Loose connections

Disconnected or broken lead wires

Nursing Action

Increase the gain (size).

Check all electrodes for proper contact.

Check all connections and tighten loose ones.

Check lead wires for damage and replace if necessary.

Reconnect lead wires if disconnected.

Change electrode sites as indicated.

STEPS FOR INTERPRETING AN ECG

A number of factors enter into the interpretation of an electrocardiogram—rhythm, rate, and the individual characteristics of the P wave, the PR interval, the QRS complex, the ST segment, and the T wave. The steps for interpreting an electrocardiogram are outlined in the Steps for Interpreting an ECG chart.

STEPS FOR INTERPRETING AN ECG (Figs. 3-4 to 3-6)

RHYTHM	Is it regular? (both atrial and ventricular)
RATE	Is it fast, normal, or slow? (both atrial and ventricular) Calculate the rates.
P WAVE	Is it present? Is it normal in shape (no more than 3 small blocks high or wide) and position (*i.e.*, upright)? Does it precede each QRS complex?
PR INTERVAL	Is it present and of normal duration (0.12–0.2 sec) in a regular pattern (*i.e.*, before each QRS)?
QRS COMPLEX	Is it present? Is it of normal height, duration (distance between onset of Q wave and completion of the S wave should not be greater than 0.12 sec), and position (usually upright, depending on lead used)? Does it have a normal and regular pattern?
ST SEGMENT	Is it depressed, elevated, or normal?
T WAVE	Is it in normal position (upright)? Is height normal (no more than 10 small blocks in chest leads and five small blocks in others)?

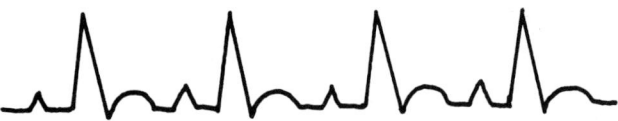

FIG. 3-4. *Normal sinus rhythm.*

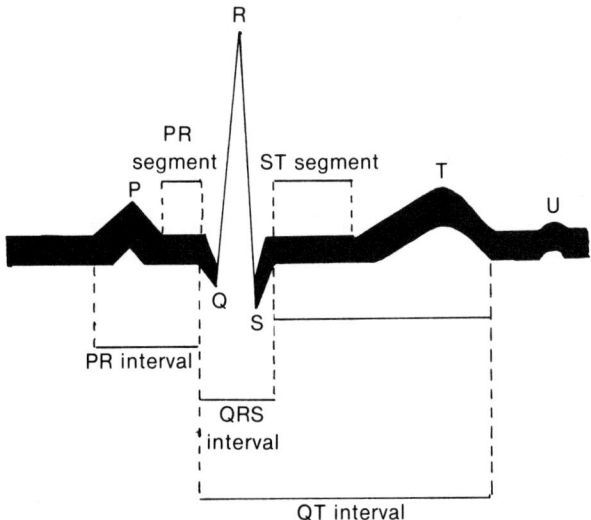

FIG. 3-5. *Normal electrocardiogram. Duration: P wave = 0.08 sec; PR interval = 0.12–0.20 sec; QRS interval = 0.07–0.10 sec; QT interval = 0.30–0.40 sec. Height: P wave = no more than 3 mm; Q wave = if present, should be less than one third the height of the QRS complex. Normally, very shallow; QRS = varies, according to specific lead; T wave = chest leads—no more than 10 mm high; other leads = no more than 5 mm high.*

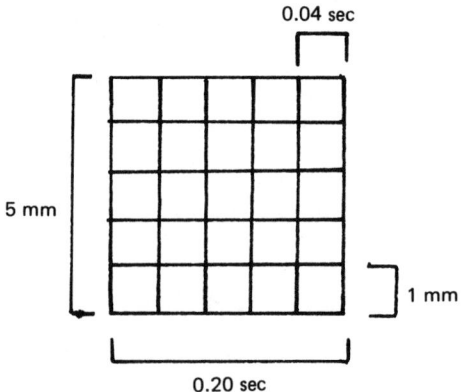

FIG. 3-6. *Interpretation of blocks on ECG paper. (Each small block is 0.04 sec wide and 1 mm tall. Each large block is 0.20 sec wide and 5 mm tall.)*

ECG INTERPRETATION

1. Look at the ECG.
2. Determine the area of the complex in which the abnormality is located (*e.g.*, P wave, PR interval).
3. Identify the abnormality (*e.g.*, P wave is out of normal position, PR interval is prolonged).
4. To determine the significance of the abnormality, consult the guide to ECG interpretation provided in Table 3-1. In this guide, possible abnormalities and their significance are listed for specific parts of the complex.

TABLE 3-1. **Guide to ECG Interpretation***

Abnormality	Significance
P Wave	
Enlarged, diphasic	Atrial enlargement (possible cause—mitral stenosis)
Sudden decrease in size, change in shape, or absence	May indicate impending atrial standstill
Abnormal position or shape	Impulse originated outside SA node (*e.g.*, nodal rhythms)
Absent and replaced with one of the following:	
Presence of fibrillatory waves, or "f" waves	Atrial fibrillation—undulating baseline, no definable P waves, variable PR interval
Sawtooth pattern (Flutter waves, or "F" waves)	Atrial flutter—characteristic sawtooth pattern, regular PR interval
"f" waves and sawtooth pattern	Flutter-fibrillation—rhythm varies from atrial flutter to atrial fibrillation
No identifiable P wave or atrial impulse	Atrial standstill—no atrial activity; lower pacemaker takes over, either nodal or ventricular; ventricular standstill may occur at any time
	Sinus block—impulse blocked from SA node for one or more beats; no P wave, QRS complex or T wave is present for those beats; interval of block is a multiple of the normal cycle length
	Sinus arrest—SA node fails to fire for a time; no P wave, QRS complex, or T wave is present during this time; interval of block is *not* a multiple of the normal cycle length
Variable shape and position	Wandering pacemaker—location of pacing stimulus varies; may originate in SA node, atria, or AV node
P wave is unidentifiable or abnormally shaped	Paroxysmal atrial tachycardia (PAT)—sudden onset and termination (usually); P wave is either

*To use the guide, refer to the specific part of the complex involved; then, in the designated columns, locate the abnormality you have identified and its significance.

(*Continued*)

TABLE 3-1. **Guide to ECG Interpretation*** (*Continued*)

Abnormality	Significance
with fast ventricular response	abnormally shaped or not visible (buried in QRS complex or T wave); impulse is from an ectopic atrial pacemaker; ventricles generally respond to each impulse; therefore, the rhythm is fairly regular PAT with block—some impulses are blocked from ventricles; may occur in a regular or irregular random pattern; ventricular rate is slower than PAT without block
Ratio of P waves to QRS complexes is greater than 1:1 (one P wave for every QRS complex); ratio may be 2:1, 3:1, 4:1, etc.; a 2:1 ratio means that there are two P waves for every QRS complex	Second degree heart block with fixed ratio
P wave with no ventricular response	Second degree heart block, Mobitz II—occurs occasionally and without warning as with other heart blocks (*i.e.*, there is no prolonged PR interval); at time of expected beat, there is no ventricular response to SA node stimulation
Inverted	Paroxysmal nodal tachycardia—ectopic pacing site is in AV node; ventricular response is rapid; inverted P wave may occur either just before or after the QRS (may not be visible if buried in QRS) Nonparoxysmal nodal tachycardia—same as paroxysmal nodal tachycardia, but the ventricular response is slower
PR Interval	

Prolonged	Arteriosclerotic heart disease
	Rheumatic fever
	    First degree heart block—prolonged PR interval is only abnormality in cycle.
	    Second degree heart block—Mobitz I (Wenckebach)—prolonged PR interval continues to increase until a QRS is dropped.

Shortened	Wolff–Parkinson–White syndrome—presence of Delta wave (slurring of upstroke of R wave) Nodal rhythms—pacing site is in AV node; P wave is usually inverted.
Variable	Complete heart block—PR interval is highly variable, showing no direct relationship between atria and ventricles (*i.e.*, atria and ventricles are beating independently of each other).

*To use the guide, refer to the specific part of the complex involved; then, in the designated columns, locate the abnormality you have identified and its significance.

TABLE 3-1. **Guide to ECG Interpretation*** (*Continued*)

Abnormality	Significance
QRS Complex	
Q wave is deep and wide	Indicates myocardial infarction
R wave	
Enlarged	Enlargement of ventricle
Decreased	Pericardial effusion, myxedema, cardiac failure, obesity, any condition causing extensive myocardial damage
QRS is widened and abnormally shaped	Bundle-branch block—each QRS preceded by a normal P wave; regular rhythm.
M shaped in Lead V_1	Right bundle-branch block
V shaped in Lead V_1	Left-bundle branch block
Widened QRS (ventricular origin) preceded by P wave	Fusion beat—a combination of a normal SA paced beat with an ectopic ventricular beat occurring at the same time; preceded by a P wave; QRS is wide although not as wide as a premature ventricular contraction (PVC)

Ventricular response preceded by long pause	Escape beats—SA node fails to pace for a period of time; one of the lower pacemakers senses this and fires an impulse as a protective measure; shape depends on location of focus
	   Atrial—abnormally shaped P wave
	   Nodal—no P wave
	   Ventricular—resembles a PVC

QRS appears before next expected beat for one cycle	Premature atrial contraction—ectopic pacemaker in atrium fires early in the cycle, before the normal SA paced beat; P wave is shaped abnormally and precedes the QRS complex Premature nodal contraction—ectopic pacemaker in AV node fires early in the cycle, before the normal SA paced beat; P wave is usually inverted and occurs either right before or right after the QRS complex (P wave may not be visible if buried in QRS)

Widened, large and deep, bizarre shape occurring early in the cycle	Premature ventricular contraction—characteristic shape; no P wave; usually followed by a compensatory pause. If not followed by a compensatory pause, contraction is called an interpolated PVC. PVCs may occur as follows:
	   Singly—random appearance of single PVC, no pattern
	   Every other beat—bigeminy
	   Every third beat—trigeminy
	   Every fourth beat—quadrigeminy
	   There may be 3 or more consecutive PVCs—ventricular tachycardia
	   PVCs may be shaped differently—multifocal PVCs

(*Continued*)

TABLE 3-1. **Guide to ECG Interpretation*** (*Continued*)

Abnormality	Significance
QRS replaced by configurations resembling a stretched coil	Ventricular flutter—ectopic pacemaker is in ventricle; ventricular response is extremely rapid; treatment same as for ventricular fibrillation
QRS replaced by chaotic pattern; no recognizable P, QRS, or T	Ventricular fibrillation—characteristic pattern; grossly irregular
Total cessation of ventricular response	Ventricular standstill—SA node may continue to fire but the impulse is blocked Asystole—complete absence of cardiac activity
ST Segment	
Elevated	Acute MI (fresh injury) usually May also indicate acute pericarditis
Depressed	Myocardial ischemia Digitalis effect
Prolonged	Hypocalcemia (chronic renal failure is usually underlying cause)
Shortened	Hypercalcemia (metastatic carcinoma is usually underlying cause)
T Wave	
Flattened	Myocardial ischemia Hypokalemia (usually the result of diuretics)
Inverted	Acute MI
Elevated, peaked	Hyperkalemia (renal disease is usually underlying cause)
QT Interval	
Prolonged	Congestive heart failure Hypocalcemia Quinidine effect Procainamide effect
Shortened	Hypercalcemia Digitalis effect
U Wave	
Visible on ECG (occurs rarely)	Hypokalemia (relationship is unknown, but if it occurs, will usually be in this setting)
RR Interval	
Irregular	Sinus arrhythmia—the complex itself is normal; only the rate and rhythm are irregular. Many arrhythmias have irregular RR intervals. See specific complex abnormality.
Rapid	Sinus tachycardia—the complex and rhythm are normal; the rate is abnormally fast.
Slow	Sinus bradycardia—the complex and rhythm are normal; the rate is abnormally slow.

CALCULATION OF THE HEART RATE ON ECG PAPER
METHODS

1. Calculate the heart rate by measuring the distance between two consecutive waves with a rate calculator.

2. Count the number of R waves in a 6-second strip of ECG tracing and multiply the result by 10.

3. Count the number of large squares between two consecutive R waves (*i.e.*, the heavy black lines) and divide the result into 300. Second R wave must fall on heavy black line. (See Table for Calculating the Heart Rate by Measuring the Number of Large Squares in the Appendix.)

4. Count the number of small squares between two consecutive R waves (*i.e.*, the smaller black lines) and divide the result into 1500. (See Table for Calculating the Heart Rate by Measuring the Number of Small Squares or Time Interval in the Appendix.)

5. Divide the time interval between R waves into 60 seconds. Time interval is determined by measuring, in seconds, the distance between R waves. Each large square is equal to 0.20 second. Each small square is equal to 0.04 second. (See Table for Calculating the Heart Rate by Measuring the Number of Small Squares or Time Interval in the Appendix.)

SPECIAL CONSIDERATIONS

In some arrhythmias, the atrial and ventricular rates differ and should be calculated separately.

1. An approximate rate will be obtained by counting the squares if the rhythm is irregular. In this case, the rate may be determined as an average of several RR intervals (i.e., using two RR intervals or three QRS complexes, count the number of squares and divide into 600).

2. To calculate the heart rate if the second R wave falls between two heavy black lines, remember that each small line is equal to 1/5 or 0.2, 0.4, 0.6, or 0.8 respectively. Use the following method to determine rate in this situation.
   - Count the heavy black lines between R waves.
   - Add to this the value, in decimals, of the small line the second R wave falls on (following the last heavy black line).
   - Add these two values together.
   - Divide into 300 to obtain rate. (See Table for Calculating the Heart Rate if the Second R Wave Falls Between Two Heavy Black Lines in the Appendix.)

4

Interpretation of Arrhythmias

In general, an arrhythmia is a disturbance of the normal rhythm of the heartbeat. The characteristics, causes, clinical manifestations, and treatment of specific arrhythmias are presented in this chapter.

SINUS ARRHYTHMIA

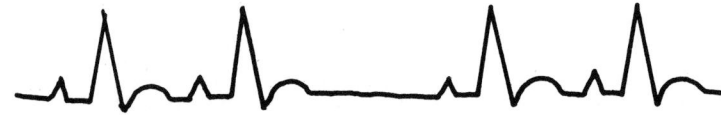

Rate	Normal (60–100)
Rhythm	Irregular
P Wave	Normal
PR Interval	Normal
QRS Complex	Normal width
Clinical Manifestations	Irregular pulse (On inspiration the rate increases; on expiration the rate decreases.)
Cause	Vagal influence, usually associated with respiration
Treatment	None (does not cause hemodynamic effects)
Comments	Common in both old and young

SINUS BRADYCARDIA

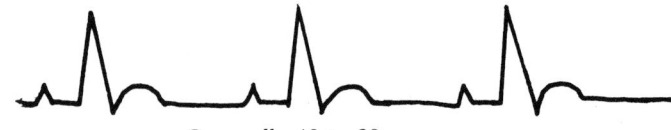

Rate	Generally 40 to 60
Rhythm	Regular
P Wave	Normal

PR Interval	Normal
QRS Complex	Normal
Clinical Manifestations	Pulse is slow. Symptoms are evident if cardiac output is adversely affected.
Cause	MI
Treatment	This condition may be normal in athletes and therefore require no treatment. In other cases, atropine and isoproterenol may be used. If drug therapy is unsuccessful, pacemaker therapy is indicated.
Comments	Do not administer drugs that have bradycardic effects.

SINUS TACHYCARDIA

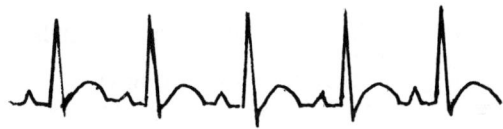

Rate	100 to 150
Rhythm	Regular
P Wave	Normal
PR Interval	Normal
QRS Complex	Normal
Clinical Manifestations	May show no symptoms Dyspnea Palpitations Rapid pulse
Causes	Hyperthyroidism Anxiety Fever Physical activity

Congestive heart failure
Pain
Anemia
Hemorrhage
Shock

Treatment   Treat underlying cause (*i.e.,* fever—antipyretics; congestive heart failure—digitalis; anxiety—tranquilizers).

Comments   When condition returns to normal it does so gradually rather than abruptly.
Sinus tachycardia may lead to cardiac decompensation.

WANDERING PACEMAKER

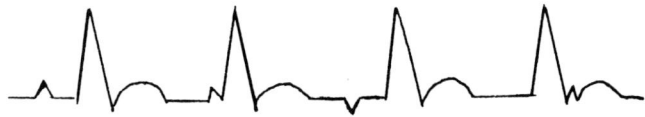

Rate   Normal (may be slow)

Rhythm   Slightly irregular

P Wave   Shape and position varies according to pacing site.

PR Interval   Varies according to pacing site

QRS Complex   Normal

Clinical Manifestations   None

Causes   Digitalis toxicity
Rheumatic carditis
Variations in vagal tone in normal heart
Associated with sinus arrhythmia

Treatment   Usually none
If patient is on digitalis, withhold it to see if it is the cause. Inform the physician.
If the AV node becomes the dominant pacemaker, atropine is administered.

Comments   Observe tracing for more serious arrhythmias (*i.e.,* AV nodal rhythm). This condition may be normal in athletes, the very young, or the elderly.

ATRIAL FIBRILLATION

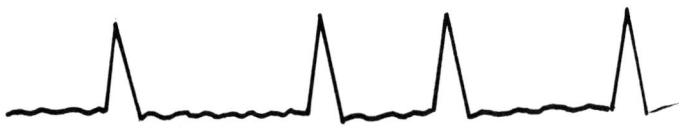

Rate	Atrial—350 to 800 Ventricular—Varies (40–160) but is irregular and slower because the AV node cannot conduct all of the atrial impulses it is receiving to the ventricles. ("fibrillation is said to be *controlled* through physiologic means or medications if the rate is 60 to 75, with the rate for *uncontrolled* fibrillation being much faster.)
Rhythm	Irregular
P Wave	None Irregular undulations occurring rapidly (called "f" waves or fibrillatory waves) are present. They vary in size, rate, and shape.
PR Interval	Unmeasurable because there are no P waves
QRS Complex	Normal (may be irregular if aberrant conduction is present)
Clinical Manifestations	Pulse deficit (peripheral rate is slower than apical) Irregular pulse (peripheral pulse may be absent if stroke volume is inadequate) Skipping of the heart or palpitations Congestive heart failure Carotid sinus massage slows the ventricular rate, although it remains grossly irregular
Causes	Arteriosclerotic or rheumatic heart disease (especially in the older patient) Thyrotoxicosis Pericarditis
Treatment	Depends on the effects of the arrhythmia Drug therapy is instituted if cardiac output is adequate. • May convert to sinus rhythm following digitalization. • Quinidine used concurrently with digitalis may convert arrhythmia to sinus rhythm when digitalis alone was not successful.

- Digitalis and propranolol (Inderol) may be used concurrently to slow the ventricular rate when digitalis alone was not successful. This combination may also convert the arrhythmia to sinus rhythm.

Diuretics such as furosemide (Lasix) may be administered if the patient is in congestive heart failure.

Emergency cardioversion (starting with 50–100 watt sec) may be used to convert the arrhythmia to sinus rhythm if complications such as left ventricular failure have developed. (This arrhythmia is more difficult to convert to sinus rhythm by cardioversion in contrast to atrial flutter.)

NOTE. Cardioversion may be dangerous in a digitalized patient (see Special Considerations, p 83).

Temporary pacemaker therapy may be instituted when a low ventricular rate resulting from block is present.

Closely monitor the patient, including vital signs. Observe closely for signs of left ventricular failure.

NOTE. Apical-radial pulses, taken simultaneously, should be checked frequently to monitor the pulse deficit (*i.e.,* the peripheral pulse is usually slower than the apical rate in the presence of atrial fibrillation).

If this arrhythmia is a problem of a long duration, the ventricular rate is normal or adequate, and the patient is tolerating it well, no treatment may be necessary. He should still be monitored closely during the hospital stay for signs of decompensation.

NOTE. Atrial fibrillation may be difficult to determine if the F waves are hidden by other waves or are too small to be seen. Remember, no P waves or flutter waves plus complete irregularity of the QRS equals atrial fibrillation.

ATRIAL FLUTTER

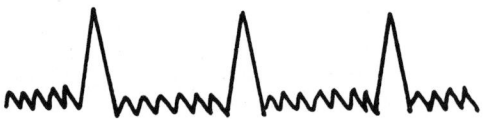

Rate	Atrial rate—250 to 350 (usually 300)
	Ventricular rate—Depends on degree of AV block (may be 1/4, 1/3, or 1/2 the atrial rate); The AV node is not able to accept and conduct each P wave.
Rhythm	Ventricular rate is usually regular, but it may become irregular, as degree of AV block varies. Irregular rhythm may mean arrhythmia is getting ready to convert to atrial fibrillation.
P Wave	P wave is in a sawtooth pattern (also called "F" waves or flutter waves). It may be partially concealed in QRS complex or T wave.
PR Interval	The PR interval is constant or variable, depending on amount of block. It is not measured in this arrhythmia.
QRS Complex	Normal
Clinical Manifestations	Clinical manifestations depend on rate of ventricular response.

Clinical manifestations depend on rate of ventricular response.

- 2:1 block (2 P waves/QRS)—ventricular response would be extremely rapid and dangerous (150). Cardiac output may be decreased and the patient may exhibit signs of palpitations, dyspnea, chest pain, or heart failure.
- 4:1 block (4 P waves/QRS)—ventricular response would be normal (75) and the patient would have no symptoms.
- 1:1 block—ventricular rate would be 300. This ventricular response is rare but possible in hyperthyroidism.

Causes

Organic heart disease
Hyperthyroidism
Neoplasm of the atria
May follow intrathoracic operations

Treatment

Drug therapy
- Digitalis is the drug of choice.
- Propranolol (Inderal) may be administered to supplement digitalis and to slow the ventricular response.
- Quinidine or procainamide (Pronestyl) may be used concurrently if digitalization alone is not successful in restoring normal sinus rhythm. These drugs may cause an abnormally rapid ventricular response (1:1) unless the patient has been digitalized.

If drug therapy fails, complications occur, or the ventricular rate is extremely rapid, the arrhythmia can be quickly terminated by cardioversion at low wattage (50 watt/sec). Digitalis and quinidine would be administered for maintenance following conversion.

NOTE. Cardioversion can be dangerous in a digitalized patient (see Special Considerations, p 83).

Rapid atrial pacing, either temporary or permanent, may be used if the arrhythmia does not respond to cardioversion or digitalis. The purpose may be to convert the arrhythmia to atrial fibrillation, which is much more responsive to drug therapy and has a slower ventricular rate.

Administration of diuretics may be necessary if symptoms of congestive failure are present (*i.e.*, furosemide or Lasix).

Treat the underlying cause (*i.e.*, hyperthyroidism).

Closely monitor the blood pressure and pulse.

Edrophonium (Tensilon) or neostigmine bromide (Prostigmin) may be administered to slow the ventricular response, but this is rare.

NOTE. Detection of atrial flutter with a 2:1 block, the most common block, is difficult because the P waves may be hidden in the T waves or QRS complex. Therefore, atrial flutter should always be suspected if a supraventricular arrhythmia with a ventricular rate of 150 (2:1) exists.

COMPLETE ATRIAL STANDSTILL

(Paced from AV node)

(Paced from site in ventricle)

Rate	Slow, depending on pacing site (AV node = 60; ventricle = 30–40)
Rhythm	Regular

P Wave	Absent (Escape beats from AV node or ventricles take over as the basic pacemaker.)
PR Interval	Absent
QRS Complex	If pacing site is in AV node, it may be normal in width. If it is paced from ventricles, it will be wide (0.12 second or greater) and distorted.
Clinical Manifestations	There are no characteristic symptoms. Ventricular standstill occurs if latent pacemakers from AV node or ventricles fail to escape.
Causes	Quinidine toxicity Digitalis toxicity Acute MI with SA node injury Vagal stimulation Hyperkalemia
Treatment	1. Withhold quinidine and digitalis, if it is causative agent. Notify the physician 2. Correct electrolyte imbalance. • If the electrolyte imbalance is hyperkalemic, withhold potassium. • Administer sodium bicarbonate or insulin and glucose to lower serum potassium. 3. Begin pacemaker therapy. 4. Treat ventricular standstill if present. 5. Monitor closely. Ventricular standstill is a serious threat.

SINUS ARREST

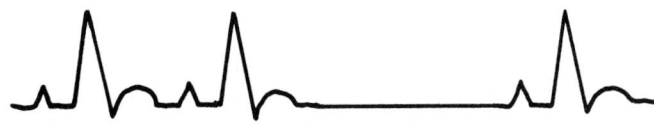

(Interval is not a multiple of the cycle length.)

Rate	Normal
Rhythm	Irregular
P Wave	Normal when present
PR Interval	Normal when present
QRS Complex	Normal when present

Clinical Manifestations	Patient may exhibit no symptoms. A prolonged pause is noted when checking pulse or heartbeat. Pause is *not* a multiple of the basic RR interval or cycle length (in contrast to sinoatrial block). Cerebral insufficiency may develop if block is prolonged or frequent.
Causes	Intense vagal stimulation Digitalis or quinidine toxicity Organic heart disease (*i.e.*, MI)

Treatment	1. Digitalis or quinidine should be withheld if it is the causative agent. Notify physician
	2. Administer atropine or isoproterenol to inhibit vagal influence.
	3. Pacemaker therapy is indicated if the arrhythmia continues.
	4. Sinus arrest may require no treatment if it occurs infrequently
	5. Monitor closely.
	    • Notify physician if frequency or length of pause increases (more than two consecutive beats).
	    • Condition may progress to complete atrial standstill.

SINOATRIAL BLOCK

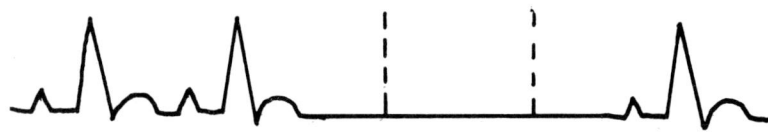

(Interval is a multiple of the cycle length.)

Rate	Varies, slow
Rhythm	Normal
P Wave	Normal, except for dropped beat(s)
PR Interval	Normal when present
QRS Complex	Normal, except for dropped beat(s)
Clinical Manifestations	May exhibit no symptoms A prolonged pause is noted when checking pulse or heartbeat. Pause is a multiple of the basic RR interval or cycle length.

Cerebral insufficiency may develop if block prolonged or frequent.

Causes Digitalis or quinidine toxicity
Organic heart disease (*i.e.*, MI)
Intense vagal stimulation

Treatment 1. Sinoatrial block may require no treatment
2. Withhold digitalis or quinidine if it is the causative agent. Notify physician.
3. Monitor closely.
   • Notify physician if block (more than two consecutive blocks) or frequency increases.
   • Sinoatrial block may progress to complete atrial standstill.
4. Administer atropine or isoproterenol (Isuprel) if the patient is symptomatic.
5. Pacemaker therapy may be indicated if drug therapy is unsuccessful.

PREMATURE ATRIAL CONTRACTION (PAC)

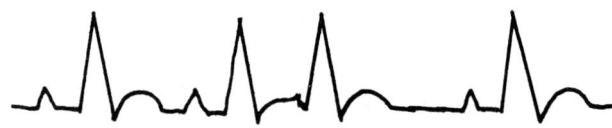

Rate Normal

Rhythm Slightly irregular

P Wave Abnormal shape (flat, inverted, notched)
Premature (may be superimposed on T wave or QRS complex)

PR Interval May be different, either shortened or longer
Depends on P wave location

QRS Complex Normal, unless aberrantly conducted

Clinical Manifestations A premature beat heard on chest auscultation. The patient may not be aware of arrhythmia or may complain of an irregular (extra) beat.

Causes Heart disease
Infections
Smoking
Digitalis
Nervous tension
Caffeine and other stimulants (tobacco)

Treatment	Treatment may not be necessary depending on cause. If more than six PACs per minute are noted, report to physician immediately. Quinidine is usually the antiarrhythmic drug ordered. If PAC is due to digitalis, especially in hypokalemic patients, withhold digitalis and correct low potassium. Notify the physician.
Comments	Pause follows PAC but it is not usually a compensatory pause. This may be a warning of more serious atrial arrhythmias (*i.e.*, atrial fibrillation, paroxysmal atrial tachycardia [PAT], especially if pause occurs frequently.

NOTE. Atrial bigeminy occurs when a PAC alternates with a normal beat. This occurs in patients with hypokalemia who are receiving digitalis.

PAROXYSMAL ATRIAL TACHYCARDIA (PAT)

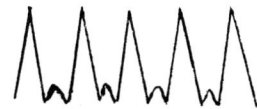

Rate	150 to 250
Rhythm	Regular
P Wave	May be abnormally shaped or buried in preceding ` QRS complex or T wave
PR Interval	Varies; may not be measurable if P wave is not visible
QRS Complex	Usually normal; may sometimes be widened
Clinical Manifestations	Rapid rate that begins suddenly and may stop just as abruptly Signs of left ventricular failure (dyspnea, angina) Fluttering sensation
Causes	Thyrotoxicosis Digitalis toxicity Fatigue Heart disease (*e.g.*, MI, rheumatic heart disease) Emotions Pregnancy Caffeine Smoking

Treatment
1. Withhold digitalis. Notify the physician.
2. Provide vagal stimulation by way of carotid massage, Valsalva maneuver, or gagging.
3. Administer edrophonium chloride (Tensilon).
4. Electrical cardioversion may be used.
5. Watch closely for signs of congestive heart failure which may develop due to the rapid rate.

NOTE. PAT with block occurs when some beats are not conducted to the ventricles. The atrial rate continues as usual (140–250), but the ventricular rate is slower. This indicates digitalis toxicity.

JUNCTIONAL RHYTHM (AV NODAL RHYTHM)

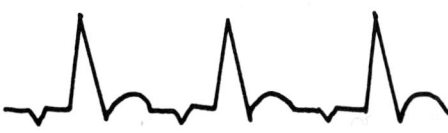

Rate
40 to 60

Rhythm
Regular

P Waves
P waves are abnormal
Depending on which site is stimulated first (*i.e.*, atria or ventricles), P waves may occur before, during, or after the QRS.
P waves occurring during the QRS are not visible.
P waves are usually inverted since the atria receive stimuli from the A-V node (retrograde stimulation).

PR Interval
Shortened or absent

QRS Complex
Normal.
AV node stimulates the ventricles in the usual fashion.

Clinical Manifestations
Patient is usually asymptomatic.
Symptoms become apparent with a very slow rate (*i.e.*, cardiac output falls with resulting cerebral or myocardial ischemia).
Pulse is regular and slow.

Causes
Digitalis or quinidine toxicity
Excessive vagal stimulation
Disease of the SA node (*i.e.*, ischemic changes)
Recent open heart surgery

Treatment

1. Withhold medication if it is the causative agent (*e.g.*, digitalis or quinidine). Discuss with physician.
2. Administer Atropine or isoproterenol (Isuprel) to increase the heart rate.
3. Pacemaker therapy may be indicated if the cardiac output is compromised or premature ventricular contractions occur. (Lidocaine is usually not effective when PVCs occur in slow rhythms.)
4. Monitor closely.
   - Slow rhythm may be suddenly replaced by a more rapid one (*i.e.*, junctional or ventricular tachycardia).
   - Notify physician if premature ventricular contractions occur.
   - Notify physician concerning sudden occurrence of nodal rhythm.
5. Closely monitor patient for signs that rhythm is not being tolerated (*i.e.*, cardiac output is compromised).
6. Administer diuretics, such as furosemide (Lasix), for symptoms of congestive failure.

PREMATURE JUNCTIONAL BEATS OR PREMATURE NODAL CONTRACTION (PNC)

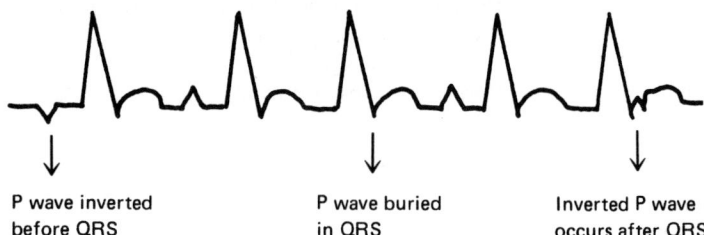

| P wave inverted before QRS | P wave buried in QRS | Inverted P wave occurs after QRS |

Rate   Normal

Rhythm   Irregular (Compensatory pause may or may not follow premature beat.)

P Wave   Varies
Inverted P wave will appear before or after QRS or may be buried in the QRS complex.

PR Interval   Shortened for PNC

QRS Complex   Normal, unless aberrant conduction occurs

Clinical Manifestations   Irregular heartbeat

Causes Organic heart disease (*e.g.*, MI)
Digitalis or quinidine toxicity

Treatment
1. Treatment may not be necessary if premature beat occurs infrequently.
2. Withhold digitalis or quinidine if it is the causative agent. Notify the physician.
3. Administer antiarrhythmic drugs such as quinidine (if not previously prescribed), lidocaine, or Pronestyl.
4. Check serum potassium levels, and administer potassium supplement if necessary. This may eliminate the premature beats.
5. Monitor closely. Notify the physician if premature beats increase (*i.e.*, more than six PNCs per minute).

NONPAROXYSMAL JUNCTIONAL TACHYCARDIA

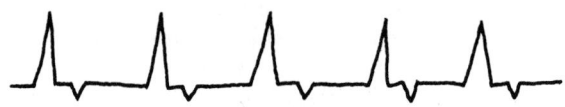

Rate 70 to 130 ventricular rate
60 to 100 atrial rate

Rhythm Regular

P Wave May be absent or occur before or after the QRS complex
Normal in shape

PR Interval Varies, may be shortened or absent

QRS Complex Normal

Clinical Manifestations May produce no clinical manifestations if cardiac output is not compromised
Occurs gradually and slows down over a period of hours or days (Note. PAT and paroxysmal junctional tachycardia have an abrupt onset and may terminate suddenly.)
Left ventricular failure

Causes Heart disease (*e.g.*, MI)
Follows open heart surgery
Digitalis toxicity

Treatment
1. Withhold digitalis preparation if it is the causative agent. Notify the physician.

2. Digitalis should be used for rapid ventricular rates in the patient who is not digitalized.
3. Pacemaker therapy may be indicated to prevent ventricles from becoming the pacing site.
4. No treatment may be necessary if the arrhythmia is well tolerated. It will eventually subside.
5. All patients should be closely monitored.

PAROXYSMAL JUNCTIONAL TACHYCARDIA (NODAL TACHYCARDIA)

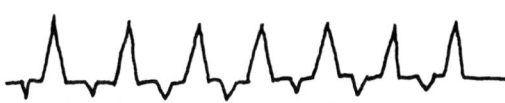

Rate	150 to 250
Rhythm	Regular
P Wave	P waves are abnormal
	Depending on which site is stimulated first (i.e., atria or ventricles), P waves may occur before, during, or after the QRS.
	P waves occurring during the QRS are not visible.
	P waves are usually inverted since the atria receive stimuli from the AV node (retrograde stimulation).
PR Interval	Shortened or absent
QRS Complex	Normal
Clinical Manifestations	Rapid rate that begins suddenly and may stop just as abruptly
	Signs of left ventricular failure (dyspnea, angina)
	Fluttering sensation
Causes	Thyrotoxicosis
	Digitalis toxicity
	Fatigue
	Heart disease (*e.g.*, MI, rheumatic heart disease)
	Emotions
	Pregnancy
	Caffeine
	Smoking
Treatment	1. Withhold digitalis. Notify the physician.
	2. Provide vagal stimulation by way of carotid massage, Valsalva Maneuver, or gagging.
	3. Administer edrophonium chloride (Tensilon).
	4. Electrical cardioversion may be used.

5. Watch closely for signs of congestive heart failure which may develop due to the rapid rate.

NOTE. Paroxysmal junctional tachycardia is very closely related to Paroxysmal atrial tachycardia.

BUNDLE BRANCH BLOCKS (BBB)

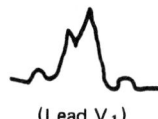

(Lead V_1)

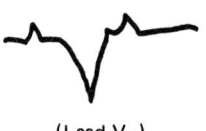

(Lead V_1)

Rate	Usually normal; may be rate dependent
Rhythm	Regular
P Wave	Normal
PR Interval	Normal
QRS Complex	Complex is always prolonged to 0.12 seconds or more and notched or slurred. Lead V_1 is the lead used to differentiate between right and left bundle block.

Right Bundle Block
- QRS is above the isoelectric line (positive deflection).
- Complex resembles an M (first upward deflection or R wave denotes activation of the left ventricle; second upward deflection, or R^1 denotes activation of the right ventricle).

Left Bundle Block
- QRS is below the isoelectric line (negative deflection).
- Complex is a deep V shape.

Clinical Manifestations   None

Causes
Hypertension
MI
Hyperkalemia
Antiarrhythmic drugs (*e.g.,* digitalis, quinidine, procainamide)
Cardiomyopathy
Pulmonary embolism
Hypoxia
Coronary artery disease

Treatment
1. Withhold antiarrhythmic drugs. Consult physician.
2. Pacemaker therapy may be indicated, especially if the arrhythmia develops abruptly.
3. Keep in mind that ventricular standstill may occur suddenly if more than one of the branches are blocked.
   - Have emergency equipment and drugs readily available.
   - Notify the physician if this condition develops.
   - Get a 12-lead ECG immediately.
   - Start resuscitation procedures if ventricular standstill occurs (see Ventricular Standstill, p 68).
4. Characteristic ECG changes of a MI are altered by a left bundle branch block.
5. Treatment may not be necessary.

FASCICULAR BLOCKS

The left bundle branch divides to form the anterior superior and the posterior superior branches. The right bundle branch and the anterior superior and posterior superior branches of the left bundle branch are called fascicles. Blocks in the fascicles are called fascicular blocks. The three types of fascicular blocks are as follows: monofascicular, one fascicle is blocked; bifascicular, two fascicles are blocked; and trifascicular, all fascicles are blocked.

HEMIBLOCKS

Hemiblocks occur when there is a block in either the anterior superior or posterior inferior branches (*i.e.,* left anterior hemiblock or left posterior hemiblock). With left anterior hemiblock ECG changes include abnormal left axis deviation, Q wave in lead I, S wave (wide or deep) in lead III, and a normal or slightly widened (0.10–0.12 sec) QRS. With left posterior hemiblock ECG changes include abnormal right axis deviation, S wave (wide or deep) in lead I, and Q wave in lead III.

FIRST DEGREE AV BLOCK

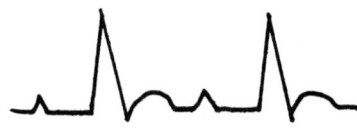

Rate   Normal

Rhythm   Regular

P Wave	Normal
PR Interval	Constant prolonged beyond the normal 0.20 second
QRS Complex	Normal
Clinical Manifestations	None (does not slow cardiac output)
Causes	Heart disease (*e.g.*, ischemia or damage of the AV node) Antiarrhythmic drugs (*i.e.*, digitalis, quinidine, or procainamide) Overactivity of vagal influence

Treatment	1. Usually treatment is not indicated.
	2. Withhold antiarrhythmic drugs (*i.e.*, digitalis, quinidine, or procainamide). Notify physician.
	3. Monitor closely.
	   • In a patient with a damaged myocardium, the condition may progress to a higher degree of block. Notify physician immediately if this occurs.
	   • Notify physician if PR interval continues to increase.
	4. Administer atropine or isoproterenol to increase AV conduction.
	5. Pacemaker therapy may be indicated if block continues to progress.

SECOND DEGREE AV BLOCK

This heart block is divided into three classifications—type I (Wenckebach or Mobitz I), type II (Mobitz II), and AV block with fixed ratio.

TYPE I (WENCKEBACH OR MOBITZ I)

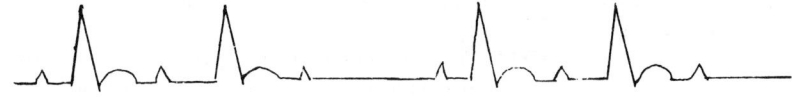

(Mobitz I or Wenckebach)

Rate	Normal but slow
Rhythm	Irregular
P Wave	More P waves than QRS complexes
PR interval	Varies, increases progressively with each beat until a dropped beat occurs
QRS Complex	Usually normal when present

Clinical Manifestations   Usually none (Symptoms appear when ventricular rate is extremely slow and cardiac output is affected.)

Causes   Organic heart disease (*i.e.*, inferior wall MI)
Medications (*e.g.*, digitalis, the most common; procainamide or quinidine toxicity
Vagal stimulation

Treatment
1. Withhold antiarrhythmic drugs (*i.e.*, digitalis, procainamide, or quinidine). Notify the physician.
2. Monitor closely.
   - Usually a transient arrhythmia causes no adverse effects on cardiac output.
   - Condition may progress to complete block. Notify physician immediately.
   - Ventricular standstill is not a common complication of this type of heart block.
3. Pacemaker therapy may be indicated if patient is symptomatic.
4. Administer isoproterenol or atropine to increase the ventricular rate.

NOTE. This type of second degree block may be described in ratio of number of P waves per QRS complexes (*e.g.*, 3:2 [3 P waves for every 2 QRS complexes]).

TYPE II (MOBITZ II)

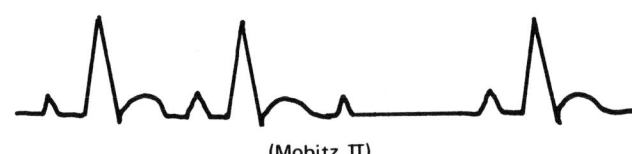

(Mobitz II)

NOTE. A QRS complex is dropped following a normal P wave. At least two P waves have been conducted prior to dropped beat. The PR interval remains constant. The dropped beat occurs without any warning.

Rate   Atrial—normal
Ventricular—varies, slower

Rhythm   Irregular due to dropped beats

P Wave   Normal

PR Interval   Constant until one P wave is blocked

QRS Complex	Widened (almost always accompanied and preceded by bundle branch block)
Clinical Manifestations	Symptoms of decreased cardiac output (*e.g.*, myocardial or cerebral ischemia)
Causes	Anterior wall MI Severe coronary artery disease

Treatment

1. Pacemaker therapy is almost always indicated due to underlying cause (organic heart disease).
   • Temporary pacemaker is inserted initially until a permanent one can be implanted.
   • Drug therapy is generally not successful in controlling this arrhythmia due to the underlying cause.
2. Monitor closely.
   • Notify physician immediately if this arrhythmia develops.
   • Prepare for pacemaker insertion.
   • Keep in mind this arrhythmia is a precursor of complete heart block (third-degree heart block).
3. Administer atropine or isoproterenol to increase heart rate while waiting for insertion of pacemaker.

NOTE. Second-degree heart block may be described in ratio of number of P waves per QRS complexes, for example, 3:2 (3 P waves for every 2 QRS complexes).

SECOND-DEGREE AV BLOCK WITH FIXED RATIO (2:1, 3:1, 4:1 Block)

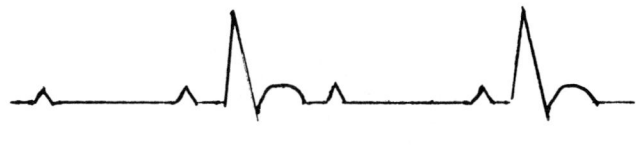

(Fixed ratio)

Rate	Slow Atrial—normal Ventricular—1/4, 1/3, 1/2 the atrial rate
Rhythm	Regular
P Wave	Normal (not always followed by QRS; may be 2, 3, or 4 P waves for every QRS)

PR Interval   Constant for conducted beats

QRS Complex   Usually normal. The width of the QRS indicates the location and seriousness of the block. Narrow QRS (less than 0.10 sec) means the block is in the AV node. Widened QRS (0.12 sec or more) means the block is below the AV node, usually below the Bundle of His or near the bundle branches, which is much more dangerous.

Clinical Manifestations   See Mobitz I in preceding section of this chapter.

Causes   See Mobitz I in preceding section of this chapter.

Treatment
1. Pacemaker therapy is indicated, especially if QRS is widened.
2. Atropine or isoproterenol (Isuprel) may be administered to increase the heart rate if the QRS complexes are narrow. (Drug therapy is not a reliable treatment when QRS complexes are wide.)
3. Monitor closely.
   • Notify physician if this condition develops.
   • Prepare for pacemaker insertion.
   • Watch closely for progression of block.
4. Keep in mind that this arrhythmia may quickly progress to complete heart block or ventricular standstill, especially when QRS complexes are widened.
5. Withhold antiarrhythmic drugs (*i.e.,* digitalis, quinidine, or procainamide). Notify physician.

COMPLETE AV BLOCK (THIRD-DEGREE HEART BLOCK)

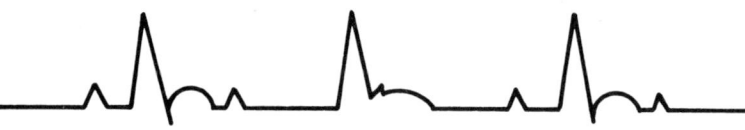

Rate   Atrial—usually normal; faster than ventricular
Ventricular—20 to 40 if block occurs low in AV node, 40 to 70 if block occurs in higher part of AV node.

Rhythm   Atrial—regular
Ventricular—regular

NOTE. Atria and ventricles are beating independently of each other.

P Wave   Normal (more P waves than QRS complexes)

PR Interval	Highly variable because of the independent beating of atria and ventricles
QRS Complex	QRS is normal if pacing site and block are near the AV node. It will be widened and distorted if below the node.
Clinical Manifestations	Patient may be asymptomatic if ventricular rate is sufficient for normal cardiac output (especially true if congenital). Slow ventricular rate will produce symptoms associated with inadequate cardiac output (*i.e.*, acute congestive heart failure, ventricular irritability, and Stokes–Adams syndrome).
Causes	Organic heart disease (especially MI) May be congenital Digitalis toxicity Vagal stimulation

Treatment	1. Pacemaker therapy (either temporary or permanent) is indicated if patient is symptomatic.
	2. Administer isoproterenol (Isuprel) while waiting for pacemaker insertion.
	3. Monitor closely.
	  • Notify physician immediately if it occurs suddenly.
	  • Complete heart block is usually preceded by other AV blocks, therefore, it is best to treat these AV blocks before they progress to complete block. (See other AV blocks in a preceding section of this chapter.)
	  • Watch closely for appearance of premature ventricular contractions, which may warn of impending ventricular tachycardia or fibrillation. (See treatment for ventricular tachycardia and fibrillation in a preceding section of this chapter.)
	  • Watch for ventricular standstill, which may occur suddenly. Start CPR. (See treatment for ventricular standstill in a preceding section of this chapter.)
	4. Withhold digitalis. Notify physician.

STOKES–ADAMS SYNDROME (OR ATTACK)

Stokes–Adams syndrome can occur in a patient with heart block. Ventricular contractions are inefficient, leading to decreased cardiac output and diminished supply of blood to the brain. This causes sudden unconsciousness that may occur with or without seizures resulting from the hypoxia. The syndrome is usually transient with ventricular action and cardiac output spontaneously returning to normal levels and the patient regaining consciousness. It will develop into cardiac arrest if ventricular action does not return to normal.

PAROXYSMAL VENTRICULAR TACHYCARDIA (FAST VENTRICULAR TACHYCARDIA)

NOTE. Ventricular tachycardia refers to a ventricular rate that is faster than the normal inherent rate (40 beats/min). In clinical practice, however, ventricular tachycardia generally refers to paroxysmal ventricular tachycardia (ventricular rate is 100–220 beats/min, or faster) as opposed to nonparoxysmal ventricular tachycardia (ventricular rate is 60–100 beats/min).

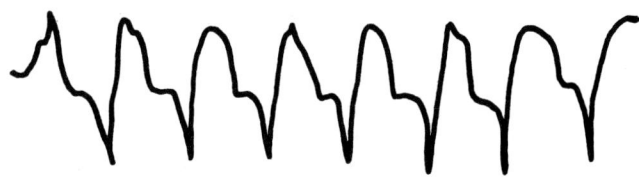

Rate	100 to 220 beats/min or faster
Rhythm	Generally regular but may be slightly irregular
P Wave	Usually not visible
PR Interval	None (Atria and ventricles are beating independently of each other.)
QRS Complex	Wide, bizarre
Clinical Manifestations	Weakness and fainting Palpitations Dyspnea Decreased cardiac output (symptoms of left ventricular failure, shock) Angina
Causes	MI Digitalis toxicity
Treatment	1. Monitor closely, including vital signs. Immediately notify physician if this arrhythmia develops.

2. Withhold digitalis. Consult physician.
3. Electrical countershock is indicated if the patient is unconscious or if drug therapy is ineffective.
4. Administer Lidocaine
   - Initially, a bolus of Lidocaine administered intravenously.
   - If IV push lidocaine is effective, connect a continuous lidocaine drip to the intravenous line.
     - Amount of solution used for continuous infusion will depend on patient's ability to tolerate intravenous fluid.
     - An infusion pump is used to administer Lidocaine at a precise rate, as prescribed by the physician.
   - If IV push lidocaine is ineffective, electrical countershock is indicated, starting at 200 watt/sec.
     - Lidocaine drip should be continued following cardioversion.
   - Lidocaine drip should be continued for at least 24 hours following termination of arrhythmia.
5. Keep in mind that this arrhythmia may quickly deteriorate into ventricular flutter or ventricular fibrillation.
   - Keep emergency equipment and drugs readily available.
   - If ventricular flutter or ventricular fibrillation occurs, treat accordingly.
6. If due to hypokalemia, correct imbalance.
   - Closely monitor serum potassium levels.
7. Monitor blood gases closely, as there may be decreased cardiac output and a possibility of lactic acidosis.
   - Administer sodium bicarbonate as indicated.
8. Procainamide is sometimes used to treat this arrhythmia when lidocaine is not effective.
   - Other antiarrhythmics may be employed for ventricular tachycardia occurring intermittently (*i.e.*, quinidine, Dilantin, or Inderal).
   - Patient should be continuously monitored.
9. Precordial thump is sometimes effective.
   - This may terminate the arrhythmia.
   - Keep in mind that it may cause ventricular fibrillation.
10. Ventricular pacing is sometimes effective.
    - This may terminate the arrhythmia.
    - It may also cause ventricular fibrillation.

NONPAROXYSMAL VENTRICULAR TACHYCARDIA (SLOW VENTRICULAR TACHYCARDIA OR ACCELERATED IDIOVENTRICULAR RHYTHM)

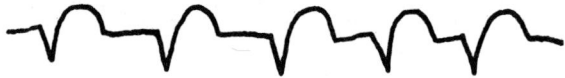

(Accelerated idioventricular rhythm)

Rate	60 to 100 (close to that of sinus rhythm)
Rhythm	Generally, fairly regular
P Wave	Usually buried in QRS complex
PR Interval	Not measurable
QRS Complex	Prolonged Usually begins and ends with a fusion beat
Clinical Manifestations	Cardiac output is usually not adversely affected because this arrhythmia is of short duration and occurs intermittently, coming and going spontaneously.
Causes	Organic heart disease (*e.g.*, MI) Digitalis toxicity
Treatment	1. Monitor closely. This arrhythmia has the potential to accelerate to a more dangerous one. 2. Withhold digitalis. Notify the physician. 3. Keep in mind that this arrhythmia usually occurs as an escape rhythm when the sinus rate slows. 4. Atropine may be administered if the patient becomes symptomatic due to poor cardiac output. This will increase the sinus rate so it can become the pacemaker. 5. Lidocaine may be administered to stop the irritable ventricular focus. 6. Usually treatment is not indicated because it is of short duration, stopping spontaneously and causing no major hemodynamic changes. Condition may last from a few seconds up to a minute.

PREMATURE VENTRICULAR CONTRACTIONS (PVC) OR BEATS (PVB)

PVCs occur prematurely or early in the cycle. They are usually followed by a compensatory pause—the interval measured from the R wave preceding the PVC to the R wave following the PVC is twice the normal RR interval (*i.e.*, the pause equals two normal beats).

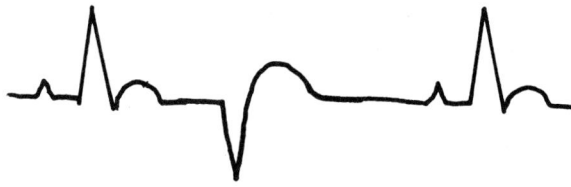

Rate	Usually normal
Rhythm	Irregular due to PVCs
P Wave	Absent in PVC
PR Interval	Absent in PVC
QRS Complex	Bizarre in shape and widened with the T wave opposite in direction
Clinical Manifestations	May be asymptomatic Feelings of heart fluttering, palpitating, flip-flopping, or skipping Angina Hypotension

Causes

Fatigue	MI
Digitalis toxicity	Alcohol
Arteriosclerotic heart disease	Coffee
Smoking	Hypokalemia

Treatment

1. Withhold digitalis. Notify physician.
2. Monitor serum potassium level, especially if patient is on diuretics.
   - If patient is hypokalemic, administer supplemental potassium.
   - Continue to monitor serum potassium.
3. Administer lidocaine to suppress PVCs
   - Initially, a bolus is injected IV push.
   - Start a continuous lidocaine drip.
   - Pronestyl IV is sometimms used.
   - Continue to monitor the patient closely during drug therapy.
4. Pronestyl or quinidine may be administered orally for long-term therapy.
5. Continue to monitor closely.
   - Notify physician if this arrhythmia develops suddenly, especially if it is one of the dangerous varieties.
   - Keep in mind that this arrhythmia may quickly progress to a life-threatening situation.

- Have emergency equipment and drug therapy readily available.
6. No treatment may be necessary if this arrhythmia occurs infrequently and is not of a dangerous variety.

TYPES OF PVCs

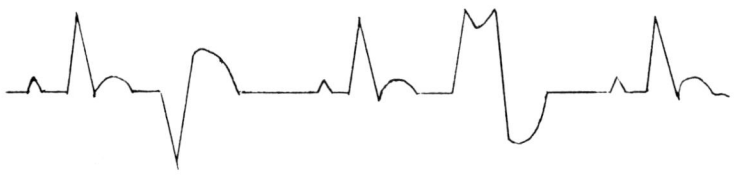

Multifocal premature ventricular contractions

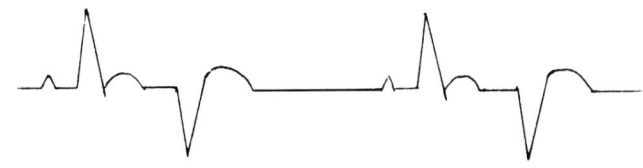

Bigeminy

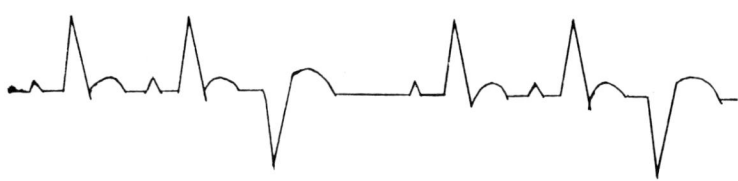

Trigeminy

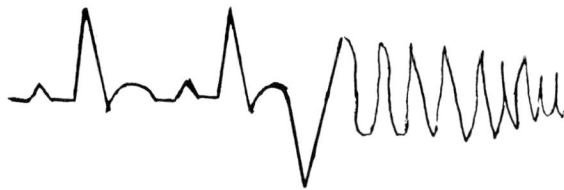

Ventricular fibrillation
R on T pattern

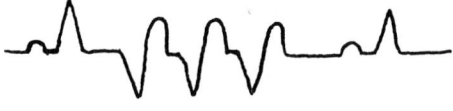

Sequential PVC's

Description by origin of beat
- Unifocal—PVCs originate from the same area of ventricle; therefore, they are alike in shape and direction.
- Multifocal—PVCs originate from different areas of the ventricle; therefore, they are of different shapes and directions.

Description by occurrence in the cycle
- Bigeminy—every second beat is a PVC.
- Trigeminy—every third beat is a PVC.
- Quadrigeminy—every fourth beat is a PVC.
- Interpolated—This type of PVC occurs between two normal beats without interrupting the rhythm (*i.e.*, no compensatory pause follows this PVC).
- Fusion beat—normal beat and PVC occur together, resulting in a widened QRS preceded by a P wave; this occurs in the normal position in the cycle and is not followed by a compensatory pause.
- "R on T" pattern—PVC hits a T wave of a normal beat, which could result in ventricular tachycardia or fibrillation.
- Grouped or sequential—two or three PVCs occur in groups.

VENTRICULAR FLUTTER

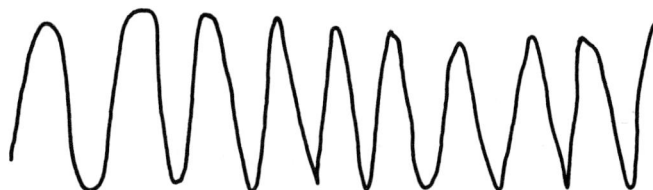

Rate	200 to 300
Rhythm	Usually regular
P Wave	Usually not visible
PR Interval	Not measurable
QRS Complex	Indistinct, prolonged, greated than 0.12 sec (resembles a stretched spring, a sine wave or the letter M)
Clinical Manifestations	Symptoms of poor cardiac output (including faintness progressing to loss of consciousness and cardiac arrest)
Causes	Occlusion of coronary artery Medications (digitalis, quinidine, potassium chloride) Electrical shock MI PVCs

Treatment

1. Begin immediate defibrillation at 400 watt/sec for adults and 200 watt/sec for children (initially).
   • This is the only treatment for this arrythmia.
   • Repeat as necessary.
2. If defibrillation is ineffective, start cardiopulmonary resuscitation and drug therapy immediately (*i.e.*, sodium bicarbonate and epinephrine) before trying defibrillation again.
3. Treat lactic acidosis.
   • Administer sodium bicarbonate initially and repeat every 5 to 10 minutes to correct this condition.
   • Monitor arterial blood gases and pH to regulate administration of sodium bicarbonate.
4. Oxygen therapy is indicated if defibrillation is unsuccessful or ineffective respirations return.
   • Intubate the patient with an endotracheal tube.
   • Ventilate.
   • Monitor arterial blood gases and pH.
5. Start patient on lidocaine drip following successful resuscitation to prevent this arrhythmia from recurring and maintain until condition is stable.
6. Administer medications intravenously.
   • Patient should already have a keep-open IV. If not, start one immediately.
   • Intracardiac injections are to be avoided if at all possible because of potential complications (*i.e.*, cardiac tamponade, laceration of a coronary artery or pneumothorax).
7. Prevention of this arrhythmia is the best policy.
   • Treat significant premature ventricular contractions and ventricular tachycardia vigorously.
   • Monitor closely.

VENTRICULAR FIBRILLATION

Rate	Not measurable
Rhythm	Completely irregular, chaotic
P Wave	None
PR Interval	None
QRS Complex	None

Clinical Manifestations	Cardiogenic shock Cyanosis Unconsciousness Convulsions Dilated pupils Pulse and blood pressure are unobtainable Clinical death followed by biological death if untreated

Causes	Occlusion of coronary artery Medications (digitalis, quinidine, potassium chloride) Electrical shock MI PVCs

Treatment

1. Immediate defibrillation at 400 watt/sec for adults and 200 watt/sec for children (initially).
   - This is the only treatment for this arrythmia.
   - Repeat as necessary.
2. If defibrillation is ineffective, start cardiopulmonary resuscitation and drug therapy immediately (*i.e.,* sodium bicarbonate and epinephrine) before trying defibrillation again.
3. Treat lactic acidosis.
   - Administer sodium bicarbonate initially and repeat every 5 to 10 minutes to correct this condition.
   - Monitor arterial blood gases and pH to regulate administration of sodium bicarbonate.
4. Keep in mind that there are two types of ventricular fibrillation—fine and coarse.
   - Fine—this type has low amplitude waves and is difficult to defibrillate. Fine should be "coarsened" with the administration of epinephrine and calcium prior to defibrillation.
   - Coarse—this type has high amplitude waves and indicates the arrhythmia is recent. Course ventricular fibrillation is much easier to defibrillate.
5. Oxygen therapy is indicated if defibrillation is unsuccessful or ineffective respirations return.
   - Intubate the patient with an endotracheal tube.
   - Ventilate.
   - Monitor arterial blood gases and pH.
6. Start patient on lidocaine drip following successful resuscitation to prevent this arrhythmia from recurring and maintain until condition is stable.
7. Administer medications intravenously.
   - Patient should already have a keep-open IV. If not, start one immediately.

- Intracardiac injections are to be avoided if at all possible because of potential complications (*i.e.,* cardiac tamponade, laceration of a coronary artery or pneumothorax).
8. Prevention of this arrhythmia is the best policy.
   - Treat significant premature ventricular contractions and ventricular tachycardia vigorously.
   - Monitor closely.

VENTRICULAR STANDSTILL (ASYSTOLE)

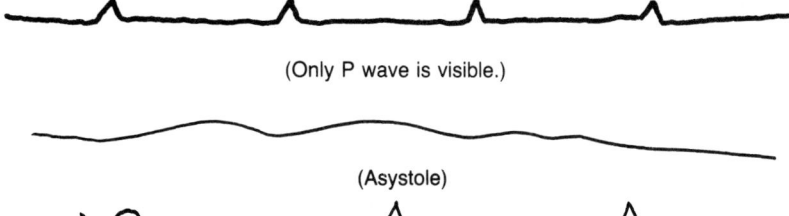

(Only P wave is visible.)

(Asystole)

(Some electrical activity in the ventricle is visible, but it is inadequate for proper myocardial stimulation and contractions.)

Rate	None
Rhythm	None
P Wave	May be present for short time; irregular
PR Interval	None
QRS Complex	None
Clinical Manifestations	(See ventricular fibrillation in a preceding section of this chapter.
Causes	Medications (digitalis, quinidine, lidocaine, pronestyl) Hypoxia (due to poor cardiac output, anesthesia, anaphylaxis, severe blood loss, drug overdose) Hyperkalemia MI Intense vagal stimulation
Treatment	1. Administer precordial thump immediately.

   - If there is no immediate response, begin CPR immediately.
   - Precordial thump is not indicated for asystole due to anoxia or exsanguination.
   - Precordial thump is not recommended for children.

2. Establish patent airway.
   - Intubate.
   - Ventilate (mechanical ventilator or Ambu bag).
   - Provide oxygen therapy.
3. Epinephrine is needed to stimulate electrical activity.
   - Administer epinephrine intravenously.
   - Avoid intracardiac injection if possible
4. Calcium may also be administered intravenously to stimulate electrical activity. Avoid intracardiac injections.
5. Administer vasopressors such as Levophed Bitartrate or Aramine.
6. Monitor closely, including vital signs.
7. Defibrillation at 400 watt/sec may be successful.
8. Correct lactic acidosis by administering sodium bicarbonate.
9. Pacemaker therapy is indicated if the patient fails to respond to the preceding treatments.

MISCELLANEOUS ARRHYTHMIAS

IDIOVENTRICULAR RHYTHM

Description   Ventricles take over pacing of heart due to blocking of the normal impulse from above the ventricles or an inadequate atrial pacemaker.

Characteristics   All complexes are ventricular in origin; therefore, they are wide and bizarre or distorted in appearance. Ventricular rate is 30 to 40.

Treatment
1. Monitor closely. Cardiac output may be adversely affected due to slow rate.
2. Treat the underlying cause, such as withholding digitalis when condition is due to digitalis toxicity.
3. Pacemaker therapy may be indicated.

SICK SINUS SYNDROME

Description   Sick sinus syndrome is a term used to describe inadequate function or failing of the SA node.

Characteristics   It is manifested as sinus bradycardia, SA block, or SA arrest. Sick sinus syndrome may also appear as alternating rapid and slow rhythms (*i.e.,* the bradycardia tachycardia syndrome).

Treatment
1. Monitor closely. Cardiac output may be adversely affected due to changes in rate.
2. Pacemaker therapy is indicated for bradycardia.

3. Drug therapy is indicated for control of tachycardia, combined with pacemaker therapy for the bradycardia in the bradycardia–tachycardia syndrome.

AV DISSOCIATION

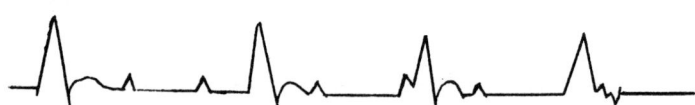

Description

Two separate pacemakers are in control; therefore, the atria and ventricles are beating independently of each other for one or more beats. This is usually a transient arrhythmia.

Characteristics

AV dissociation is used to describe several variations.
- Atrial pacing slows excessively, which allows junctional or ventricular beats (pacemakers) to escape.
- Atrial impulses are intermittently blocked, which allows escape rhythms of junctional or ventricular origin to occur. (Complete heart block is a type of AV dissociation.)
- Rapid rhythms of junctional or ventricular origin occur as a result of irritability of an ectopic site in either area.

NOTE. In AV dissociation, the atria are controlled by the atrial pacemaker and the ventricles are controlled by the escape focus of junctional or ventricular origin.

Treatment

1. Monitor closely. Cardiac output may be adversely affected due to changes in rate.
2. Withhold digitalis, as this is a frequent cause of the arrhythmia. Notify the physician.
3. Pacemaker therapy may be indicated. (See complete heart block on p 58.)

WOLFF–PARKINSON–WHITE SYNDROME

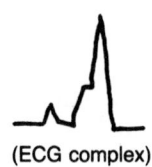

(ECG complex)

Description

A preexcitation syndrome, congenital in origin, in which the atrial impulse is transmitted through an abnormally shortened pathway to the ventricles. In this manner, the AV node is bypassed.

Characteristics

The following are characteristics of Wolff–Parkinson–White syndrome in the presence of sinus rhythm.
- PR interval is shortened (less than 0.12 second).
- QRS complex is widened (greater than 0.12 second).
- Delta wave (*i.e.*, a slurred upstroke of the QRS complex) is present.
- There are secondary S-T segment and T wave changes.

Important Variations

Some patients exhibit the characteristic ECG changes only intermittently, changing back and forth from normal to Wolff–Parkinson–White beats, with the delta wave varying in size.

PR interval may not be present if the delta wave begins before the ending of the P wave.

The characteristic widening of the QRS with the accompanying delta wave usually disappears during attacks of tachycardia; therefore, Wolff–Parkinson–White syndrome cannot be diagnosed until the tachycardia stops.

NOTE. Wolff–Parkinson–White syndrome is associated with recurrent paroxysmal tachycardia; therefore, the condition should be suspected in this type of arrhythmia. During periods of atrial fibrillation or flutter, the bypass tract may allow 200 or more impulses to stimulate the ventricles (*i.e.*, the bypass tract has a shorter refractory period than the AV node). Very rapid ventricular response interferes with the cardiac output and may lead to loss of consciousness, cardiogenic shock, ventricular fibrillation, or sudden death.

Treatment

1. Monitor closely. Cardiac output may be adversely affected by the tachycardia.
2. Quinidine therapy may be effective. Pronestyl may also be considered.
3. Digitalis alone is contraindicated because it may increase the ventricular rate.
4. Digitalis combined with quinidine may successfully treat atrial flutter or fibrillation.
5. Lidocaine may be administered to slow the rapid ventricular rate.

6. Surgery may be necessary where the accessory pathway is interrupted.
7. Extremely rapid ventricular rhythms may require electrical countershock.

NOTE. The ECG of Wolff–Parkinson–White syndrome may be misleading. It may mask other diseases or may be misinterpreted (*e.g.*, MI, bundle branch block). It is extremely important to correctly diagnose this condition. Conventional therapy may be ineffective and sometimes dangerous (*i.e.*, the use of digitalis alone).

LOWN–GANONG–LEVINE SYNDROME

Description   Lown–Ganong–Levine syndrome is another type of preexcitation syndrome. Although the AV node is bypassed, the accessory pathway enters the Bundle of His, resulting in normal ventricular conduction.

Characteristics   The following are characteristic of Lown–Ganong–Levine syndrome in the presence of sinus rhythm.
• PR interval is shortened (less than 0.12 second).
• Delta wave is absent.
• QRS complex is normal.

NOTE. Supraventricular tachycardia may be associated with this syndrome.

PARASYSTOLE

Description   In parasystole an ectopic pacemaker (usually ventricular) fires at a fixed rate, functioning independently of the basic rate.

Characteristics   Parasystole may appear as fusion beats or other random beats. The complex has a different configuration than the basic rhythm.

Treatment   See the treatment for premature beats (atrial, nodal or ventricular), depending on the origin in a preceding section of this chapter.

ESCAPE BEATS (or rhythm)

Description   An escape beat is a back-up system that is activated when the normal pacemaker fails to fire for one or more beats. The escape beat may be atrial, nodal or ventricular in origin.

Characteristics

The following are characteristics of each type of escape beat.

- Atrial—P wave is abnormally shaped, but the QRS complex is normal.
- Nodal—QRS complex is normal, and the normal P wave is absent.
- Ventricular—an escape beat originating in the ventricle resembles a PVC.

Treatment

Treatment depends on the cause (*i.e.*, some degree of block in the SA or AV nodes; extremely slow basic rhythm).

5
Cardiac Trauma

Early detection of cardiac trauma may be essential to the patient's survival. Some of the most common conditions seen in the critical care unit are discussed in this chapter—myocardial contusion, penetrating cardiac wound, ruptured aorta, and cardiac tamponade.

Basic Information

Types of cardiac trauma
- *Penetrating*—trauma caused by a knife, bullet, fractured rib
- *Nonpenetrating*—blunt trauma caused by indirect pressure or force
- *Iatrogenic*—trauma caused by cardiopulmonary resuscitation, cardiac catheterization and other procedures

Effects of cardiac trauma
- Arrhythmias
- Coronary artery injury (may be accompanied by MI)
- Cardiac tamponade
- Aneurysm formation
- Emboli
- Bacterial endocarditis
- Pericarditis
- Myocardial contusion
- Myocardial laceration
- Myocardial rupture
- Septal defects
- Valve injury
- Great vessel injury
- Papillary muscle injury
- Injury of the chordae tendineae

MYOCARDIAL CONTUSION (CARDIAC CONTUSION)

Description

Bleeding in the myocardium due to trauma may involve a small area or may be extensive. Decreased cardiac output and resulting necrosis may follow an extensive contusion.

Cause

Nonpenetrating trauma (*e.g.*, from steering wheel injury)

Clinical Manifestations

May be asymptomatic

Transient angina located retrosternal (unless atherosclerotic coronary artery disease present)

Pericardial friction rub

Bruise on chest wall

Arrhythmias (any type of atrial or ventricular arrhythmias)

May not appear for several hours or days and may be masked by other injuries

Diagnostic Tests

ECG changes—tachycardia; changes consistent with myocardial infarction; varying arrhythmias

Serum enzymes—elevated but not a specific diagnostic tool here because of soft tissue injury (*i.e.*, elevations are associated with soft tissue injury, also)

Should be suspected with any major anterior chest wall contusion

Isoenzymes MB—CPK will help differentiate cardiac from soft tissue injuries

Treatment and Nursing Actions

1. Monitor continuously. Treat arrhythmias according to conventional methods.

2. Promote rest. Bed rest and restriction of activities are indicated.

3. Be alert for complications such as cardiac rupture, aortic rupture, congestive failure or aneurysm.

4. Closely observe any patient with major trauma of the anterior chest wall, especially sternal injuries, for several days for this condition. Notify physician immediately if condition is suspected.

5. Have emergency equipment and drugs readily available. Complications such as cardiac tamponade or life-threatening arrhythmias (*i.e.*, ventricular tachycardia or fibrillation) could develop at any time.

6. Keep in mind that the irritability of the myocardium is increased. Avoid drugs, including general anesthesia if possible, that could compound this problem.

7. Assist physician with insertion of a Swan–Ganz catheter to monitor wedge pressures. Monitor closely.

8. Keep in mind that hypervolemia and hypovolemia are equally dangerous.

PENETRATING CARDIAC WOUND

Description

A penetrating cardiac wound is a wound in which an object has entered the interior of the heart.

Causes

Sharp object (*e.g.*, knife, icepick)

Missile (*e.g.*, bullet, shrapnel)

Clinical Manifestations

Hemorrhage (external or internal)

Chest pain

Change in level of consciousness (*i.e.*, from confused or drowsy to unconscious)

Symptoms of cardiac tamponade

Chest wound (either anterior or posterior)

Hemothorax

Pneumothorax

Patient may be agitated or combative

Cardiac arrest

Diagnostic Tests

Pericardiocentesis—confirms the diagnosis of tamponade

Chest x-ray film

Treatment and Nursing Actions

1. Attach patient to monitor and watch closely.
2. Check vital signs and level of consciousness frequently.
3. Prevent any further damage and bleeding
   - If the object is still in place when patient is admitted to the hospital, do *not* remove it. Secure it with sterile dressing to prevent any futher movement. Removal of the object is the physician's responsibility and will be done in the operating room.
   - If the object has already been removed, apply direct pressure to the wound, using a sterile dressing.
4. Assist with insertion of hemodynamic monitoring devices and watch pressures closely.
5. Administer oxygen.
   - Method (*i.e.*, mask, intubation) depends on patient status
   - Check blood gases.
6. Prepare for and assist with pericardiocentesis.

7. Prepare for and assist with thoracentesis or chest tube insertion.
8. Prepare patient for emergency surgery (*i.e.*, type and crossmatch blood, prep)
9. Keep emergency equipment and medications readily available, including respirator and defibrillator.
10. Provide emotional support.
    - If patient is drowsy or unconscious, provide protective measures (*i.e.*, raise side rails or apply stretcher belt).
    - If patient is agitated or combative, protect him from further injury (*i.e.*, pad side rails, apply body restraints).
    - Explain what is being done. (Keep in mind that fear increases anxiety and agitation.)
11. Start an IV in a large vein and replace volume as necessary.
12. Administer medications as ordered.
13. Initiate resuscitation techniques if patient has cardiac arrest.
14. Insert Foley catheter and attach it to drainage bag.
15. Monitor intake and output closely.
16. Examine closely for other injuries (both anterior and posterior surfaces)

NOTE. Security provisions should be made for safeguarding the object causing the trauma after its removal until it can be given to law enforcement personnel. Follow hospital policy.

RUPTURED AORTA

Cause

Trauma (*i.e.*, sudden deceleration as in auto accident, compression injury from high fall, penetrating wound)

Clinical Manifestations

Pain in chest or back, not influenced by respiration

Weakness in extremities or paraplegia

Weak, thready pulse

Dyspnea (may be due to pressure of the left main bronchus)

Sensorium changes (*i.e.*, drowsiness, loss of consciousness)

Hemothorax

NOTE. In some patients, the following clinical manifestations may be detected. There may be elevated blood pressure and pulse amplitude in the upper extremities or decreased blood pressure and pulse amplitude in the lower extremities.

Diagnostic Tests

Chest x-ray film—shows widening of the mediastinum

Retrograde aortogram—confirms the diagnosis

NOTE. If the tear is partial (*i.e.*, the outer layer is intact), the patient may survive until surgical intervention may be arranged. If the tear is complete or full-thickness, death usually ensues immediately due to exsanguination.

Treatment and Nursing Actions

1. Monitor closely, including vital signs. This condition is very unstable.
2. Have emergency equipment and medications readily available, including a respirator and defibrillator.
3. Administer oxygen.
   - Method depends on patient status.
   - Check blood gases.
4. Prepare patient for emergency surgery (*i.e.*, type and crossmatch blood, prep). Immediate surgical resection and grafting are indicated.
5. Start an IV in a large vein and replace volume as necessary.
6. Insert Foley catheter and attach to drainage bag.
7. Closely monitor intake and output.
8. Administer medications as ordered, including antihypertensives such as Nipride if hypertension is present.

CARDIAC TAMPONADE

Description

Cardiac tamponade is a progressive condition that results from the escape of excess fluid into the pericardial space. The type of fluid (*i.e.*, purulent, hemorrhagic, serous) depends on the cause. Normally, only a small amount of fluid is present (approximately 25–30 ml). In tamponade, excessive amounts of fluid accumulate in the pericardial space. Accumulation may occur slowly or rapidly, depending on the underlying cause. This causes an increase in intrapericardial pressure, resulting in marked interference with ventricular diastolic filling.

Causes

The collection of fluid causing tamponade is called pericardial effusion. Some of the conditions that result in pericardial effusion of sufficient degree to cause tamponade include the following:

Trauma to the great vessels or heart (either direct or indirect)

Postmyocardial infarction syndrome (Dressler's syndrome)

A primary or metastatic tumor involving the pericardium

Rupture of the great vessels or heart

Anticoagulant therapy when given in the presence of pericarditis

Nonspecific pericarditis

Pericarditis resulting from infections (*i.e.*, acute rheumatic fever, pyogenic infections, tuberculosis)

Postthoracotomy syndrome

Uremia

Connective tissue disease

Clinical Manifestations

Distended neck veins

Dyspnea

Orthopnea

Faint heart sounds

Elevated venous pressure

Low arterial blood pressure with narrowed pulse pressure

Low cardiac output

Paradoxical pulse

Possibility of sinus tachycardia or supraventricular tachycardia

Shock

Cyanosis

Change in level of consciousness

Fast, thready pulse

A conscious patient may complain of pain over the precordium that varies with respiration or posture usually described as tearing or sharp

Patient characteristically sits upright and leans forward

Diagnostic Tests

X-ray films—both invasive and noninvasive methods are used. The chest x-ray film shows an enlarged heart and clear lung fields. More sophisticated x-rays may confirm the presence of a pericardial effusion. These include echocardiography, radioisotope cardiac scanning angiocardiography, and a chest x-ray film following the intravenous injection of CO_2 with the patient lying on his left side.

Possible ECG changes
- Complete electrical alternans—a decrease in the amplitude or size of the P wave, QRS complex, and T wave with alternate beats
- A generalized lessening in voltage
- Show ST-segment elevation with or without inversion of the T wave.
- ECG may remain normal

Treatment

• Pericardiocentesis is the immediate treatment for cardiac tamponade. In this procedure, fluid is removed from the pericardium by way of needle aspiration (see procedure.) Repeated aspirations may be necessary. The patient may need surgical intervention if pericardiocentesis is unsuccessful or complications develop.

Complications

Arrhythmias

Laceration of the ventricle

Cardiac arrest

Laceration of a coronary artery

Hydropneumothorax

Puncture of liver, lung, or stomach

Air embolism

Infection

Recurring cardiac tamponade

PERICARDIOCENTESIS

Description

Fluid is removed from the pericardium by means of needle aspiration to relieve cardiac tamponade.

Equipment

Sterile pericardiocentesis tray

Sterile gloves

ECG machine

Defibrillator equipment

Sterile alligator clips and ground wires

Antiseptic skin preparation (povidone-iodine preparation)

Local anesthesia

Crash cart

Specimen containers for lab analysis (if applicable)

16–18 gauge short bevel needle

50-ml syringe

3-way stopcock

Hypodermic syringe with needle

Sponges and compresses

Solution container

Preliminary Actions

1. Premedicate patient as ordered to allay apprehension (meperidine, morphine, barbiturates). Obtain written consent if time permits.
2. Place patient in semirecumbent position.
   - Elevate head at a 60° angle.
   - This position facilitates insertion of the needle.
3. Apply limb leads of the ECG.
   - Constant ECG monitoring is necessary during the procedure.
4. Prepare emergency equipment and medications. (Turn on defibrillator and have anti-arrhythmic agents ready to administer.)

   ALERT. Complications may occur at any time.

5. Monitor the CVP (if line is present), the blood pressure, cardiac rhythm, and pulse before and during the procedure. Also, monitor respirations and general condition of patient.

Procedure

1. Using aseptic technique, open tray.
   - Assist physician.
   - After connecting the wire to the sterile needle, using the alligator clips, the physician will pass it to the nurse, who attaches the wire to the precordial or V-lead wire of the ECG.
   - Monitoring the entrance of the pericardial needle by way of ECG aids in safe positioning and helps prevent puncturing of the heart.
2. Observe monitor during insertion of the needle.
   - Notify the physician immediately of any adverse effects.
   - Normally, there is a short increase in the QRS complex when the pericardial sac is entered.
   - Penetration of the myocardium is indicated by marked elevation of the ST segment, PR segment elevation, and arrhythmias. If any of these ECG changes occur, the needle should be withdrawn a few millimeters until they are no longer visible.
3. Observe patient for effect of procedure.
   - Note the fluid aspirated; it may be cloudy, clear, or bloody. Normally, pericardial blood does not clot. (Accidental puncture of the heart will yield blood that does clot.)
   - In conditions in which bloody pericardial fluid is present, it is important to be aware of the needle position, as evidenced by ECG, to be sure that a heart chamber has not been entered.
   - If the procedure is unsuccessful, or clotting blood is present in the pericardial fluid (*i.e.,* trauma), immediate surgery is indicated.
4. Label specimen and send to lab.
   - Diagnostic studies are sometimes ordered by the physician.

5. Observe patient closely following procedure.
   - Monitor CVP, rhythm, pulse, and blood pressure for 24 hours.
   - Recurring cardiac tamponade is a genuine possibility. Repeated aspirations may be necessary.
   - Surgery is indicated if the procedure is unsuccessful, fluid continues to accumulate, or complications develop.
6. Protect the site against infection after the procedure.
   - Cleanse with antiseptic preparation.
   - Apply bandage.

6

Electrical Countershock

Electrical countershock (cardioversion and defibrillation) is frequently used in the treatment of specific arrhythmias. These procedures and associated nursing responsibilities are described in this chapter.

Complications of Electrical Countershock

Cardiac
- Arrhythmias
- Arrest
- Hypotension

Pulmonary
- Edema
- Arrest
- Emboli

Systemic emboli

Skin burns

Death

DEFIBRILLATION

Description

Emergency therapy

Unsynchronized charge

Charge is delivered by way of paddles applied externally to the chest wall or internally applied directly to the myocardium.

Purpose

To terminate ventricular fibrillation

Equipment

Defibrillator

ECG monitor

Paddles (external and sterilized internal paddles)

Conductive gel or saline pads

Equipment for oxygen therapy

Equipment for emergency pacing

Crash cart with emergency drugs, airway, resuscitator bag, endotracheal tubes and equipment necessary for insertion

Nursing Actions

1. Correctly diagnose ventricular fibrillation.
   - Check the monitor.
   - Check the patient.
2. Turn power on and make sure the machine is properly grounded.
3. Set the discharge energy at 400 watt/sec (adult).
4. Depress the charge button to charge the unit.
5. Turn the switch to defibrillation.
6. Be sure the synchronizer switch is turned off.
7. Apply conductive jelly to entire surface of paddles.

   NOTE. Moistened saline gauze pads placed in the proper position on the chest may also be used. Never use alcohol soaked pads. Remove any excess electrode gel that may be present on the chest, especially after repeated "shocks," to prevent electrical arcs. Electric arcs not only decrease the electric current delivered to the heart but may result in burns for both the patient and the person defibrillating him.

8. Make sure all personnel are clear of the bed.
   - Give the order to clear.
   - Visually check to make sure all are clear.
9. Cut off oxygen during defibrillation.
10. Firmly depress the discharge button on the machine or simultaneously depress the buttons on the paddles until the full charge is delivered.
11. Observe the monitor and patient for effectiveness.
12. Immediately prepare machine for possible reuse.
13. Be prepared to support the patient with (CPR) and emergency drug therapy.
14. Oxygen therapy is usually indicated.

Aftercare

1. Closely monitor the patient's vital signs, heart and lung sounds, and sensorium.
   - Check every 15 minutes or less for the first hour post defibrillation.
   - If stable, check every hour, eventually progressing to checks every 4 hours as the condition permits.
2. Observe the ECG continuously.

3. Prepare the machine for possible reuse. Remove all conductive jelly from paddles with soap and water.

4. Remove all conductive jelly from the patient's chest with soap and water and check for skin burns. Treat according to physician's orders.

Special Situations
Internal Defibrillation

1. Have sterile prepared tray readily available for opening the chest (should be kept on crash cart).

2. Sterile internal defibrillation paddles are placed over sterile saline pads against the myocardium.

3. Electrical current is usually set at 15 (or less) to 30 watt/sec (joules).

The Patient with a Pacemaker

1. Turn off temporary external pacemaker before defibrillating.

2. If the patient has a permanent pulse generator, do not place paddles over the generator.

Infants and Children

Use smaller appropriate size paddles available for this age group for the transverse position.

Anterior-posterior paddles may be used.

The amount of current suggested for this age group (following correction of acidosis) is as follows:
- Neonate—10 to 25 watt/sec
- Infant—25 to 50 watt/sec
- Children (12–25 kg)—50 to 100 watt/sec
- Older Children (25–50 kg)—100 to 200 watt/sec[1]

CARDIOVERSION

Description
Elective therapy

Charge is synchronized to the patient's R wave

Charge is delivered via paddles applied to the external chest wall

Purpose
To terminate ventricular and atrial tachyarrhythmias

Equipment
Cardioverter

ECG monitor

External paddles

Conductive gel or saline pads

Equipment for oxygen therapy

Equipment for emergency pacing

Crash cart with emergency drugs, airway, resuscitator bag, endotracheal tubes, and equipment necessary for insertion

Preliminary Actions

Sedate patient prior to the procedure.

Patient is not allowed anything by mouth for at least 6 hours prior to the procedure.

Nursing Actions

1. Establish an IV.
2. Monitor vital signs, ECG, and sensorium to establish baseline. Arterial blood gases should also be checked.
3. Support the patient emotionally.
   - Reinforce physician's explanation of procedure.
   - Answer questions.
   - Stay with patient.
   - Explain what is going on, especially the function of any equipment.
4. Remove dentures and make-up (including nail polish).
5. Administer oxygen prior to cardioversion to improve oxygen supply to the myocardium and discontinue when electrical charge is delivered.
6. Attach patient to monitor.
7. Have cardioverter and emergency drugs readily available.
8. Sedation is administered intravenously just prior to procedure to lessen any discomfort as well as to relax the patient. Valium or Brevital are most commonly used.
9. Prepare the machine for cardioversion.
   - Turn power on. Make sure the machine is properly grounded.
   - Turn the synchronizer switch on.
   - Set the discharge energy at the amount ordered by the physician. Low voltages are initially used (50–100 watt/sec at a time).
   - Depress the charge button.
   - Apply conductive jelly to entire surface of paddles (see Defibrillation Nursing Actions #7 in a preceding section of this chapter).
   - Make sure the machine is properly synchronized to the R wave (indicated by the machine). If the R waves are not large enough to trigger the discharge of electrical current, increase the gain. If still unsuccessful, change leads.
10. Place the paddles appropriately on the chest. Make sure they are firmly in contact with the skin surface.
11. Make sure all personnel are clear of the bed.
    - Give the order to clear.
    - Visually check to make sure all are clear.

12. Cut off oxygen during discharge of current.

13. Firmly depress the discharge button on the machine or simultaneously depress the buttons on the paddles until the full charge is delivered.

14. Observe the monitor and the patient for effectiveness.

15. Immediately prepare machine for possible reuse.

16. Be prepared to support the patient with antiarrhythmic drugs if PVC's occur, or CPR and emergency drugs if ventricular fibrillation occurs. Be sure to turn machine back to defibrillation (synchronizer is turned off) if this complication occurs. (See Defibrillation, p 79.)

17. Oxygen therapy may be indicated. Drugs used for premedication can result in respiratory depression causing hypoxia.

18. Care following the procedure (See Defibrillation, Aftercare, pp 80–81.)

Special Considerations
- Digitalis preparations are usually withheld several days prior to the procedure to prevent death-producing arrhythmias caused by digitalis toxicity. Digitalis level should be checked prior to procedure if possible.
- Hypokalemia also predisposes the patient to dangerous arrhythmias. Therefore, potassium level should be checked, and if abnormal, corrected prior to the procedure.
- Have the patient empty his bladder prior to the procedure.

REFERENCE
1. Oakes Annalee R (ed): Critical Care Nursing of Children and Adolescents. Philadelphia: WB Saunders, 1981

7
Pacemaker Therapy

The insertion of a pacemaker is a frequent emergency necessity. Temporary and permanent pacemakers and the nursing responsibilities associated with them are presented in this chapter.

Description and Purpose
A pacemaker is a device that delivers electrical stimulation by way of electrodes placed within the heart to improve rate. This stimulation either augments the inherent cardiac pacemaker or takes over the pacing function.

General Information
- Mercury zinc batteries are most commonly used as the power source. Others currently in use are nickel cadmium, lithium iodide, and nuclear powered devices.
- Pacemaker may be temporary or permanent.

ALERT. Care of pacemaker during defibrillation is as follows.

1. Turn off the pacemaker.
2. Disconnect wires from battery pack.
3. Avoid any contact of defibrillator paddles with wires.

Components of the Pacemaker
Pulse generator—this is a power source, which is usually battery powered.

Cable wire (bridging cable)—this extension is sometimes used to connect the electrodes and the pulse generator.

Electrodes—they carry the information from the area to be paced back to the pulse generator, and then transmit the electrical impulse from the pulse generator back to the area.
- Unipolar electrode—negative pole is located within the heart; a wire suture, which is placed in the skin on the chest wall serves as the positive pole.
- Bipolar electrode—both positive and negative poles are located on the tip of this electrode about 1 cm apart.

Pacing Methods

External pacing—this is the original method of pacing, whereby an electrode is placed on the chest wall. The external pacing method is for temporary use only and is no longer used.

Direct pacing—one of the following methods may be used.

- A small electrode is passed through the venous system and into the right ventricle, in contact with the endocardium.
- The electrodes are inserted by way of a thoracotomy or midline mediastinal incision and attached to the cardiac epicardium. This method may be for temporary or permanent use.

Transthoracic pacing—a needle electrode is inserted through the chest wall into the myocardium. Transthoracic pacing is used for emergency resuscitation and is for temporary use only.

TYPES OF PACEMAKERS
ASYNCHRONOUS PACEMAKER
(continuous, set, or fixed-rate pacing)

Leads   One, either an atrial or a ventricular lead

Function   This pacemaker continuously fires at a preset rate without regard to the cardiac rhythm that may be present (Figs. 7-1 and 7-2).

SYNCHRONOUS PACEMAKER (P wave or QRS triggered)

Leads   Atrial—2 leads (1 in atrium and 1 in ventricle)
                   Ventricular—1 lead

Function   Senses when the pacemaker should fire
                   - Atrial—atrial lead senses atrial contraction; information is transmitted to pulse generator; following

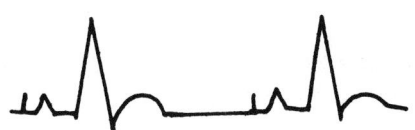

FIG. 7-1. *Asynchronous pacemaker, atrial lead.*

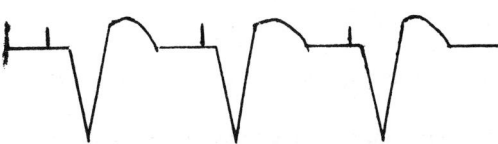

FIG. 7-2. *Asynchronous pacemaker, ventricular lead.*

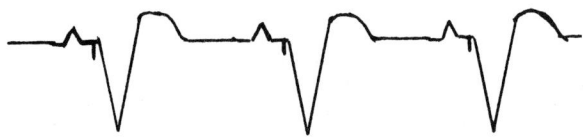

FIG. 7-3. *Synchronous pacemaker, atrial lead.*

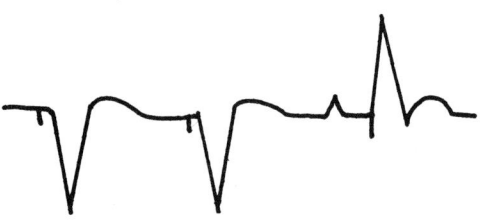

FIG. 7-4. *Synchronous pacemaker, ventricular lead. (Pacemaker fires continuously, even during the normal QRS.)*

a short pause (equivalent to PR interval), ventricles are stimulated; built-in safeguards prevent ventricular rate from going above preset rate in response to tachyarrhythmias by blocking excess stimulation (Fig. 7-3).

- Ventricular—ventricular lead will stimulate a contraction when the rate drops below the preset rate and fires within the QRS complex when the patient's rate exceeds that of the pacemaker (Fig. 7-4).

DEMAND PACEMAKER (Ventricular or QRS-Stimulus Inhibited)

Lead   One ventricular lead

Function   Pacemaker fires only when necessary or on demand, that is, when the patient's rate drops below the preset rate (Fig. 7-5).

SEQUENTIAL DEMAND PACEMAKER (Bifocal Demand)

Lead   One atrial and one ventricular lead

Function   When the patient fails to pace on his own, this pacemaker operates on demand, that is, the atrial electrode will pace the atria, and the ventricular electrode will pace the ventricles if necessary (Fig. 7-6).

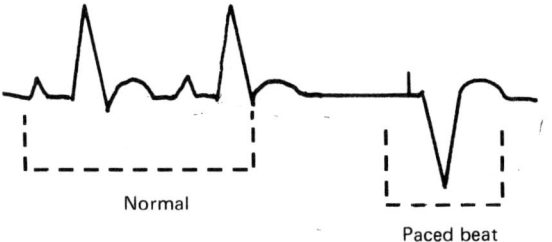

FIG 7-5. *Demand pacemaker.*

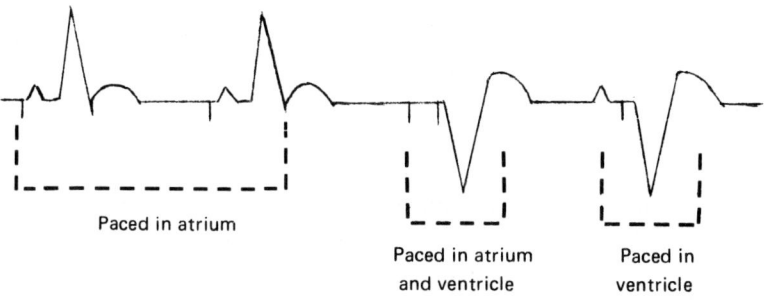

FIG. 7-6. *Sequential AV pacing.*

PACEMAKER INSERTION

NOTE. Before beginning, make sure new battery is working properly.

Temporary Pacemaker
Preoperative Nursing Actions

1. Explain the procedure, equipment to be used, and purpose. If possible, obtain a signed consent form.

2. Connect the patient to a properly grounded ECG monitor.
   • Disconnect other electrical equipment.
   • Monitor continuously.
   • If the pacing catheter is to be positioned with the aid of ECG monitoring, attach the limb leads to all extremities and after insertion, attach the chest (V) lead to free end of the electrode (using an alligator clamp).

3. Check vital signs and monitor closely.

4. Start an IV or check the patency of the established one in case emergency drug therapy is necessary.
   - Crash cart and emergency equipment should be readily available.
   - Have a syringe filled with Lidocaine readily available.

ALERT. Ventricular premature beats or fibrillation may occur when the catheter tip is threaded through the ventricles.

5. Sedate the patient as ordered.

6. This is a sterile procedure; personnel in contact with patient should wear gloves, gown, and mask.

7. Prepare the skin by cleaning with a solution of povidone-iodine.

8. Have the patient lie flat to prevent air embolism.

Nursing Actions During Insertion

1. Continuously monitor the patient throughout the procedure.

2. Watch for the following ECG changes as the catheter enters the heart and is correctly positioned.
   - Small, inverted P waves; amplitude of P waves and QRS about the same in the vena cava
   - Tall, biphasic P waves in the right atrium (Amplitude of QRS increases and P wave decreases as the catheter approaches the right ventricle.)
   - Large QRS and P waves that grow progressively smaller in the right ventricle
   - Elevated ST-segment (current of injury pattern)—catheter is wedged against right ventricular wall.

3. Watch for PVC's or ventricular fibrillation as the catheter is threaded into the ventricle.
   - Notify the physician immediately of this occurrence and treat accordingly.

4. When the catheter is positioned correctly (against the ventricular wall), the free end of the pacing electrode is connected to the pacemaker by the physician in the following manner
   - The external pacemaker is turned on.
   - The pacemaker is adjusted until effective capture is obtained (*i.e.*, a ventricular response follows each pacemaker impulse).
   - The electrode wire is sutured at the insertion site. Any exposed electrode wire should be covered by a rubber glove.

ALERT. Never touch exposed wire with bare hands.

For a summary of ECG changes observed when a standard catheter or a flow-directed (balloon-tipped) catheter is used during pacemaker insertion, see Intracavitary ECG Monitoring chart.

INTRACAVITARY ECG MONITORING

During pacemaker insertion, using a standard pacing catheter or a flow-directed (balloon-tipped) catheter, the following ECG changes should be observed:

1. As the tip of the catheter is directed into the vena cava, the P wave will appear small and inverted.
2. When the catheter passes into the right atrium, the following should appear:
   • *High*—P wave is very tall, dwarfing the QRS.
   • *Middle*—P wave is still very tall, but the QRS equals it in size.
   • *Low*—P wave becomes much smaller; QRS increases in size.
3. When the catheter passes into the right ventricle
   • *High*—QRS suddenly becomes very large.
   • *Against the ventricular wall*—the "current of injury" pattern (*i.e.*, ST segment) is markedly elevated.
4. At this point, the pacing catheter will be positioned properly.
5. After the pacemaker is connected to the battery source and turned on, the ECG will show the standard tracing for a paced heart, depending on the type of pacing method used (demand, fixed-rate).

Postoperative Care

ALERT. It is essential for the nurse to know the type of pacing used, the set rate, and the type of ECG tracing a properly functioning pacemaker will exhibit. This information should be recorded on the kardex and the chart.

1. Monitor the ECG closely.
   • Observe closely for arrhythmias such as ventricular tachycardia or fibrillation and treat accordingly.
   • Make sure that the pacemaker is functioning properly.
   • Watch closely for pacemaker malfunction.
   • Check the threshold every 8 hours at least.
   • Run a rhythm strip every hour for 48 hours, as necessary, as ordered, or if any abnormality is detected.
2. The external battery pack must be covered with a plastic cover to prevent the dials from being changed inadvertently.
3. Following the procedure, the electrode position is checked by obtaining a 12-lead ECG and chest x-ray film.
4. Maintain electrical safety precautions.

- The patient's bed should be nonelectric.
- Keep the patient and his environment dry (*i.e.,* change gown and linen if they become wet).
- Make sure that all electrical equipment in use is properly grounded.
- Make sure that all exposed connections are covered by a rubber glove. Never touch exposed wires with bare hands; wear rubber gloves.
- Prevent outside electrical interference by restricting the use of the following equipment near the patient: microwave ovens; diathermy equipment; electrocautery and electrocoagulating equipment; electric toothbrushes, radios, and shavers.

NOTE. Battery-operated devices may be used.

5. Secure the free end of the pacing catheter to prevent it from being inadvertently dislodged.
   - Tape catheter securely to the skin, being careful to prevent any tension. Apply armboard to keep the arm straight.
   - Secure (with tape) the battery pack either to the bed or to the patient.
   - Encourage the patient to minimize movement as much as possible for 24 hr to 48 hr following insertion to prevent displacement of the catheter tip.
   - Position patient on back or left side. Keep off of right side.
6. Check insertion site and treat site daily.
   - Keep area dry. Apply sterile dressing.
   - Clean site with povidone-iodine.
   - Prevent rubber glove (covering wire) from touching skin and from being dislodged by placing sterile gauze pads underneath and on top. Secure sterile gauze pads with tape.
   - Secure area with a sterile dressing.
7. Keep emergency drugs and equipment (*i.e.,* crash cart and defibrillator) readily available in case dangerous arrhythmias occur.
8. Check vital signs at least four times a day, including temperature. Temperature elevation should be reported to the physician immediately.
9. Serum electrolytes should be closely monitored because abnormalities may cause cardiac irritability.

PERMANENT PACEMAKER
Preoperative Nursing Actions

1. See preoperative care for insertion of temporary pacemaker in a preceding section of this chapter.
2. Patient teaching concerning the procedure will vary according to the approach used (*i.e.,* since endocardial implantation uses the transvenous route, local anesthesia is used; epicardial implantation involves either a thoracotomy or a midline mediastinal incision—the pleural cavity is not entered—hence general anesthesia is used).

Nursing Actions During Insertion

1. Permanent pacemaker insertion performed in the operating room under strict aseptic technique.

2. Insertion of a permanent pacemaker is the same as for a temporary pacemaker, with the exception that the pacemaker generator is inserted under the skin in the deltopectoral area (transvenous approach) or the left upper quadrant of the abdomen (epicardial approach).

Postoperative Care

1. If general anesthesia is used, provide care for surgical patient who has undergone general anesthesia and a thoracotomy (*i.e.*, chest tubes and suction).

2. Monitor the ECG closely (See step 1 of Postoperative Care for the Temporary Pacemaker, p 89.)

3. Prevent electrical interference by utilizing safety measures discussed in postoperative care of temporary pacemaker insertion.

4. Keep IV patent in case administration of emergency drugs is necessary and, also, as routine therapy following chest surgery.

5. Keep emergency drugs and equipment readily available.

6. Check site for pacemaker generator and pacing catheter insertion or incision for chest surgery and pacemaker generator site.
   • Care for site daily or as necessary using sterile technique.
   • Site should be cleaned with povidone-iodine.
   • Secure area with a sterile dressing after it has been cleaned.

7. Check vital signs at least 4 times a day, including temperature. (Vital signs should be checked every 4 hours if chest surgery was performed.)

8. Administer analgesics as ordered for pain.

9. Administer antibiotics as ordered to prevent infection.

Patient Teaching

1. Begin teaching both patient and family members a program for home care.
   • Teach patient to check pulse.
     • Check pulse daily.
     • Make sure patient knows the preset rate.
     • Caution him to notify physician if pulse rate is below or above set rate.
   • Instruct patient to wear an identification bracelet designating the necessary information—type of pacemaker, brand, rate, physician, and the hospital where procedure was performed.
   • Advise patient of safety methods to prevent electrical interference.
     • Avoid areas of high voltage—TV; radio or radar transmitters and towers (not home television antennas); microwave ovens; ignition systems (working directly over); diathermy; electrocautery; faulty or poorly grounded electrical equipment; arc welders; theft protection devices in stores (the detection area).

- Inform dentist that you have a pacemaker; electric drill may affect pacemaker.
- Avoid the use of or contact with any electrical device that causes dizziness or light-headedness.
- Check with physician concerning devices that may have an effect on your specific pacemaker. Many are resistant to electrical interference, with some exceptions.
  - Advise patient to protect the pacemaker site.
  - Avoid sports or other activities in which a sudden blow might be delivered to this area.
  - Wear loose fitting clothing over the site.
- Identify the physical signs and symptoms that indicate pacemaker failure (*i.e.*, fainting, dizziness, chest pain, palpitations).
- Instruct patient about proper cleaning of the site.
- Advise patient to notify the physician immediately if he observes any signs of infection (swelling, redness, pain or tenderness, drainage) or if the pacemaker is protruding through the incision.
- Stress the need for follow-up care with the physician.
  - Check with physician regarding the desired schedule for regular examinations and ECG. Examinations are needed to determine pacemaker function, need for battery replacement, and patient response.
  - Give patient a copy of his ECG to keep, along with pacemaker information (brand, type, serial number, rate, physician, hospital).
2. Check with physician concerning initiation of passive and active range of motion exercises (usually permissible 24–48 hr following insertion).

COMPLICATIONS OF PACEMAKER THERAPY

Complications may be associated with any of the following factors.

PACING ELECTRODE WITHIN THE BODY

Physical problems
- Perforation of ventricular wall by the catheter tip

NOTE. A very small amount of bleeding occurs; therefore, tamponade does not usually result unless the patient is on anticoagulants.

- Skin infection or thrombophlebitis at insertion site
- Ventricular irritability leading to dangerous arrhythmias resulting from stimulation by the catheter
- Pulmonary emboli resulting from blood clot formation on catheter tip
- Pulmonary air embolism
- Structural complications within the heart (*e.g.*, endocarditis, trauma to the chordae tendineae of the tricuspid valve)
- Escape of pacing impulse to noncardiac areas (*i.e.*, contractions of the chest wall or diaphragm, hiccups)
- Breaking off (fracture) of the catheter, with segments becoming an embolus

Mechanical problems
- Fracture of wire
- Malposition
- Dislodgement
- Poor pacemaker connection
- Break in insulation

Problems accompanying general anesthesia and chest surgery

PERMANENT PACEMAKER

Physical problems
- Protrusion of the battery through the incision
- Infection
- Hematoma

Mechanical problems
- Power depletion
- Short circuit between pacemaker terminals
- Seal broken, allowing body fluids to enter pacemaker
- Component failure

PACEMAKER FUNCTION

Improper release of stimulus
- Loss of pacemaker spike, occurring intermittently or constantly
- Acceleration of the pacing rate (runaway pacemaker)
  - Failure to sense—pacemaker fails to sense the QRS complex and fires without regard for the patient's own rhythm (competition)
  - Loss of capture—pacing spike fails to produce QRS (ventricular pacemaker) or P wave (atrial pacemaker)

PACEMAKER MALFUNCTION

Clinical Signs

Fainting

Dizziness

Memory loss

Convulsions

Stokes–Adams attack

Congestive heart failure

Palpitations

Chest pain

Pulse changes (apical rate is faster or slower than set rate)

Hiccups or twitching of abdominal muscle

Second heart sound becomes widely split

Sudden death

Nursing Actions for External Pacemaker Malfunctions
Loss of Pacing Spike

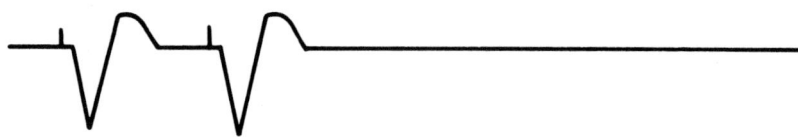

1. Check battery pack. See if needle is fluctuating back and forth. Replace battery if depletion is the problem.
2. Evaluate patient's rhythm and its effectiveness.
3. Check all connections.
4. Keep Isuprel drip on standby.
5. Turn milliampere (Ma) dial up to highest setting if patient is symptomatic and emergency condition exists.
   • Turn back to original setting if there is no improvement.
6. Begin emergency measures immediately.
7. Notify physician.

Failure to Sense (Competition)

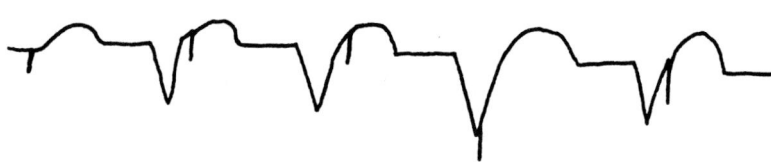

1. Evaluate patient's rhythm and its effectiveness.
2. Check battery pack.
   • Turn off pacemaker if patient's rate is effective.
   • Increase the sensitivity by turning clockwise as far as it will go if patient's rate is not effective.
   • Turn the Ma as high as it will go if increasing the sensitivity is not effective.
   • Return both Ma and sensitivity to normal settings if raising the Ma is not effective.
3. Reposition the patient or limb (if pacing catheter was inserted here).
4. Begin emergency measures immediately.
5. Notify physician.

NOTE. Occasionally a pacing stimulus will fall on the T wave, possibly resulting in ventricular fibrillation.

Loss of Capture (Heart is not responding to pacing stimuli)

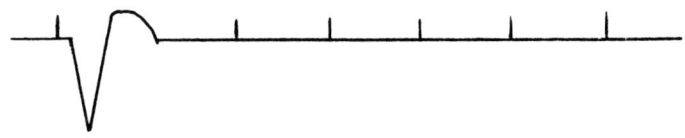

1. Evaluate patient's rhythm and its effectiveness.
2. Begin emergency measures immediately if patient loses consciousness.
3. Reposition the patient or limb (if pacing catheter was inserted here).
4. Notify physician.
5. See also Nursing Actions for Loss of Pacing Spike, p 94.

Nursing Actions for Permanent Pacemaker Malfunction

Since the pacemaker and electrodes are located within the body, nursing actions for malfunction of the permanent pacemaker are as follows.
1. Evaluate patient's rhythm and its effectiveness.
2. If patient is symptomatic and an emergency condition exists, begin emergency measures immediately, as follows.
    • Stabilize inherent cardiac rate with drug therapy
    • Begin CPR.
    • Defibrillate if indicated.
3. Notify the cardiologist immediately.

NOTE. The nurse supports the inherent cardiac rate and treats the symptoms resulting from permanent pacemaker malfunction until the cardiologist can assess the problem and intervene.

8

Cardiopulmonary Resuscitation

It is imperative that the nurse be certified in the performance of cardio-pulmonary resuscitation (CPR) for all age groups. This chapter describes CPR procedures for the adult and older child and for the infant and younger child.

CPR FOR ADULT OR OLDER CHILD (9 years and up)

Preliminary Actions

1. Make sure patient is in arrest by shaking, calling by name, and checking for carotid pulse, respirations, and pupil size. Clinical signs of arrest are unresponsiveness, no carotid pulse, no breathing, dilated pupils (takes 45 seconds following arrest before this occurs).

2. Call for assistance.

3. Note time.

Procedure

1. Begin CPR.

2. Position patient flat on a firm surface.

3. Tilt the head and lift the neck; or tilt the head and lift the chin (unless contraindicated).

4. Pinch the nostrils closed.

5. After taking a deep breath, the rescuer places his mouth around the edges of the victim's mouth and "breathes" for the patient. (Mouth to nose technique may be used.)

6. During lung inflation, the rescuer must watch the chest wall to make sure the chest rises.

7. Deliver four quick breaths as quickly as possible, without allowing full lung deflation between each one.

8. Check the carotid pulse again.

9. If no response, begin compressions.

10. Place hands on lower half of sternum (avoiding the xiphoid process) and depress 1½ inches to 2 inches (4–5 cm).

11. If only one rescuer is present, 15 consecutive compressions are performed. This ratio of 15:2 is continued with a compression rate of approximately 80 per minute.

12. If two rescuers are present, 5 consecutive chest compressions are performed, with one lung inflation quickly interposed between the fifth compression and the first of the next series. This ratio of 5:1 is continued with a compression rate of approximately 60 per minute.

CPR FOR INFANT OR YOUNGER CHILD

Preliminary Actions

1. Make sure patient is in arrest by shaking, calling by name, and checking for brachial pulse in infant and carotid pulse in child, respirations, and pupil size. Clinical signs of arrest are unresponsiveness, no pulse, no breathing, and dilated pupils (occurs several seconds following arrest).

2. If in arrest, call for assistance.

3. Note time.

Procedure

1. Begin CPR.

2. Position patient.
   - *Infant*—place in supine position with firm support (rescuer's hand may be used) under the back. A small folded blanket may also be used.
   - *Younger child*—position flat on a firm surface.

3. Tilt the head and lift the neck; or, tilt the head and lift the chin (unless contraindicated).

ALERT. Do not exaggerate the head tilt. This will occlude the airway.

4. *Infant*—the rescuer covers the mouth and the nose with his mouth and breathes for the patient with just enough air to make the chest rise.

5. *Younger child*—if the mouth and the nose can be covered with the rescuer's mouth, continue as for infant. If not, pinch the nostrils closed, and place your mouth around the edges of the victim's mouth and breathe for the patient, once again with just enough air to make the chest rise.

6. During lung inflation, the rescuer must watch the chest wall to make sure the chest rises.

7. Four quick breaths are delivered as quickly as possible without allowing full lung deflation between each one.

8. The pulse is checked again.

9. If no response, begin compressions.
- Infant—place 2 or 3 fingers on the middle of the sternum (between the nipples) and depress ½ inch to 1 inch (1.3–2.5 cm).
- Larger infant or child—the rescuer places the heel of his hand on the lower half of the sternum and depresses 1 inch to 1½ inches (2.5–3.8 cm).

10. Five consecutive chest compressions are followed by one quick lung inflation. This is done at a faster rate.
- Infant—20 lung inflations/min (one inflation every 3 sec) to 100 compressions/min
- Child—15 lung inflations/min (one inflation every 4 sec) to 80 compressions/min

11. The 5:1 ratio remains the same for one or two rescuers.

Special Considerations

Do not compress the xiphoid process.

Compression should be smooth and rhythmic.

Only the heel of the hand should touch the chest wall. Keep fingers off the rib cage.

When pressure is completely released, the hand or fingers should keep contact with the chest wall.

If a cervical spine injury is suspected, support the head in normal body alignment and lift the lower jaw up forward (rescuer places hands on either side of lower jaw at the angle) to open the airway. If this is not successful, the head is tilted back ever so slightly before artificial respirations are attempted.

The pulse should be checked periodically to make sure that adequate compressions are being delivered, especially the first minute following the initiation of CPR, every few minutes throughout the procedure, and following change of rescuers.

If the patient is being monitored in the intensive care setting, begin treatment for the specific arrhythmia immediately (*e.g.*, immediate defibrillation for ventricular fibrillation).

The precordial thump (the rescuer delivers a blow with the fleshy part of his fist to the midsternum from a height of 8–12 in or 20–30 cm) is to be used only on monitored patients in the intensive care unit in the following situations: ventricular tachycardia, ventricular fibrillation, or asystole (ventricular) caused by heart block (until pacemaker can be inserted). Contraindicated in children. Use with care in the elderly.

When performing chest compressions on the newborn or infant, to prevent damage to the spinal cord do not encircle the chest with the rescuer's hands.

The decision to stop CPR is a medical one.

If the physician desires a "No Code" (no cardiopulmonary resuscitation), he must write it on the physician's order sheet.

For problems associated with CPR and the actions called for, see Table 8-1.

TABLE 8-1. **Problems of Cardiopulmonary Resuscitation**

Problem	Action
Pulse present but no respirations	This is respiratory arrest. Administer artificial respiration until spontaneous and effective respirations return or advanced life support is begun. **NOTE.** Continue to check for presence of pulse. If absent, begin cardiac and pulmonary resuscitation.
No pulse	Artificial respirations and chest compressions are initiated.
Distended abdomen	1. Check inflation technique and position of patient. Avoid excessive pressure in breathing (breathe just enough to make the chest rise). 2. Do not attempt to relieve distention unless it is severely inhibiting respirations. 3. If distention must be relieved, turn patient on side and apply gentle pressure over the epigastrium. This may have to be repeated to prevent long interruptions in CPR.
Regurgitation	Turn patient to side, clean out the mouth (manually or by suctioning) and turn back to supine position to continue CPR. Severe abdominal distention may be the cause.

Obstructed Airway	1. Turn patient on side and deliver four quick back blows (between shoulder blades).
	 2. Administer four quick abdominal or chest thrusts.
	   • Abdominal—place fist (thumb side toward body) halfway between waist and rib cage and place the second hand on top of the first. Then deliver four quick compressions using an inward and upward approach. Avoid compression of the rib cage. Turn the head to the side.
	   • Chest—place the heel of the hand over the lower half of the sternum, and place the other hand on top of this one. Deliver four quick compressions. Avoid compression of the rib cage. Turn the head to the side.
	
	 NOTE. If conscious, the rescuer stands behind the patient, bringing his arms under the axillae and placing his hands midsternal.
	
	   • The rescuer relieves obstruction by using fingers in a sweeping motion to manually clean out the mouth.

(Continued)

TABLE 8-1. **Problems of Cardiopulmonary Resuscitation** (*Continued*)

Problem	Action
Patient with a tracheostomy tube or who has had a laryngectomy	Tracheostomy tube—inflate cuff and begin CPR. If tracheostomy tube has no cuff, close off the mouth and the nose with hand and use the mouth-to-stoma method. Laryngectomy patient—use the mouth to stoma method. Remember, this is patient's only airway. There is no connection between the mouth and the trachea.

Respiratory Nursing

9
Acute Respiratory Failure

Acute respiratory failure is an extreme emergency. It is caused by and associated with many different clinical conditions. The general aspects of acute respiratory failure, its treatment, and associated nursing considerations are discussed in this chapter. Specific underlying conditions are described in chapter 10.

Description

In acute respiratory failure the normal arterial blood gases can no longer be maintained (usually a $pO_2 < 50$ mm Hg or a $pCO_2 > 50$ mm Hg).

Causes

Trauma (*e.g.*, ruptured diaphragm, flail chest, pneumothorax, hemothorax)

Drugs (narcotics, tranquilizers, sedatives, anesthetic overdose, antibiotics—neomycin, kanamycin, streptomycin)

Neuromuscular disease (myasthenia gravis, Guillain-Barré syndrome, poliomyelitis, multiple sclerosis)

Pneumonia

Atelectasis

Toxins (*e.g.*, botulism, tetanus)

Airway obstruction (*e.g.* pulmonary edema, chronic obstructive lung disease, asthma, croup, near-drowning, burns of the airway, ruptured bronchus or trachea)

Pulmonary emboli

Acute respiratory distress syndrome

Restriction of the thorax by nonrespiratory causes (*e.g.*, abdominal surgery, peritonitis, obesity)

Oxygen therapy—improperly administered

Restriction of the thorax (*e.g.*, thoracic surgery)

Pulmonary tumors

Clinical Manifestations

Hypoxia

Increased respirations

Shortness of breath

Yawning

Use of accessory muscles of respiration

Flared nostrils

Central or peripheral cyanosis (late)

Tachycardia

Hypertension, initially (if uncorrected, will become hypotensive)

Restlessness

Impaired judgment

Anxiety

Confusion

Agitation

Delirium

Arrhythmias

Unconsciousness

Death

Hypercarbia (CO_2 Narcosis)

Headache

Drowsiness

Dizziness

Confusion

Unconsciousness

Hypertension

Tachycardia

Sweating

Papilledema

Reddening of skin (also, sclera and conjunctiva)

Apnea

Death

Diagnostic Test

Arterial blood gases

Treatment and Nursing Actions

Improve and Support Respiratory Function

1. Provide adequate oxygenation.

- Administer oxygen as ordered.
- Oxygen should be humidified.
- Closely monitor flow rate and patient's response to therapy.
- Be constantly alert for signs of hypoxia or hypercarbia.
- Closely monitor arterial blood gases.
- Intubation and mechanical ventilation may be necessary to assist ventilation (by way of endotracheal or tracheal intubation).

2. Administer oxygen with extreme caution to the acutely ill patient who has had chronic respiratory failure.
   - Remember that the hypoxic drive (*i.e.*, low arterial oxygen stimulates the chemoreceptors in the aorta and carotid bodies, resulting in increased respirations) is crucial to this patient to maintain respirations.
   - Oxygen administered improperly will lessen and eventually "knock out" this hypoxic drive, resulting in hypoventilation, CO_2 narcosis, and, without treatment, death.
   - Arterial blood gases should be monitored closely and frequently.

3. Maintain patent airway.
   - Encourage patient to cough and breathe deeply if possible.
   - Suction secretions as necessary (oropharyngeal, and endotracheal or tracheal).
   - Administer medications as ordered (bronchodilators, mucolytic agents)
   - Prevent airway obstruction due to improper positioning. Keep airway straight.
   - Change position frequently (at least every 2 hours).
   - Perform chest physiotherapy.

Improve and Support Cardiac Function

1. Monitor ECG closely for arrhythmias.
   - Arrhythmias may occur due to hypoxia or disturbance in acid-base balance.
   - Treat underlying cause (*i.e.*, restore blood gases to near normal or normal). This may be the only treatment necessary.
   - Antiarrhythmic drug therapy may be necessary.

2. Treat existing cardiac disease as ordered (*e.g.*, congestive heart failure).

3. Venesection is in order if the hematocrit is above 60 (to prevent sludging of the blood).

Closely Monitor Vital Signs and Levels of Consciousness

1. Pay close attention to quantity and quality of respirations.

2. Auscultate heart and lung sounds.

3. Notify physician of adverse changes.

Closely Monitor Laboratory Values
(*i.e.*, arterial blood gases, hematocrit, electrolytes)

1. Notify physician of any adverse change.

Promote and Maintain Fluid and Electrolyte Balance
1. Monitor electrolytes and hematocrit level closely.
2. Keep an accurate record of intake and output.
3. Weigh daily if condition permits.
4. Check skin turgor.
5. Administer intravenous fluids, as prescribed.
6. Correct deficiencies as indicated by lab data.

Prevent or Treat Infection
1. Administer antibiotics as ordered to prevent infection or treat one that is already present.

Provide Emotional Support
1. Stay with the patient.
2. Remember that the patient in acute distress may be extremely anxious and fear an impending catastrophe.
3. Reassure him that measures will be performed to assist his breathing.
4. Explain procedures.

Promote Comfort
1. Place patient in comfortable position.
   • Usually, high-Fowler's (sitting upright) and leaning forward with support is the preferred position.
2. Instruct in proper breathing techniques that may be less tiresome and more effective.

Avoid the Use of Drugs That May Depress Respirations or Coughing
1. Narcotics and sedatives are generally contraindicated in this patient.
2. If ordered, have resuscitative equipment readily available (*i.e.*, respirator, respiratory stimulants, narcotic antagonists, suction and oxygen apparatus, equipment for intubation).
   • Use resuscitative equipment with extreme caution.
   • Monitor respiratory response closely.
   • Treat respiratory depression immediately.
   • Notify physician of adverse changes.
3. Sedation may be ordered if the patient is being mechanically ventilated.
   • Have emergency drugs and suction and oxygen apparatus readily available.

10

Conditions Causing Acute Respiratory Failure

Several important underlying causes of acute respiratory failure are discussed in this chapter—pulmonary embolus, acute pulmonary edema, pneumothorax, hemothorax, mediastinal shift, ruptured bronchus or trachea, fractured larynx, ruptured diaphragm, flail chest, and acute respiratory distress syndrome (ARDS).

PULMONARY EMBOLUS

Description
Pulmonary embolus is any obstruction of the pulmonary artery or one of its branches by a blood clot or foreign substance. If necrosis of lung tissue occurs due to the embolus, pulmonary infarction is said to occur.

Causes
Dislodged thrombus originating from the following sites
- deep veins of the legs (most commonly)
- pelvic veins
- right heart

Any foreign substance
- Amniotic fluid emboli forced into the circulation during complicated deliveries or following the complications of pregnancy itself
- Tumor emboli originating from either primary or metastatic sites
- Air emboli caused by the injection of air into a body cavity during procedures or intravenously as a result of poor technique
- Fat emboli which especially follow the fracture of long bones within 48 hours, other types of trauma (*e.g.,* burns, closed-chest massage in CPR), liver disease, nephritis

Clinical Manifestations
Most pulmonary emboli are small and produce no clinical signs or symptoms, many times going undetected. A large embolus usually produces clinically detectable manifestations, including the following.

Sudden chest pain—crushing in quality increased by respiration; described as stabbing or sharp; located in left or right side of chest or substernally; does not generally radiate to arms or jaw (helps distinguish it from pain of an MI)

Dyspnea that occurs suddenly

Hypoxia

Cyanosis due to decreased pO_2

Coughing

Wheezing

Marked anxiety and apprehension

Symptoms of right heart failure (indicates involvement of major pulmonary artery)

Petechiae over chest and shoulders accompanied by above symptoms is characteristic of a fat embolus

Shock (indicates massive pulmonary emboli)

Sudden death (indicates complete obstruction of a major pulmonary artery)

NOTE. If infarction has occurred, moderate temperature elevation (101° F–102° F or 38.3° C–38.9° C), cough with hemoptysis (small or large amounts), transient friction rub over the affected area, or pleuriticlike chest pain may occur.

Diagnostic Tests

ECG changes—the ECG may be perfectly normal or show sinus tachycardia and ST segment or T wave changes that are nonspecific. Pulmonary embolus should be suspected, however, when any of the previously mentioned clinical manifestations, especially sudden shortness of breath, are accompanied by one or more of the following ECG changes.

• Right axis deviation that occurs suddenly
• New complete or incomplete right bundle branch block
• ST segment depressions and T wave inversions in leads V_1 to V_3
• Large Q wave and T wave inversion in lead III, and large S waves in leads I and V_6

Lung scan—following the IV injection of a radioactive isotope, scanning the lungs will identify the oxygen deprived area affected by the embolus.

Chest x-ray film—This is not necessarily reliable immediately following the event. If pulmonary embolism is present, the x-ray film may show decreased vascularity, pulmonary arteries that are dilated, and an elevated diaphragm. If pulmonary infarction is present, the x-ray film will show a wedge-shaped opacity.

Pulmonary angiogram—contrast medium is injected through a catheter that is inserted into an arm vein and passed into the right side of the heart and up into the pulmonary artery to detect the area of reduced blood flow caused by the emboli. This is the most effective diagnostic tool for detecting pulmonary embolism.

Arterial blood gases—initially, the pCO_2 is increased but later decreases as a result of overcompensating hyperventilation. The pO_2 is decreased.

Serum enzymes—LDH is frequently elevated.

Treatment and Nursing Actions

1. Administer anticoagulants. IV heparin is used initially.
   - An oral agent (usually Coumadin) is used after improvement is shown on lung scan.
2. Administer oxygen therapy, possibly positive pressure.
3. Promote bed rest, with head elevated.
4. Prepare for possible surgery for embolectomy from pulmonary artery if indicated. Vena cava interruption is performed (by way of plication or ligation of the inferior vena cava just below the renal veins or insertion of an umbrellalike prosthesis positioned in the lumen of the inferior vena cava) if patient continues to have pulmonary emboli despite treatment or if anticoagulation is contraindicated.
5. Administer sedation to lessen pain and anxiety. Morphine and meperidine (Demerol) have hypotensive effects and are usually avoided for that reason.
6. Start intravenous therapy.
7. Closely monitor vital signs, arterial blood gases, and ECG.
8. If shock is present, treat accordingly (see Cardiogenic Shock, Chap. 20).
9. Provide constant emotional support. Stay with patient.

Prevention

Patient should do passive or active exercises as the condition warrants and as ordered. Encourage movement of feet and legs. A footboard would be valuable.

Avoid placing any pressure behind the knee, from improperly fitted elastic hose or bandages, gatching the foot of the bed too severely, or placing pillows under the knee.

Advise use of properly fitted antiembolic hose. They should extend well above the knee.

Proper hydration to prevent increased viscosity of blood.

Administer anticoagulant therapy prophylactically.

Caution patient not to strain at stool.

Increase level of activity gradually and monitor effects closely.

ACUTE PULMONARY EDEMA

Description

Acute pulmonary edema is a condition in which lung congestion causes the escape of serous fluid from the capillaries into interstitial tissues or the alveoli (*i.e.*, pulmonary edema).

Causes

Acute left ventricular failure is the most common cause

NOTE. This is the most extreme form of left ventricular failure.

Infections (due to toxins)

Uremia

Liver diseases

Mitral or aortic valve disease

Congestive heart failure following MI

Inhalation of chemical irritants (*e.g.*, sulfur dioxide, ammonia, chlorine)

Chest trauma

Burns of respiratory tract (*i.e.*, following inhalation of hot gases)

Fluid overload (intravenous infusions, blood transfusions)

Complication of pregnancy (Prenatal and postnatal)

Clinical Manifestations

First Stage (Fluid has escaped from the capillaries into the pulmonary interstitial spaces)—beginning pulmonary edema
- Dyspnea on exertion
- Orthopnea
- Persistent cough (patient may complain of a "cold")
- Restlessness.
- Anxiousness
- Ventricular gallop may be heard
- Rales may be auscultated at the bases of the lungs
- Hyperventilation
- pCO_2 decreases
- pO_2 slightly below or near normal

Second Stage—advanced pulmonary edema
(Fluid moves into the alveoli)
- Respiratory distress
  - Acute shortness of breath
  - Hyperventilation
  - Labored respirations
  - Audible rales and wheezing
  - Incessant coughing that produces large amounts of frothy, blood-tinged sputum
  - Cyanosis
- Profuse sweating
- Skin becomes clammy and cold
- Hypotension
- Tachycardia

- Arrhythmias may be detected
- Both pCO_2 and pO_2 decrease significantly
- *p*H is increased

Third Stage—Acute Pulmonary Edema
(Fluid moves into the bronchial tree)
- Acute respiratory distress intensifies
- Rales become coarse and bubbling
- Level of consciousness decreases
- Symptoms of cardiogenic shock present
- Ventricular arrhythmias may be present
- Breath sounds diminish
- Death is imminent unless treatment is immediately implemented
- pO_2 decreases severely; pCO_2 increases significantly
- A state of metabolic and respiratory acidosis

Treatment and Nursing Actions

1. Observe patient closely for symptoms of impending pulmonary edema; try to catch in beginning stage. Pulmonary edema can progress rapidly from one stage to another. The more quickly it is detected, the better the chance of survival.

2. Administer morphine immediately, either IM or IV. Watch closely for signs of respiratory depression. Keep morphine antagonist by bedside.

3. Administer high-concentration oxygen therapy using intermittent positive-pressure apparatus delivering 100% oxygen (humidified) by face mask with a nonrebreathing bag.

   NOTE. Nasal cannulas or catheters are the least desirable methods for administering O_2, since their O_2 concentration is only 30% to 40%.

4. Support left ventricular function as follows.
   a. Administer a rapid-acting digitalis preparation for less severe stage. Usually digoxin is given orally for less severe stage and IV for acute stage.
   b. Administer aminophylline IV. Give slowly. Watch for hypotensive effects.
   c. Patient is digitalized over a period of time until maximum cardiac effects are obtained or maximum dosage is achieved. The patient is then maintained on a smaller daily maintenance dose.

5. Administer rapid-acting diuretics. Usually ethacrynic acid (Edecrin), or furosemide (Lasix), is given IV. The patient may show dramatic improvement within minutes. Insert an in-dwelling catheter to take care of the tremendous amount of diuresis. Notify the physician if the diuretic is not effective (*i.e.,* if urinary output does not increase or begins to decrease). Watch the patient closely for signs of urinary obstruction.

6. Perform the procedure of rotating tourniquets (*i.e.,* bloodless phlebotomy).

7. Prepare for phlebotomy. Usually 500 ml of blood is removed. This method is seldom used, except where the condition is caused by over-administration of blood or fluid.

8. Stay with the patient to help allay apprehension. This condition is very frightening to both patient and staff. Appear confident. Anxiety increases respirations, and this only intensifies the condition.

9. Facilitate breathing by elevating the patient's head. Provide support with pillows. Position for comfort.

10. Prevent exertion—provide for plenty of rest.

11. Have a suction catheter and suction apparatus available for nasopharyngeal aspiration or endotracheal aspiration if the patient is intubated.

12. Record precise intake and output.

13. Watch the cardiac monitor for presence of arrhythmias and treat accordingly.

14. Start an IV for emergency drug route.

15. Draw arterial blood gases and monitor closely.

16. Monitor vital signs and general appearance closely.

17. Restrict sodium.

18. Weigh the patient when condition permits and keep record to check for effectiveness of therapy.

PNEUMOTHORAX

Description

Pneumothorax is the collection of air in the pleural cavity causing some degree of lung collapse, depending on the amount of air that escapes from the lung. It may occur as a result of trauma or spontaneously (without trauma).

Causes

Trauma—penetrating chest injury, fractured ribs, violent cough, fall

Disease
- Degenerative (e.g., rupture of emphysematous bleb)
- Infectious—lung abscess

Thoracic surgery (entering the pleural cavity)

Complications from thoracentesis, pericardiocentesis, catheterization of the subclavian vein

Positive-pressure ventilation causing alveolar rupture

Sometimes occurs without reason in people who were previously healthy

Types

Open pneumothorax (sucking chest wound). Air passes freely in and out through an opening in the chest wall (bullet wound, knife wound).

Closed pneumothorax. Air enters the pleural space internally. There is no communication with the outside (ruptured bronchus).

Tension pneumothorax. A variation of a closed pneumothorax; air enters the pleural cavity and is trapped, causing a tremendous build-up of pressure in the pleural space (Fig. 10-1) (An open chest wound may be converted to a tension pneumothorax by sealing of the chest wound.)

Hydropneumothorax. Air and serous fluid are present in the pleural cavity (*e.g.*, rupture of a tuberculous bleb).

Hemopneumothorax. Air and blood are present in the pleural cavity.

Clinical Manifestations

Sharp, constant chest pain, occurring suddenly—usually limited to the affected side

Apprehension

Dyspnea

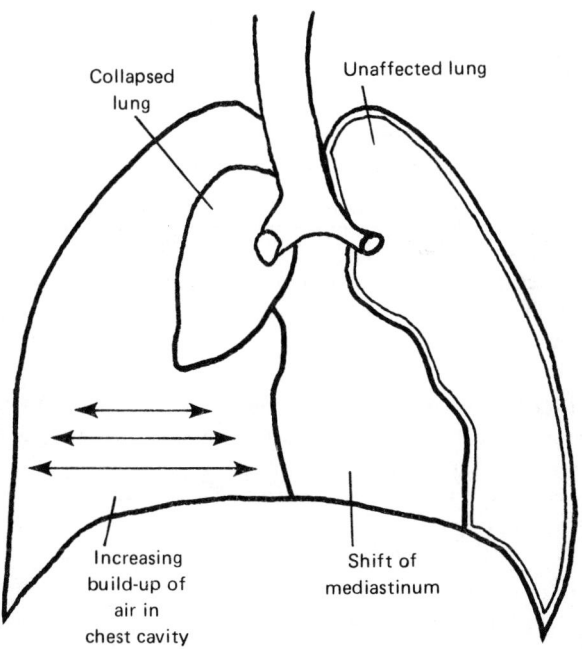

FIG. 10-1. *Tension pneumothorax. Air enters the chest cavity on inspiration and is unable to escape. Each inspiration adds more air, which causes further lung collapse, mediastinal shift, and encroachment on unaffected lung. Tension pneumothorax occurs when a bleb is ruptured in the lung, a chest wound opens on inspiration and seals itself on expiration, or a chest wound is sealed with a dressing while a large internal air leak is present.*

Hypoxia

Cyanosis

Distant or absent breath sounds over the affected area

Acute respiratory distress (especially with tension pneumothorax)

Audible passage of air during inspiration and expiration (with open pneumothorax)

Nonproductive cough

Hyperresonance or tympany over the affected area

Mediastinal shift may be present

Trachea may be displaced to opposite side

Fall in blood pressure

Weak, rapid pulse

Shock

No symptoms in a small percentage of patients

Diagnostic Tests

A chest x-ray film definitely establishes the diagnosis of pneumothorax—there are no lung markings at the periphery of the involved side. If any doubt exists or the condition is suspected, an x-ray study should be done on moderate expiration.

Treatment and Nursing Actions

1. Stay with the patient. Explain what is going on.
2. Notify the physician immediately.
3. Elevate the head of the bed to facilitate the patient's breathing.
4. Carefully monitor vital signs until the emergency is over and the patient has stabilized (every 10–15 min or less depending on the patient's condition), and attach patient to monitor. Watch for symptoms of mediastinal shift.
5. Administer oxygen therapy as ordered.
   - Use oxygen with extreme caution if patient has a history of chronic pulmonary disease or insufficiency.
   - Use mechanical ventilation, if necessary.
   - Observe safety precautions.
   - Carefully monitor arterial blood gases.
6. Prepare for emergency thoracentesis.
   - Have tray at bedside.
   - Explain procedure to patient.
7. Prepare for chest tube insertion.
   - Have equipment at bedside, including suction and drainage system.
   - Explain procedure to patient.
8. Prepare for thoracotomy in the following order.
   - Obtain signed consent form for surgery.

- Prep patient.
- Administer premedication as ordered.
9. Start an IV or ensure the patency of one in place for emergency drug route.
10. Administer pain medication as ordered by the physician.
11. Treat shock as indicated.
   - Have crash cart and emergency drugs at bedside.
   - Begin cardiopulmonary resuscitation if the patient goes into cardiac or pulmonary arrest.
12. Encourage bed rest until the patient's condition has stabilized.

Special Considerations

Do not remove impaled objects (*e.g.*, ice pick, knife). This is the responsibility of the surgeon and is done in the operating room. Secure with sterile dressing to prevent further trauma.

If patient presents with an open pneumothorax (sucking chest wound), proceed as follows:
- Instruct patient to exhale forcefully.
- Place an occlusive dressing (sterile Vaseline gauze covered by sterile dressings) over the entrance wound.
- Make wound as airtight as possible by sealing with tape.
- If patient shows signs of acute respiratory distress rather than improvement following application of occlusive dressing, remove the dressing and notify the physician immediately (see Tension Pneumothorax, p 113).

If a tension pneumothorax has occurred, immediate relief may be accomplished by insertion of a large-bore needle (14–16 gauge) into the pleural cavity. Decompression in this manner can be continued by attachment of a flutter valve (tying of a perforated finger cot) to the needle until more definitive therapy (chest tubes attached to water-seal drainage) can be instituted.

Hemothorax and pneumothorax frequently occur together (hemopneumothorax).

HEMOTHORAX

Causes

Disease

Trauma

Chest surgery

Clinical Manifestations

Chest pain

Dyspnea

Cyanosis

Fast, thready pulse

Hypotension

Rapid, shallow respirations

Breath sounds decreased or absent over affected area

Frothy or bloody sputum

Bruising over affected area

Shock

Possible mediastinal shift

Limited chest excursion (depending on amount of blood in the pleural space)

Treatment and Nursing Actions

See Pneumothorax, Treatment and Nursing Actions, pp 114–115.

Special Considerations

An emergency thoracentesis may be performed as a diagnostic measure. Blood aspirated from the pleural space indicates hemothorax.

Closely monitor amount of drainage.

- Carefully mark level of drainage in collection bottle or measure aspirate following first evacuation of blood.
- Carefully monitor and measure blood loss every 15 min to 30 min until the patient stabilizes.
  - Notify the physician if drainage is above or below the set rate for a specific period of time.
  - Immediate thoracotomy is indicated if the initial blood drainage is over 1000 ml.

Blood replacement therapy may be indicated.

- Hemoglobin and hematocrit should be closely monitored.

Continued bleeding is suggested by a rising pulse rate and a falling blood pressure.

- Notify the physician.

MEDIASTINAL SHIFT

Description

Mediastinal shift is a condition in which the contents of the mediastinum shift or are pushed toward the unaffected side (*i.e.*, opposite tension pneumothorax or hemothorax).

Causes

Usually follows tension pneumothorax

Hemothorax

Clinical Manifestations

Severe dyspnea

Trachea and larynx displaced from their midline position toward the un-affected side

Distended neck veins

Cyanosis

Increased pulse and respiratory rates

Change in position of cardiac apex beat

Severe hypotension

Shock

Cardiac arrhythmias

Danger

Return of blood to the heart and cardiac output are severely impeded.

The unaffected lung may be compressed.

Treatment and Nursing Actions

1. Immediately treat underlying cause.
2. Monitor ECG closely.

RUPTURED BRONCHUS OR TRACHEA

Cause

Chest trauma—crushing or blunt (suspect if fractures of the upper ribs are present)

Clinical Manifestations

Acute respiratory distress

Hemoptysis

Massive subcutaneous emphysema

Pneumothorax (with symptoms of a major air leak)

NOTE. Respiratory distress is not relieved by chest tube insertion or me-chanical ventilation.

Treatment

Surgical repair

FRACTURED LARYNX

Cause

Trauma

Clinical Manifestations

Obstruction of upper airway

Voice changes

Dyspnea

Subcutaneous emphysema

Hemoptysis

Difficulty in and pain upon swallowing

Treatment

1. Prepare patient for immediate tracheostomy.
2. Surgical repair may be indicated.

RUPTURED DIAPHRAGM

Causes

Chest trauma

Abdominal trauma

Multiple trauma (suspect if there is thoracic injury)

Clinical Manifestations

May be asymptomatic initially, but with the stomach and bowel becoming distended, acute respiratory distress may present.

Acute respiratory distress
- Dyspnea
- Cyanosis
- Acute chest pain (may be referred to shoulder or abdomen)
- Absent or diminished breath sounds over affected area
- Mediastinal or tracheal shift may occur
- Dullness and tympany over affected side
- Bowel sounds may be auscultated on affected side (if viscera have herniated)

NOTE. Usually occurs on left side (the liver protects right side)

Treatment

Surgical repair

FLAIL CHEST

Cause

Chest trauma

Clinical Manifestations

Paradoxical respirations (Fig. 10–2)

Chest pain

Cyanosis

Dyspnea

Subcutaneous emphysema

A

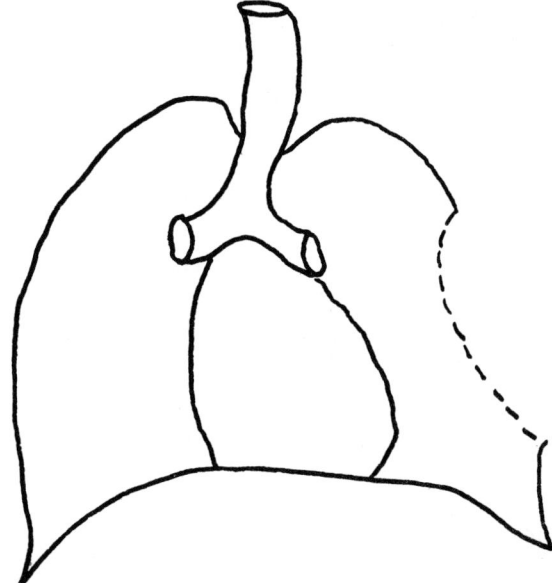

B

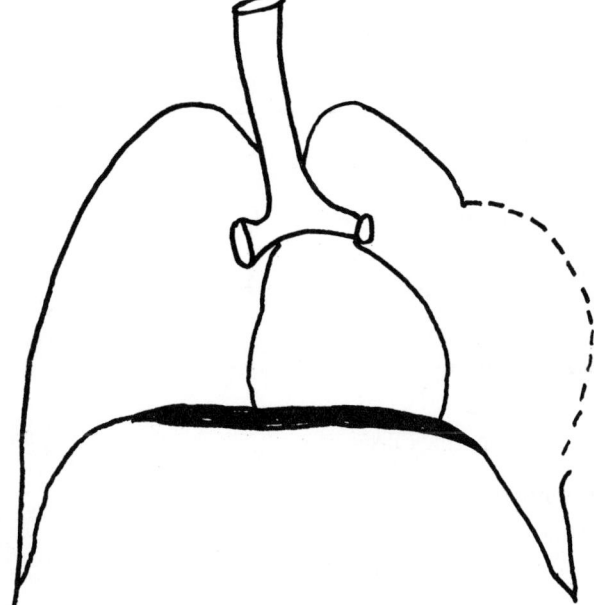

FIG. 10-2. *Paradoxical respirations.* (A.) *Upon inspiration, flail segment goes in.* (B.) *Upon expiration, flail segment bulges out.*

Treatment and Nursing Actions

1. Temporary stabilization of the chest wall is needed immediately.
   - Apply pressure to affected area with hands, sandbag, folded blanket, or pillow.
   - Place patient on affected side; use a folded blanket or sandbag to provide compression.
2. Tracheal intubation (endotracheal intubation may be used initially) with a volume-control ventilator is the treatment of choice.
3. Surgical stabilization of the chest wall may be performed if the trauma is extensive (*e.g.*, a large flail segment).

ACUTE RESPIRATORY DISTRESS SYNDROME

Description

Acute respiratory distress syndrome (ARDS) is a severe respiratory disorder that results in acute respiratory failure.

Synonyms

Adult hyaline membrane disease

Shock lung

Traumatic wet lung

Causes

The most common causes are the following:

Pulmonary surgery

Pulmonary trauma

Shock

Fat emboli

Aspiration and viral pneumonia

Cardiopulmonary bypass

Toxins—inhaled or ingested

Oxygen toxicity

Massive head injuries

Septicemia

There may be no specific cause

Clinical Manifestations

Severe dyspnea

Cyanosis and hypoxemia (respond poorly to oxygen therapy)

Tachypnea

Rales

Pulmonary edema (not of cardiac origin)

Noisy or grunting respirations

Respiratory distress grows progressively worse without treatment

Treatment and Nursing Actions

1. Closely monitor vital signs, with special attention to quantity and quality of respirations and heart and lung sounds.
2. Provide support of the respiratory system.
   - Administer oxygen therapy as ordered.
   - Mechanical ventilation is indicated.
     - High inspiratory pressure
     - Large tidal volume
     - Positive end expiratory pressure (PEEP)
   - Closely monitor arterial blood gases.
3. Notify physician immediately if this disorder is suspected.

ALERT. Death follows acute respiratory failure if ARDS is undetected and untreated (see Acute Respiratory Failure, pp 103–106).

11

Special Procedures

Special procedures and nursing considerations associated with acute respiratory failure are presented in this chapter.

PHLEBOTOMY (THERAPEUTIC)

Description

Phlebotomy, or venesection, involves cannulation of a vein for withdrawal of blood.

Purpose

A phlebotomy is performed to reduce the volume of circulating blood and decrease intravascular pressure. Phlebotomy is used chiefly in the treatment of pulmonary edema resulting from over-administration of blood or fluid.

Equipment

Tourniquet

Blood collection tubing

Large-bore needle (16-, 18-, or 19-gauge needles)

Sterile collection bottle (500-ml capacity) containing anticoagulant to prevent clotting of blood

Sterile 2 × 2s

Nonallergenic tape

Povidone-iodine prep swabs (and ointment)

NOTE. It is necessary to have a physician's order to begin procedure. The order should state the amount of blood to be removed.

Preliminary Actions

1. Explain procedure to patient.

2. Check vital signs to establish baseline readings.

3. Set up equipment.
   - Check collection bottle for presence of vacuum (no splashing sounds audible upon shaking) and possible air leak (no bubbles visible with bottle inverted) after tubing is inserted and clamp closed.
   - If bottle is not intact, discard.
   - Prepare dressing.
     - Open 2 × 2s, maintaining sterility.
     - Tear strips of tape of appropriate length.
     - Open povidone–iodine swabs, maintaining sterility.
   - Apply small amount of povidone-iodine ointment to a sterile dressing (if it is hospital practice to cover a needle puncture site with this type of dressing).

Procedure

1. Apply tourniquet.

2. Select a large vein.

3. Cleanse the site with povidone-iodine swabs.

4. Insert needle.

5. Depress flashbulb of tubing for blood return.

6. Open clamp on tubing.

7. Secure needle with tape and cover with sterile dressing with povidone-iodine ointment.

8. Lower collection bottle below insertion site (approximately 6–12 in).

9. Gently rotate collection bottle at frequent intervals throughout procedure to ensure proper mixing of blood and anticoagulant.

10. Continue to monitor vital signs, electrocardiogram (ECG), and patient response throughout procedure. Notify physician immediately concerning adverse effects.

11. Discontinuing the procedure
    - Clamp tubing when amount of blood ordered by physician has been removed.
    - Remove needle.
    - Apply sterile pressure dressing to site and secure with tape.
    - Invert collection bottle and rotate gently.
    - Send to laboratory if possibility of readministering to patient in shock. Must be refrigerated immediately.
      - Label properly.
      - Maintain sterility of the system.

12. Continue to monitor vital signs and ECG postprocedure until patient is stable.

13. Check insertion site to make sure bleeding has stopped. Reapply sterile dressing as necessary.

ROTATION OF TOURNIQUETS (BLOODLESS PHLEBOTOMY)

Description
Bloodless phlebotomy is the application of tourniquets or inflating cuffs to the extremities according to a consistent pattern and timetable.

Purpose
Rotation of tourniquets is performed to retard venous return to the heart.

Equipment
Compression devices (any one of the following types may be used)
- 4 tourniquets, *or*
- 4 blood pressure cuffs, *or*
- automatically inflated/deflated cuffs (Danzer apparatus)

4 small towels

Watch (for timing of rotation)

Chart for recording time of rotation

Preliminary Actions

NOTE. It is necessary to have a physician's order before starting procedure.

NOTE. This procedure must not be performed on a patient in shock.

NOTE. A tourniquet must not be applied to an extremity that has an intravenous (IV) line in place. Consult with physician. (A central line may be established as an alternative for emergency drug administration.)

1. Explain the following to the patient if time and conditions permit. If the patient is in acute distress, explain as you perform the procedure.
   - Purpose of the procedure
   - Temporary skin changes (mottling or skin discoloration) that will occur as a result of the procedure
   - That there may be discomfort and that pain medication will be administered
2. Take blood pressure to obtain a baseline reading.

Procedure
1. Apply tourniquets, cuffs, or Danzer apparatus
   - Tourniquets
     - Place tourniquets under each extremity.
     - Apply 3 tourniquets as high as possible on 3 extremities.
     - To lessen discomfort, apply tourniquets over gown or small towel.
   - Blood pressure cuffs or Danzer apparatus
     - Place cuffs as high as possible on each extremity.
     - Inflate 3 of the cuffs to a pressure just above diastolic pressure.

NOTE. One extremity does not have a tourniquet or cuff applied.

2. Monitor arterial pulse. Arterial pulse should be present in all extremities *at all times.*
   • Check immediately following application of tourniquet or cuff and throughout the procedure.
   • If not palpable, reapply tourniquet or deflate cuff until pulse can be palpated.

ALERT. The purpose of this procedure is to retard venous return to the heart. *Arterial flow should not be impeded.*

3. Rotate Tourniquets. Starting in a clockwise or counterclockwise direction (either direction may be used, provided that it is followed consistently), at intervals of 15 min, maintain the following pattern.
   • Apply tourniquet to (or inflate cuff on) the free extremity.
   • Remove another tourniquet.

NOTE. The new tourniquet should be applied to the free extremity before the other tourniquet is removed.

   • Establish a rotation schedule.
     • Keep a chart at the bedside and record the time and sequence of rotation (see sample chart below).
   • The maximum time a tourniquet should be applied to an extremity is 45 minutes.
   • Always continue in the same direction (either clockwise or counterclockwise) once the procedure has been started. Changing direction will lengthen the maximum time a tourniquet is applied to an extremity and will compromise circulation.

NOTE. Tourniquets may have to be rotated more frequently (every 5 min) in the case of elderly patients or if circulatory impairment is present.

METHOD FOR RECORDING ROTATION OF TOURNIQUETS (Clockwise Direction)

Start			
Off	Off	Off	Off
R.A.	R.L.	L.L.	L.A.
1:00	1:15	1:30	1:45
2:00	etc.		

An easy (and handy) method of keeping up with clockwise rotation of tourniquets is presented above. Write down initials of each extremity and "off" over each one. Start with the right arm (R.A.) as the extremity without a tourniquet and write the time at which the procedure was started underneath. Continue in this manner, rotating the tourniquets in a clockwise manner every 15 minutes.

4. Closely monitor blood pressure throughout the procedure.
   • Check every few minutes for hypotension, which sometimes occurs as a result of the procedure.
   • Notify the physician of adverse effects.
5. Closely monitor urinary output.
   • Check whether output is significantly decreased by hypotension.
   • Check for effectiveness or response to therapy if rapid-acting diuretics have been administered.
   • Use in-dwelling urinary catheter.
6. If normal color and temperature do not return to the extremity shortly after removal of the tourniquet or if an arterial pulse is not palpable, report to the physician immediately.
7. Discontinuing the procedure
   • Obtain a physician's order.
   • Continuing the established pattern, remove one tourniquet every 15 min until all have been removed.
   • Check respiratory rate and quality and blood pressure following release of each cuff. If respiratory distress or significant blood pressure change occurs, notify the physician immediately (before removing any more cuffs) and prepare for possible reinstitution of the procedure.

ALERT. Do not remove all tourniquets at one time. A sudden increase in circulating volume may cause pulmonary edema or circulatory overload.

8. Carefully monitor patient response following the procedure. If symptoms of pulmonary edema or circulatory overload reoccur, the procedure may have to be reinstated.

THORACENTESIS

Description
Thoracentesis is the aspiration of fluid from the pleural space.

Purpose
The procedure is carried out to collect a specimen or as a therapeutic measure.

Equipment
Sterile thoracentesis tray, containing
- Towels and drapes
- Needles (22- and 26-gauge; 16-gauge, 3″)
- 2 × 2s and 4 × 4s
- Specimen container
- Syringes (5-, 20-, 50-ml)
- 3-way stopcock with tubing
- Hemostat
- Kelly clamp

- Solution cup
- Biopsy needle, if requested
- Local anesthetic
- Povidone–iodine swabs or solution
- Sterile gloves
- Sterile collection bottle
- Tape

Preliminary Actions

1. Explain procedure to patient. Obtain signed consent form.
2. Prepare equipment.
   - Open sterile tray.
   - Pour povidone-iodine solution in solution cup for skin preparation.
3. Place patient in appropriate position as requested by physician.
   - Semi-Fowler's, with arm on affected side raised over head
   - Sitting on side of bed, leaning on over-bed table
   - Straddling a chair
   - Lying on unaffected side if unable to sit up
   - Affected area exposed

Procedure

1. Assist the physician with procedure.
2. Continously monitor the patient throughout procedure, including pulse and respirations.
   - Instruct patient to breathe shallowly.
   - Caution patient not to cough or move.

NOTE. Above measures may help prevent trauma to the lung.

3. Properly label specimen container if laboratory analysis is desired. Protect container from damage.
4. If a large amount of fluid is to be removed, connect drainage tubing to stop-cock, and collect fluid in specimen container.
5. Following removal of needle, apply firm pressure over the insertion site, and tape a sterile dressing securely in place.
6. Note and document the quantity and quality of the drainage. Specimens should be sent to the lab immediately.
7. Place the patient on bed rest.
8. Continue to monitor patient closely following procedure, including bilateral breath sounds.
9. Possible complications include pneumothorax and tension pneumothorax. Pulmonary edema and cardiac distress may follow removal of large amounts of drainage owing to mediastinal shift.
10. Prepare the patient for a chest x-ray study immediately following the procedure (to rule out pneumothorax).

INSERTION OF CHEST TUBES

Description and Purpose

Chest tubes (catheters) are positioned in the pleural space to remove residual air and fluid from the pleural or mediastinal space; they are connected to some type of sterile drainage system (designated by the physician). Insertion is usually performed during surgery under strict aseptic conditions. The emergency procedure is described here.

Equipment

Local anesthetic (1% xylocaine)

Povidone–iodine solution or swabs

Sterile solution cup (for povidone–iodine solution)

Sterile drapes

Sterile gloves

Sterile dressings—2 × 2s, 4 × 4s

Sterile occlusive dressing (Vaseline gauze)

Sterile scissors

Tape—adhesive or nonallergenic

Chest tubes and obturators (different sizes; check with physician concerning his preference)

Sterile equipment for actual insertion
• Scalpel (handle and blade)
• Hemostats
• Forceps
• Suture material (check with physician)

Covered Kelly clamp (two, or four if two tubes are used)—should always be kept taped to head of bed

Sterile drainage system as ordered by physician with connecting tube and connectors (straight connector for one tube; Y connector if two chest tubes are inserted) (Figs. 11-1, 11-2, and 11-3)

Suction as ordered by physician

Sterile water (large bottle)

Face masks

Preliminary Actions

1. Explain procedure to patient. Obtain signed consent form.
2. Prepare drainage system as ordered by physician.
3. On work area, set up sterile field and prepare equipment, maintaining sterility.
4. Check suction to ensure proper function.
5. Position patient as specified.
   • Supine (most common)
   • On side

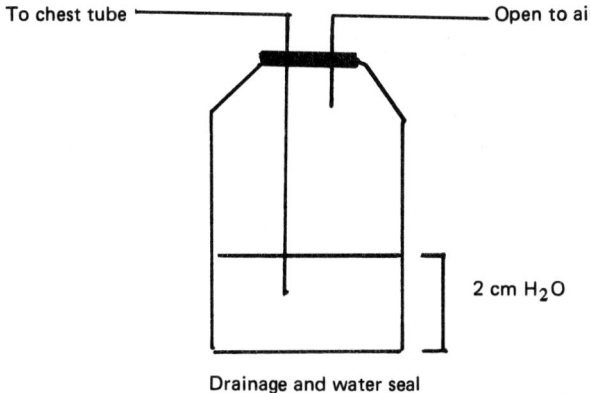

To chest tube   Open to air

2 cm H_2O

Drainage and water seal

FIG. 11-1. *One-bottle method of underwater seal chest drainage.*

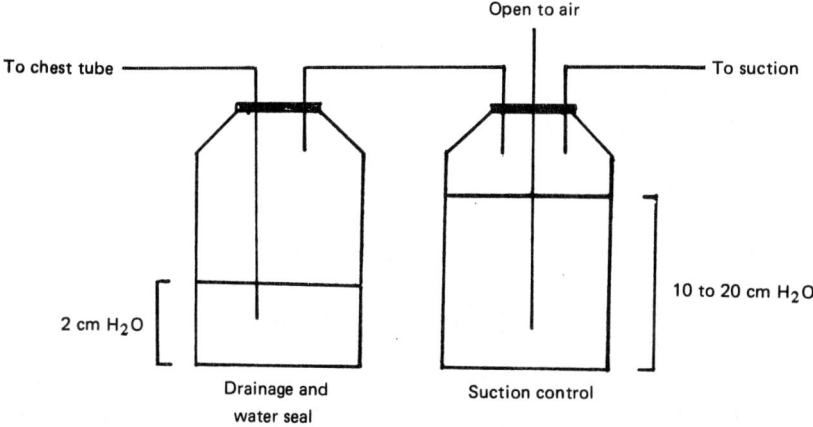

Open to air

To chest tube   To suction

10 to 20 cm H_2O

2 cm H_2O

Drainage and
water seal

Suction control

FIG. 11-2. *Two-bottle method of underwater seal chest drainage.*

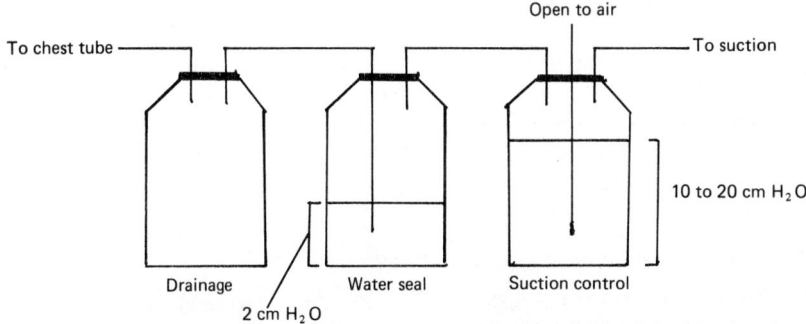

Open to air

To chest tube   To suction

10 to 20 cm H_2O

Drainage   Water seal   Suction control

2 cm H_2O

FIG. 11-3. *Three-bottle method of underwater seal chest drainage.*

Procedure

1. Assist the physician with procedure. (Nurse usually assumes the circulating rather than the sterile role.)

2. Following insertion of chest tube(s), attach tubing to drainage system.
   - Insert one end of clear connector (straight or Y shaped) into chest tube(s) and other end into drainage tubing.
   - Tape both connections securely with adhesive to prevent separation and air leaks.
   - Do not cover middle of plastic connector with tape. It must remain clear so that drainage may be observed. Tape it only where it connects to tubing.

3. Turn on suction, if ordered.
   - Connect suction tube to suction source.
   - Adjust level of suction appropriately.

4. After suturing the chest tube in place, the physician will apply an occlusive dressing around the site of insertion. Cover with sterile 4 × 4s and tape over dressing and all edges securely.

5. Measure amount of drainage following procedure. Time and amount of drainage should be marked on drainage bottle or chamber.

GENERAL CARE FOR THE PATIENT WITH CHEST TUBES

Nursing Considerations

Monitoring the Drainage System

Monitor drainage system closely throughout treatment (at least hourly for the first 24 hours after insertion).

There should be continuous moderate bubbling in the suction control bottle or chamber.

The level in the water-seal bottle or chamber should fluctuate on inhalation and exhalation.

- Pleur-evac—the level in the water-seal chamber should rise on inspiration on the right side of the chamber and fall during expiration on the left side.
- Bottle suction—the level of fluid in the glass rod, rises during inspiration and falls during expiration.
- Bubbling means there is an air leak, usually internal. This is an indication for chest tube and water-seal therapy.

ALERT. Excessive bubbling in water-seal bottle or chamber can mean either of the following.
- An air leak in the chest (internal)
- An air leak in the system (external)

ALERT. Notify the physician immediately.

Monitoring Chest Drainage

Monitor quantity and quality of chest drainage frequently (every hour the first 24 hours; every 2 hours thereafter if stable).

Quality is noted by observation of chest drainage through plastic connector attached to chest tube.

Quantity is noted by checks of level of drainage in drainage chamber or bottle

- For bottles, place strip of tape on side of bottle at initial reading and mark time and amount of drainage at each reading.
- For Pleur-evac, mark time and amount of drainage on Pleur-evac on piece of tape at each reading.

Total the amount of drainage at the end of each shift. This should be taken into account with other output.

Drainage should begin to decrease after 24 hours.

Obtaining Specimen of Chest Drainage

Pleur-evac—aspirate specimen from self-sealing diaphragm in collection chamber.

Bottle suction—specimen must be obtained from drainage bottle; check with physician concerning clamping of chest tube to obtain specimen.

Moving Patient

Bottles and Pleur-evac should always be kept lower than the chest.

NOTE. The Pleur-evac contains a valve that prevents siphoning of fluid and air into the pleural space if it is inadvertently raised higher than the patient's chest.

Preventing Inadvertent Disconnection of Tubing

Make sure *all connectors* are wedged firmly into tubing before taping.

Tape *all connections* securely with 1-inch adhesive tape.

Loop a rubber band around the tubing and pin the rubber band to the bed. Give tubing enough slack so that patient can move without danger of causing tension on chest tube or tubing.

If the chest tube is inadvertently pulled out, take the following steps.
- If a small air leak is present, use Vaseline gauze (kept by the bedside at all times) as an occlusive dressing, covered with 4 × 4s and taped securely.
- If a large air leak is present, do not apply an occlusive dressing.

ALERT. In either case, notify the physician STAT and prepare for reinsertion of chest tubes.

- If tension pneumothorax occurs following application of occlusive dressing, remove dressing immediately.

Providing Security for the System.

Prevent tension on chest tube and tubing at all times.

Pleur-evac
- Hang on bed frame using hangers provided, *or*
- Place in Pleur-evac floor stand.

Glass bottles
- Place in a safe area (never under the bed), *or*
- Tape to the floor (Write "Do Not Remove" on tape), *or*
- Place in rack.

Raising and lowering of bedrails should not affect the system. All personnel (including housekeeping) should be made aware of these safeguards.

Maintaining Patency of Chest Tubes

Keep chest tube patent either by milking or stripping tubing every hour to prevent accumulation of clots, fibrin, or drainage (this should be done in the direction of the drainage system) or by preventing kinks or undue pressure on tubing.
- Stripping
  - Lubricate tubing with water-soluble jelly.
  - Starting at proximal end of tubing (just below connector), pinch the tubing with one hand while sliding the other hand down the tube a short distance distally.
  - While pinching the distal end, slide the first hand down the tubing.
  - Repeat this process the full length of tubing down to the drainage container.
  - Do not release the proximal pinching of the tubing until the distal part is pinched off.
- Milking
  - Fold tubing into several layers.
  - Squeeze or "milk" the folded tubing.

Keep tubing free of kinks.

Do not tape tubing across or through side rail of bed.

Always check to make sure patient is not lying on tubing, especially when position is changed.

Positioning the Patient

Place patient in position of comfort.
- Semi-Fowler's position aides in drainage and comfort.

Change patient's position at least every 2 hours.

It may be necessary to administer pain medication prior to changing patient's position.

Put shoulder on affected side through range of motion exercises several times a day.

NOTE. For actions to take if the chest tube is inadvertently pulled out, see Nursing Actions for Problems Associated with Chest Tubes, p 133.

Discontinuing Suction

The physician usually orders suction to be discontinued for a trial period prior to removal of chest tubes.

Make sure the air vent in the water seal bottle or chamber is open to allow air from the chest to escape.

Continue to monitor patient for signs of tension pneumothorax.

Clamping Chest Tube

The physician usually orders chest tube to be clamped for 24 hours prior to removal.

Continue to monitor patient for signs of tension pneumothorax.

Unclamp tubes immediately if symptoms of tension pneumothorax occur, and notify physician.

ALERT. Notify physician immediately if bubbling is noted in water-seal chamber.

If air leak in chest is not sealed, chest tubes with water-seal drainage continue to be needed.

Nursing Actions for Problems Associated with Chest Tubes

Problem	Nursing Action
Tension pneumothorax	1. Notify physician immediately. 2. If chest tube clamped, remove clamp (see Pneumothorax)
Cessation of bubbling or fluctuation in water-seal chamber or bottle	1. Check tubing for kinks or undue pressure. Straighten or relieve pressure (*e.g.*, from patient lying on tubing). 2. If clots are observed in tubing, change patient's position and have him cough. This may dislodge the obstruction. 3. Make sure suction is working properly. 4. Notify the physician if above measures fail. **NOTE.** If this occurs soon after insertion, an obstruction or other problem is the most likely cause. If it occurs sometime later after insertion, it may indicate that lung reinflation has occurred.
Excessive bubbling in water-seal chamber or bottle	Notify the physician. There may be an external or internal leak in the system.
Cessation of bubbling in suction chamber	1. Check suction for proper function. 2. Check suction connection to suction source and drainage system to ensure proper connection. 3. Notify the physician if above measures fail. (Suction may have to be increased.)
Chest tube inadvertently removed	1. If small air leak is present • Occlude opening immediately, ideally with sterile Vaseline gauze and dressing. If these are not available, use 4 × 4s or a towel. Tape securely.

- Notify the physician immediately.
- If symptoms of tension pneumothorax occur, remove dressing immediately.
2. If large air leak is present
   - Do not apply an occlusive dressing. Sealing large air leak will cause a tension pneumothorax.
   - Notify the physician immediately.
3. Prepare for reinsertion of tube.
4. Do not leave patient unattended.

Excessive drainage (over 100 ml/hr) or bright red drainage (occurs suddenly or does not clear up following surgery) in tubing or drainage system

1. Notify physician immediately.
2. Monitor vital signs and ECG closely.

Excessive drainage or bleeding on dressing

1. Mark borders of area.
2. Reinforce dressing.
3. Notify physician.
4. Continue to mark borders and note time to determine rate of drainage.

NOTE. Do not remove dressing. This is the physician's responsibility.

Disconnection of chest tube from tubing or tubing from Pleur-evac *or* breaking of water-seal or chest drainage bottle

1. Reconnect tubing immediately if you are there when it happens and tubing is not contaminated.
2. If not possible to reconnect, follow the guidelines as listed below.
   - If large air leak is present
     - Do not clamp chest tube for any reason. Tension pneumothorax will result if tube is clamped.
     - Notify physician immediately.
     - Obtain new equipment and prepare for immediate attachment to the system.
   - If small air leak is present, chest tube may be clamped for a short time in an emergency.

NOTE. Tension pneumothorax is still a potential danger.

   - Clamp with covered Kelly clamps (facing away from each other) as close to chest wall as possible.
   - Notify the physician immediately.
   - Obtain new equipment and prepare for immediate attachment to the system.

- Do not leave patient unattended while chest tube is clamped. Observe constantly for tension pneumothorax. If it occurs, unclamp the tube immediately. Problem must be corrected immediately.
- If in doubt as to size of air leak, *do not clamp tubes.* Clamping the chest tube for any reason may result in a tension pneumothorax.
- Notify the physician immediately.

REMOVAL OF CHEST TUBES

Equipment
Sterile suture set
- Scissors
- Forceps

Vaseline gauze

Sterile 4 × 4s

Tape

2 Kelly clamps

Sterile gloves

Preliminary Actions
1. Explain procedure to patient.
2. Position patient appropriately (check with physician).
3. Prepare equipment.
   - Open sterile equipment
   - Open sterile 4 × 4 and Vaseline gauze. Place vaseline gauze on 4 × 4 using gloves.

Procedure
1. Assist physician with procedure.
   - Physician clamps tube and removes dressing.
   - Physician puts on sterile gloves and removes suture.
   - Nurse holds Vaseline gauze dressing over (but not in contact with) site.
   - Patient is instructed to take a deep breath and hold it while physician quickly removes tube.
   - Nurse immediately applies Vaseline gauze dressing to site and tapes it securely (entire area and all edges must be covered).

NOTE. If a purse-string suture is in place, it will be pulled closed and tied immediately following chest tube removal and then covered with the occlusive dressing.

2. Reinforce dressing as necessary.

NOTE. Physician may change dressing several days following removal.

12

Chest Physiotherapy

Chest physiotherapy is indicated in the prevention and treatment of conditions such as acute respiratory failure that may lead to pulmonary complications. Properly performed chest physiotherapy is extremely important in preventing severe pulmonary complications. Commonly used measures are postural drainage, chest percussion and vibration, rib springing, coughing maneuvers, breathing exercises, and manual hyperinflation.

POSTURAL DRAINAGE

Description

The patient is positioned in such a way that gravitational force will facilitate drainage of a certain area or areas of the lung. (See illustrated chart.)

Special Considerations

Monitor vital signs and ECG before, during, and after the procedure.

Have suction equipment readily available.

Provide sputum cup and tissues for secretions. Take protective precautions for your own safety (*i.e.*, instruct patient to cough away from you and into tissues; do not come in direct contact with sputum).

Do not administer this therapy immediately after patient has eaten (may cause vomiting and aspiration).

If there is a localized area, begin therapy with that section and then progress to other areas.

Patient should be kept in a comfortable position throughout the procedure.

Watch patient closely for signs of fatigue. This is hard work and may be exhausting to the critically ill patient. Discontinue temporarily if patient is tired.

Encourage deep breathing and coughing at regular intervals.

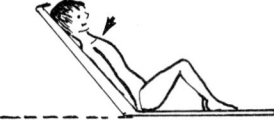

Postural drainage — Upper lobes (right and left apical segments).

Percussion — Clap under collar bone.

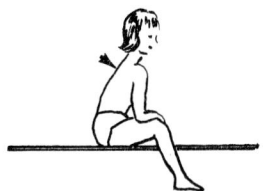

Postural drainage — Upper lobe (right and left apical segments).

Percussion — Clap under collar bone.

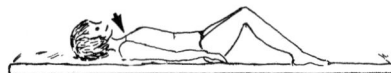

Postural drainage — Upper lobes (anterior segment).

Percussion — Clap under collar bone.

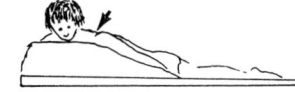

Postural drainage — Upper lobes (left posterior segment).

Percussion — Clap over shoulder blade.

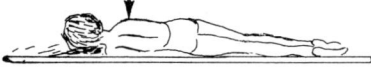

Postural drainage — Upper lobes (right posterior segments).

Percussion — Clap over shoulder blade.

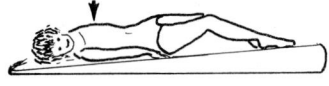

Postural drainage — Left lingular.

Percussion — Clap over nipple area.

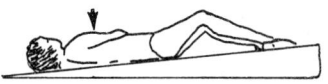

Postural drainage — Right middle lobe.

Percussion — Clap over nipple area.

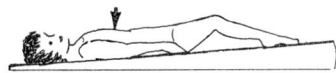

Postural drainage — Lower lobes (right and left anterior basal segments).

Percussion — Clap over ribs.

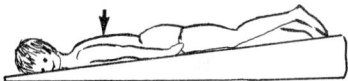

Postural drainage — Lower lobes (right and left posterior, basal segments).

Percussion — Clap over ribs.

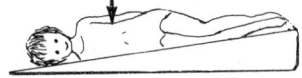

Postural drainage — Lower lobes (left lateral basal segment).

Percussion — Clap over lower ribs.

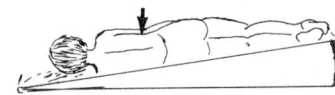

Postural drainage — Lower lobes (right lateral basal segment).

Percussion — Clap over lower ribs.

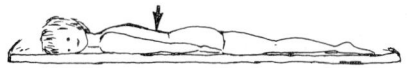

Postural drainage — Lower lobes (superior segments).

Percussion — Clap over ribs (1 inch above bottom of rib cage).

Contraindications

Unconsciousness of unknown etiology

Head injury

Intracranial hemorrhage

Cerebral aneurysm

Intrathoracic bleeding

Flail chest

Fractured ribs

Untreated pneumothorax

Active tuberculosis (or other localized infections)

Hemoptysis

Dyspnea

Severe cardiac arrhythmias

Positional hypotension

Congestive heart failure

Pulmonary edema

Nausea

CHEST PERCUSSION (CLAPPING), VIBRATION, AND RIB SPRINGING

Percussion

With the hand in a cupped position, clap the chest wall in a rhythmical manner while the patient is in the position for postural drainage.

Administer pain medication prior to procedure as ordered to lessen discomfort.

Percuss for 3 to 5 minutes over affected area.

Individualize amount of force exerted.

Do not percuss on bare skin (thin clothing or towel is indicated).

Do not percuss over bony prominences (*e.g.*, spine), female breasts, kidneys, or areas of infection or malignancies.

Encourage patient to deep breathe and cough between position changes.

Vibration

Place hands flat over appropriate area. Using minimal to moderate pressure (for vigorous vibration), vibrate quickly throughout expiratory phase.

Vibration is usually done in conjunction with postural drainage.

Vibrate for 3 to 5 minutes over affected area.

Vibrate as patient exhales.

If patient receiving mechanical ventilation, vibrate during passive expiratory phase.

NOTE. See Percussion for other guidelines, p 138.

Rib Springing

Place hands flat over the appropriate area. On exhalation, apply and then release pressure intermittently 3 or 4 times (like a spring). Perform only during exhalation.

NOTE. See Percussion for other guidelines, p 138.

Contraindications for Percussion, Vibration, and Rib Springing

Flail chest

Rib fractures

Hemoptysis

Infection or malignancy

Pain

Degenerative bone disease

Unstable cardiac status

Anticoagulant therapy (continuous IV administration of heparin)

BREATHING EXERCISES

Description

Diaphragmatic breathing. Breathing from the diaphragm.

Segmental breathing (costal). Following inspiration, pressure is applied over the affected area during expiration.

Pursed lip breathing. Following normal inspiration, the patient purses his lips and exhales slowly.

Special Considerations

Administer pain medication as prescribed prior to procedure.

Monitor patient closely for signs of fatigue or dyspnea. Discontinue exercise temporarily if this occurs.

Use exercises in conjection with postural drainage.

Contraindications

None

COUGHING

Description

The patient inspires slowly and deeply, holds his breath momentarily, and coughs deeply.

Special Considerations

Administer pain medication as prescribed prior to the procedure.

Perform in conjunction with postural drainage.

Splint surgical incisions with pillows or by holding them during coughing.

Avoid strenuous coughing.

Monitor patient's cardiac status (may impair venous return).

Use precautions in patient who may not tolerate an increase in intracranial pressure (*e.g.*, due to aneurysms).

Apply pressure on the diaphragm during exhalation if the patient is unable to cough or exhale forcibly.

Contraindications

Lack of tolerance of increase in intracranial pressure (check with physician if in doubt)

MANUAL HYPERINFLATION

Description

For the patient who is receiving mechanical ventilation or has a tracheostomy or endotracheal tube, an Ambu or manual resuscitator bag is attached to the tubing, and the lungs are hyperinflated.

Special Considerations

On inspiration, compress the bag slowly with both hands, hold it a few seconds, and then quickly release it.

Perform procedure in conjunction with postural drainage.

Vibration may be performed by a second nurse during expiration.

Perform suction as necessary.

Repeat for several breaths before reinstituting normal volume.

Closely monitor cardiac status.

Sometimes 2 ml to 3 ml of sterile saline are injected into tube prior to hyperinflation.

Contraindications

Untreated pneumothorax

13
Methods of Oxygen Administration

Many methods of oxygen administration are available. The method used depends on the patient's condition, his age (*e.g.*, a pediatric patient), the oxygen concentration desired, and the physician's preference. The most commonly used methods are described in this chapter, and safety precautions are noted.

NASAL CATHETER

Description
The nasal catheter delivers low to moderate concentrations of oxygen.

Percentage of oxygen delivery is reliable; even mouth breathers receive oxygen by this method.

Special Considerations
To determine depth of catheter for insertion, do the following.
• Measure catheter from tip of nose to earlobe.
• If catheter is visible beside uvula following insertion, pull back slightly until no longer visible.

Change catheter and insert in opposite nostril every 8 hours.

Improper placement may result in gastric distention.

Arterial blood gases should be closely monitored.

Problems
Nasal irritation

Nose bleed

NASAL CANNULA

Description
It delivers low to moderate concentrations of oxygen.

Although more comfortable than the nasal catheter, the nasal cannula is easily displaced, and the percentage of oxygen delivery is not as reliable.

NOTE. Mouth breathers receive very little oxygen by this method.

Special Considerations

Tips of cannula are inserted in nostrils.

Arterial blood gases should be closely monitored.

Problems

Nasal irritation

Nose bleed

Frontal sinus pain (high flow rates)

VENTURI MASK ("VENTI-MASK")

Description

The venturi mask precisely delivers low to medium oxygen concentrations.

It is primarily used in patients with chronic obstructive lung disease.

Special Considerations

Vent holes in plastic face mask must be open to prevent rebreathing of carbon dioxide and resulting hypoventilation.

Mask should be closely molded to patient's face.

Arterial blood gases should be closely monitored.

Problems

Tight fitting mask may cause the following.
• Pressure necrosis of the skin
• Aspiration of vomitus

OXYGEN MASK

Description

There are many types of oxygen masks with different features.

Special Considerations

The mask should be closely molded to the face in order to ensure delivery of high oxygen concentration.

The mask should be removed and the skin dried whenever necessary.

Arterial blood gases should be closely monitored.

Problems

Tight-fitting mask may cause a pressure necrosis of the skin

Aspiration of vomitus is a potential problem due to the tight fit

Poor patient toleration of mask

Discomfort owing to tight fit necessary for proper function

TYPES OF MASKS

Simple mask (without bag)
• This type of mask delivers a high concentration of oxygen.
• It is usually used with acutely ill patients with cardiac disease.

Mask with partial rebreathing bag
• Bag acts as oxygen reservoir, which permits patient to inhale oxygen at moderately high concentrations.
• It is useful when there is a need to raise the level of arterial O_2.
• Bag should be filled with oxygen prior to placing on patient.
• Bag should not completely collapse during inspiration.

Mask with nonrebreathing bag
• Bag acts as oxygen reservoir, which permits patient to inhale oxygen at high concentrations.
• Mask with nonrebreathing bag differs from mask with partial rebreathing bag in that it has flap valves between bag and mask, and on exhalation ports on mask that are one way (*i.e.,* on inspiration, patient breathes in high concentration of oxygen from reservoir bag; on expiration, one-way valve between bag and mask closes, and air is exhaled through exhalation ports where the one-way valves are now open.)
• Bag should be filled with oxygen prior to placing on the patient.
• Bag should not completely collapse during inspiration.
• Be sure flap valves are working properly.

Aerosol mask
• Aerosol mask delivers high concentration of oxygen with high degree of humidity.
• Mist should be visible at all times.
• Monitor tubing closely for excess moisture buildup and empty as needed.

FACE TENT

Description

A face tent delivers high humidity (primary purpose); oxygen concentration is more variable than with face mask (concentration is more reliable if an ultrasonic nebulizer is used.)

It is generally used by the patient who needs a smaller amount of oxygen and is well tolerated.

Special Considerations

Mist should always be visible.

Monitor tubing closely for excess moisture buildup and empty as needed.

Arterial blood gases should be closely monitored.

TRACHEOSTOMY COLLAR OR MASK

A tracheostomy collar or mask delivers oxygen and humidity to the patient with a tracheostomy (or who has had a laryngectomy).

This method is generally well tolerated by the patient.

Special Considerations

Percentage of oxygen delivered depends on oxygen flow and type of collar.

Mist should be visible at all times.

Monitor tubing closely for excess moisture buildup and empty as needed.

Heating the mist is recommended. Monitor temperature of steam closely to prevent burns (tracheal and possibly pulmonary).

Monitor position of collar closely to make sure it is properly placed over the tracheal opening.

These devices are useful in weaning patient from respirator.

They must be kept clean.

Arterial blood gases should be closely monitored.

Problems

Possible burns if steam is used (see above)

Infection

Possibility of excess moisture collected in tubing being inadvertently dumped into tracheostomy.

T-TUBE
Description

The T-tube delivers oxygen and high humidity (concentration of oxygen is more reliable if an ultrasonic nebulizer is used).

Special Considerations

This device attaches directly to endotracheal or tracheal tubes.

Monitor tubing closely for excess moisture buildup and empty as necessary.

Monitor position of T-tube to make sure it has not become disconnected.

Mist should be visible at all times (from open end).

Heating the mist is recommended. Monitor temperature of steam closely to prevent burns (tracheal and possibly pulmonary).

Arterial blood gases should be monitored closely.

Problems

Burns may develop if steam is used (see above).

Overhydration and infection may develop.

Excess moisture collected in tubing may be inadvertently dumped into tracheostomy.

OXYGEN TENT
Description

The oxygen tent delivers low to moderate concentration of oxygen high humidity, and cooled air (about 6° lower than room air) or high humidity and cooler air alone.

Special Considerations

The tent should be flushed with oxygen prior to placing the patient in it.

The sides of the canopy must be tucked firmly under the mattress and secured across the patient's legs with bed linen to ensure a tight seal and prevent air leaks.

Bed linen and clothing become damp or drenched from the moisture and should be changed as needed.

Sometimes the patient's head and shoulders are covered to keep them dry and comfortable.

The oxygen concentration drops significantly every time the tent is opened.

Nursing care should be carefully planned and performed in such a way as to disturb the patient as little as possible.

Oxygen tents are very infrequently used for adults. It is primarily used as croupette for infants and children.

An oxygen analyzer should be used frequently to determine oxygen concentration in the tent.

Arterial blood gases should be monitored closely.

Problems

Oxygen may cause fire if oxygen is used.

Carbon dioxide may accumulate if oxygen flow is low.

Oxygen level drops to that of room air every time the canopy is opened.

Patient toleration of oxygen therapy is poor in an enclosed space.

Moisture rich environment keeps the patient, clothes, and bedding uncomfortably damp or wet.

CROUPETTE (CROUP TENT OR AEROSOL TENT)
Description

The Croupette is an effective method for administration of high humidity, with or without oxygen, and cooler air (same as for regular oxygen tent) when the younger patient has a poor tolerance of other methods.

Special Considerations

Cracked ice is added to the ice chamber and the nebulizer reservoir is filled with sterile distilled water to produce a cool mist in the tent.

The tent is flushed with oxygen prior to placing the patient in it.

Friction toys are not allowed in the tent.

See Oxygen Tent in the preceding section for additional information.

HEAD HOOD
Description

The head hood delivers oxygen, humidity, and warmed air if a radiant warmer is used.

It is used with cooperative infants and young children.

IPPB

Description

IPPB delivers oxygen or air on inspiration under increased pressure at a preset rate and volume.

There are several purposes for this treatment—aids in lung expansion and increases alveolar ventilation; used for administration of aerosol medications; used as prophylactic treatment to prevent complications associated with serious illness or after surgery (hypoxia, hypercapnia, atelectasis); temporarily reduces the workload of breathing and increases the quality of respirations at the same time.

Special Considerations

The patient should be sitting in an upright, or semi-Fowler's position.

Mask or mouthpiece may be used. If mouthpiece is used, nose clip must be placed on nostrils. (To be effective, a closed circuit must be made.)

If medication is used, it is placed in the nebulizer.

Pulse, respirations, and blood pressure should be checked, and the lungs auscultated before beginning IPPB. Vital signs should be monitored throughout and following the procedure.

The machine is adjusted for the individual patient's needs.

IPPB is contraindicated in the treatment of pneumothorax, unless chest tube has been inserted, and in wound dehiscence.

Problems

IPPB may cause hemoptysis, hypo- or hyperventilation, overoxygenation, or pneumothorax.

Intracranial pressure increases.

Cardiac output decreases (from an increase in intrathoracic pressure).

SAFETY PRECAUTIONS TO BE OBSERVED DURING OXYGEN THERAPY

Smoking is not permitted in area of oxygen use.
- Post NO SMOKING—OXYGEN IN USE signs where they will be visible to staff and visitors.
- Explain rule to patient.
- Remove cigarettes, cigars, pipes, and matches or lighters from area.

Open flames or sparks are not permitted in area of oxygen use. (Maintenance department should be made aware of this.)

Ungrounded electrical equipment is not permitted in area of oxygen use.
- Frayed electrical cords should not be used.
- Extension cords should not be used.

Electric shavers should not be used.

Oils or oil-base products should not be used on the patient or equipment.

Flammable solutions (*e.g.*, alcohol) should not be used on the patient.

Take precautions to eliminate static electricity.
- Do not allow friction toys in oxygen tent with child.
- Substitute cotton blankets for wool.

14

Intubation Procedures

Intubation, either endotracheal or tracheal, is used to maintain a patent airway, relieve or bypass obstruction, prevent aspiration, and facilitate suctioning. When mechanical ventilation is employed, intubation provides the means of connecting the patient to the ventilator. Procedures and nursing responsibilities for intubation, suctioning, weaning, and extubation are described in this chapter. Emergency airways (esophageal obturator and cricothyroid stab) are also presented.

ENDOTRACHEAL INTUBATION

Description

Endotracheal intubation is the insertion of an endotracheal tube through the mouth or nose into the trachea.

Equipment

Laryngoscope with various sized blades (curved and straight)

Endotracheal tubes of various sizes (cuffed and uncuffed)

Topical anesthetic (indicated if patient is conscious)

Suction

Sterile suction catheters

Sterile gloves

Sterile normal saline solution (for clearing tubing)

10-ml syringe

Water-soluble lubricating jelly

Ambu bag

Plastic airway

Metal stylet or guide may be used to facilitate insertion

Magill forceps

Adhesive tape

Respirator

Preliminary Actions

1. Check the cuff to see that it inflates properly (i.e., inflate the cuff and either immerse it in sterile saline or observe for several minutes).
2. Check laryngoscope batteries and bulb to see if they are working properly.
3. The respirator should be tested for proper function.
4. Wash hands.

Procedure

1. Attach proper blade to laryngoscope handle.
2. Select endotracheal tube.
3. Place patient in supine position.
   - In adults, hyperextend neck with head positioned slightly above shoulders.
   - In infants and children, extend the head and keep the neck straight.
4. Remove dentures or other removable dental devices.
5. Preoxygenate the patient with 100% oxygen.
6. Apply topical anesthetic to the larynx and trachea if the patient is conscious. (Muscle relaxants may be given if necessary to facilitate intubation.)
7. With thumb and index finger of dominant hand, open the patient's jaw and insert the blade, using the nondominant hand along the right side of the mouth. The tongue moves to the left as the blade is placed in the middle. (Orotracheal intubation is preferred over nasotracheal intubation.)
8. The blade is lifted slightly (about 45°) as it is advanced until the epiglottis is visible.
9. The lubricated endotracheal tube with cuff deflated is then inserted along the right side of the mouth and through the glottis until the cuff is no longer visible. This is best performed during inspiration.
10. Remove the laryngoscope.
11. Inflate the cuff according to one of the following techniques:
    - Minimal air leak
    - No-air leak
    (See techniques for cuff inflation in a latter section of this chapter.)
12. Tape in place.
13. Suction secretions in tube if necessary, using sterile technique.
14. Administer 100% oxygen to patient immediately following procedure while auscultating both sides of the chest. Breath sounds should be heard bilaterally and be of equal intensity.
15. Attach to preset ventilator. (Set ventilator according to physician's specifications.)
16. Place airway in mouth beside tube. Tape in place.

17. Endotracheal tube should be marked at level of the mouth to check for proper positioning.
18. Position of tube should be checked by x-ray (tip is radiopaque).

Problems

Trauma to lips, tongue, larynx, vocal cords, teeth, and trachea

Cardiac arrhythmias (*e.g.*, bradycardia, PVC's)

Vomiting and aspiration

Hypoxemia

Hypercapnia

Improper positioning (in one bronchus or esophagus)

ENDOTRACHEAL EXTUBATION

Equipment

Have emergency equipment including Ambu bag, mask, and equipment necessary for reintubation readily available.

Preliminary Actions

Check arterial blood gases prior to beginning extubation.

Suction the mouth and trachea before deflating the cuff.

Preoxygenate with 100% oxygen.

Procedure

Remove endotracheal tube on inspiration or cough.

Suction if necessary.

Watch patient closely for several hours following extubation to see how he tolerates breathing on his own.

Closely monitor arterial blood gases.

Follow these basic guidelines.
• Keep NPO until normal reflexes return (may be several hours).
• Observe for signs of laryngeal edema (respiratory stridor or hoarseness)
• Administer humidified oxygen through mask as ordered.

EMERGENCY TRACHEOTOMY

Description

Tracheotomy (surgical opening into trachea at the level of the second tracheal ring) is usually an elective procedure performed in the operating room under strict surgical asepsis. In an emergency, however, it may be performed at the bedside. The following procedure refers to an emergency tracheotomy.

CUFFING

Cuff inflation is indicated for the following:
• Mechanical ventilation
• IPPB treatments
• Situations where there is a danger of aspiration (feedings or administration of medications, either oral or through a levine tube; the unconscious patient)

NOTE. Cuff is generally kept inflated for 30 minutes following ingestion of food, fluids, or medications to lessen the danger of aspiration.

Cuff deflation is indicated when the following attachments are used:
• Tracheostomy plug
• Tracheostomy talk device
• Aerosol T-tube (to assist in weaning from the respirator)

TECHNIQUES FOR CUFF INFLATION

Minimal Air Leak
1. Place stethoscope, using diaphragm, over trachea.
2. Inject air into inflating tube and cycle the ventilator. (No air will be felt from mouth or nose.)
3. Patient will be unable to talk. Remove 0.5 cc of air from the tubing and listen for small air leak at end of inspiration.
4. This procedure is repeated and the cuff is slightly deflated until small air leak is heard.
5. As an added safeguard, the tubing is clamped with a mosquito or Kelly clamp. This prevents a possible leak.

NOTE. Ventilators must be adjusted to compensate for small air leak. Used with positive end expiratory pressure (PEEP) and continuous positive airway pressure (CPAP).

No-Air Leak
1. Repeat steps 1 and 2 of above procedure.
2. Listen at end of inspiration. (No air leak should be heard.)
3. This procedure is repeated and the cuff is slightly inflated until no air leak is heard.

NOTE. Cuff pressures should be measured and monitored closely, especially with no-air leak method.

Equipment

Sterile tracheotomy tray (see sterile tracheotomy tray list)
Povidone-iodine solution
Sterile gloves
Sterile water
Silk suture (3-0 and 4-0)
Local anesthetic
Suction source
Sterile suction catheters
Sterile saline
Sterile solution bowl or cup (for clearing suction tubing)
Face masks
Sterile gowns (may be worn if time permits)

Preliminary Actions

1. Explain procedure to patient. Obtain signed consent form.
2. Prepare equipment.
   • Open sterile tray.
   • Pour povidone-iodine solution in solution cup.
3. Position the patient properly, as listed below.
   • Place flat on his back.
   • Hyperextend the neck by placing a small rolled towel under the shoulder blades.
   • Be sure the head and neck are in normal body alignment.
4. Make sure the area is well lighted.
5. Remove the headboard.
6. Check vital signs and ECG tracing to establish a baseline, and continue to monitor throughout the procedure.

Procedure

1. Assist physician as he performs procedure.
2. Keep resuscitative equipment, including mechanical ventilation, readily available.
3. Following the procedure, closely monitor the site for excessive bleeding, both external (on dressing) and internal (secretions from stoma).

ALERT. Notify physician immediately if excessive bleeding occurs.

STERILE TRACHEOTOMY TRAY
Scalpel (#11 and #15 blade)
Tissue forceps (with and without teeth)
Dissecting scissors
Suture scissors
Hemostats or mosquitos (curved and straight, 4 each)
4 Kelly clamps (straight)
Tracheotomy hook
Tracheotomy spreader
Needle holder
2 rake retractors
2 vein retractors
2 allis clamps
2 sponge forceps
4 small towel clips
Tracheostomy tubes (various sizes; adult and pediatric)
Syringes
Needles (25-gauge and 20-gauge, 1½-in)
4 × 4s without cotton batting
2 × 2s without cotton batting
Ties
2 medicine glasses
4 towels
1 fenestrated towel
Suction tip

4. Continue to monitor vital signs and ECG (as normal postoperative care) until stable.

TYPES OF TRACHEOSTOMY TUBES
General characteristics (See Table 14-1)
Special features and problems (See Table 14-2)

TABLE 14-1. **General Characteristics of Tracheostomy Tubes**

Material	Comments
Metal (silver or stainless steel)	Parts are usually not interchangeable Parts are not disposable
Plastic	Parts are usually interchangeable Most parts are disposable

Parts	
Outer cannula only	Especially used with pediatric patients
Outer and inner cannula	Inner cannula may be removed for cleaning **NOTE.** Outer cannula is *never* removed for cleaning
Obturator	Obturator usually used for insertion; some tubes used for newborns or small infants may not have obturator

Cuff	
Uncuffed tube	Children generally do not require cuffs; (older children may); used for patient requiring long-term therapy
Cuffed tube	Used for patient who requires mechanical ventilation; also used if there is danger of aspiration

TABLE 14-2. **Special Features and Problems of Tracheostomy Tubes**

Type	Material	Cuff Pressure	Comments	Problems
Uncuffed	Metal or plastic	None	Most commonly used for children Possibility of tracheal necrosis greatly reduced Used in adults requiring long-term therapy	Prevents mechanical ventilation in adult Danger of aspiration is greater in adults
Cuffed	Plastic	Low	Most commonly used Possibility of tracheal necrosis is greatly reduced Cuff does not have to be deflated periodically Cuff is bonded to tube	Relatively problem-free
	Plastic	High	Cuff is bonded to tube	Possibility of tracheal necrosis is greater Cuff should be periodically deflated

(Continued)

TABLE 14-2. **Special Features and Problems of Tracheostomy Tubes**
(Continued)

Type	Material	Cuff Pressure	Comments	Problems
	Metal	Low or high	May be sterilized for reuse because cuff is removable	Cuff can easily slip, obstructing the airway.
				NOTE. Cuffed metal tubes are not generally used for this reason.
Uncuffed, fenestrated	Plastic	None	Has tracheostomy plug that occludes the fenestration of the tracheostomy tube, allowing the patient to breathe normally through the larynx; patient is able to speak (used for weaning)	If mechanical ventilation is required, this system must be removed and replaced by one with a cuffed cannula
Cuffed, fenestrated	Plastic	Low	Has two inner cannulas used for different purposes Shorter cannula—occludes fenestration (window) in tracheostomy tube, allowing patient to breathe on his own; patient is able to speak (used for weaning) Longer cannula—must be used when mechanical ventilation is used; cuff is inflated.	Cuff must be deflated when shorter cannula is inserted; failure to do so totally obstructs the airway

TRACHEOSTOMY CARE

Equipment
Sterile disposable or hospital prepared tray containing the following:
- Towel or drape
- Pipe cleaners
- Tracheostomy brush
- Ties (½ in linen tape)

- Gloves
- 4 × 4s without cotton batting
- Cotton swabs
- Two sterile bowls
- Forceps

Sterile water or saline

Hydrogen peroxide

Sterile suction catheters

Suction

Povidone-iodine solution

Sterile Kelly clamp or tracheal dilator (should be taped to head of bed and kept there at all times)

Extra sterile tracheostomy tube (should be taped to head of bed and kept there at all times)

HOW TO CLEAN THE INNER CANNULA OF A TWO-CANNULA TRACHEOSTOMY TUBE

Procedure

1. Wash hands.
2. Prepare equipment.
   - Open sterile tray using aseptic technique.
   - Pour sterile solutions (hydrogen peroxide, sterile saline, or water) into separate sterile bowls.
   - Open sterile towel or drape for work surface.
   - Open sterile 4 × 4s and cotton swabs and drop on drape if not pre-packaged on tray.
   - Prepare suction equipment.
     - Attach sterile suction catheter to suction tubing.
     - Turn on suction.
3. Using forceps, remove soiled dressing.
4. Put on sterile gloves.
5. Suction the inner cannula, if necessary, prior to beginning the procedure. (Be sure to preoxygenate the patient prior to suctioning.)
   - Flush tubing with sterile saline.
   - Discard.
   - Attach fresh suction catheter.
   - Change gloves.
6. Remove inner cannula with dominant hand.
   - Prevent tracheostomy tube from moving by applying gentle pressure to flanges with nondominant hand.
   - Place inner cannula in basin containing hydrogen peroxide, bottom end first.
   - If patient is on ventilator, reconnect to outer cannula by using a tracheostomy care adapter.

- If adapter is unavailable, second nurse should hold ventilator tubing in place.

NOTE. Dominant hand is considered clean. Nondominant hand is considered contaminated.

7. Thoroughly clean the inner cannula as follows.
   - Pick up the cannula with the nondominant hand at the top (part that is outside the trachea).
   - Using dominant hand, insert sterile pipe cleaner or brush at the bottom of the cannula (part that is inside the trachea) and gently remove any crust formation or mucus as it is advanced through tube and out the top. (This method prevents secretions from the most contaminated area or top of the cannula from being forced into the least contamminated part or bottom of the cannula.)
   - Rinse by immersing in bowl of sterile water or saline, bottom first.
   - Holding top part down, allow excess moisture to drop off by gently shaking.
   - Place on sterile drape until ready for reinsertion.
   - Clean flanges of outer cannula using sterile 4 × 4s (without cotton batting) moistened with peroxide or sterile saline or water.
8. Suction outer cannula, if necessary, prior to reinsertion of inner cannula, using sterile technique.
9. Reinsert inner cannula while applying gentle pressure to the flanges of the outer cannula to prevent unnecessary movement and possible trauma.
   - Lock in place.
   - Reconnect the ventilator or other oxygen tubing to the tracheostomy tube.
10. Using forceps, clean the skin around the tracheostomy tube with sterile 4 × 4s (without cotton batting) moistened with povidone-iodine (peroxide, sterile saline or water may be used).
    - Clean from the stoma outward.
    - Heavy encrustations may be removed by leaving moistened 4 × 4s over the affected area for several minutes.
    - Dry, using sterile 4 × 4s.

TRACHEOSTOMY DRESSING

1. Dressing should fit around tracheostomy tube.
2. Precut dressing (with ends selvaged) may be used (provided on some disposable trays).
3. Sterile 4 × 4 (without cotton batting) may be used. (See Fig. 14-1)
4. Do not cut slit in 4 × 4 to fit around tube because fluff or unraveled threads may be aspirated in trachea.

1. Open gauze square (without cotton batting).

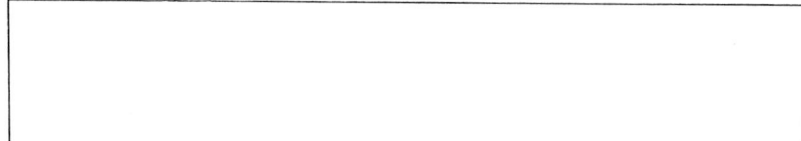

2. Fold gauze in half.

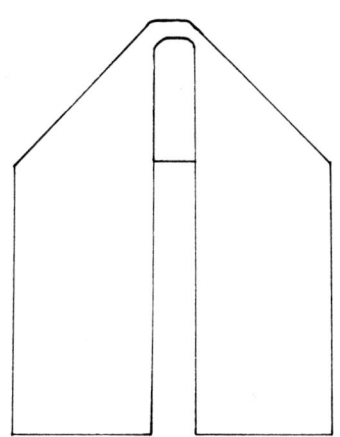

3.

a. Starting at center, fold each side in a downward direction.

b. Slip the dressing under the flanges of the tracheostomy tube (folded edges away from patient) and pull gently into place.

FIG. 14-1   *Tracheostomy dressing*

TIES

1. Change ties if soiled or wet.

2. Apply new ties and secure in place before removing old ones.

3. Cut one tie shorter than the other.

4. Fold over 1 in of one end of tie and make a cut about ¼ in long in center lengthwise. Repeat with other tie.

NOTE. Make sure cut area will not unravel.

5. Insert uncut end of tie through flanges and gently pull through, being careful not to move the tracheostomy tube.

6. Pull uncut end through notch in tie gently until it fits snugly against flange. (Once again, make sure notched area is secure and will not unravel.)

7. Repeat this procedure with other tie.

8. Tie should not be secured to flange with a knot (causes unnecessary and uncomfortable pressure on the skin).

9. When both ties are securely attached to the tracheostomy tube, bring the longer end around the back of the neck to the side and connect with the shorter end by tying a knot. (Do not connect the two at the back of the neck as this is uncomfortable.)

10. Check to make sure that the ties are fitting properly before tying a knot.
    - Tape should fit snugly against skin but not cut into it.
    - The nurse should be able to fit two fingers under the ties.
    - The tracheostomy tube should not be sliding in and out with respirations. If this is noticed, the ties are not tight enough.

NOTE. If old ties are removed before applying new ones, a second nurse must be present to hold tracheostomy tube in place throughout the procedure. This method is not recommended.

ONE-CANNULA TRACHEOSTOMY TUBES

1. Clean the flanges of the cannula and the skin around it.

2. Replace the dressing if wet or soiled.

3. Change the ties if necessary. (See above procedure for changing ties.)

TIME SCHEDULE FOR TRACHEOSTOMY CARE

Immediately following tracheostomy procedure—perform tracheostomy care as needed (every 30 min to 1 hr), depending on amount of secretions.

NOTE. Patient should not be left alone during this period until amount of secretions has lessened.

When secretions have lessened, for the first 24 hours following surgery—perform tracheostomy care every 2 to 4 hours, depending on amount of secretions.

After the first day—perform tracheostomy care at least every 8 hours or as needed

Special Considerations

Never remove the outer cannula of a one-cannula or a two-cannula tracheostomy tube.

If the inner cannula is inadvertently contaminated, replace with a sterile one.

Significant bleeding around or aspirated from the stoma at any time should be reported to the physician immediately.

Suspect a tracheal-esophageal fistula if coughing occurs following ingestion of food or fluids either orally or by tube feeding or if food or fluids are aspirated from tracheostomy. Report to physician immediately.

EMERGENCY REINSERTION OF TRACHEOSTOMY TUBE

If the tracheostomy tube is accidentally removed, insert a sterile tracheostomy tube which should be kept taped to head of bed, or reinsert the dislodged tube if it is not contaminated.

Equipment

Sterile tracheostomy tube and obturator or dislodged tracheostomy tube and obturator

Sterile gloves

Ties

Sterile 4 × 4s (without cotton batting)

Syringe (for inflating cuff)

NOTE. Make sure cuff is completely deflated on dislodged tube.

Procedure

1. Explain procedure to patient.
2. Wash hands.
3. Put on sterile gloves.
4. Remove inner cannula and insert obturator in outer cannula. (If a one-cannula tracheostomy tube is being used, the obturator fits directly into this cannula because there is no inner cannula.)
5. Gently insert tracheostomy tube into the stoma, aiming the tube back and downward.
6. Remove obturator as soon as tube is in place, and insert inner cannula, locking it in place.
7. Inflate cuff.
8. Attach ties and secure tube in place.
9. Auscultate both sides of the chest to make sure that both are being aerated.
10. Administer oxygen if patient needs it.

NOTE. If hospital policy does not permit the nurse to reinsert a tracheostomy tube, use a curved Kelly clamp or tracheal dilator (kept at the bedside) to maintain the tracheostomy opening until a physician or respiratory therapist arrives.

HOW TO WEAN PATIENT FROM TRACHEOSTOMY TUBE

1. Explain procedure to patient.
2. If it is not already in place, a fenestrated tracheostomy tube is inserted by a physician, respiratory therapist, or an RN who is specially trained in this procedure.
3. Plug the tube if the patient experiences no respiratory problems for approximately 12 to 24 hours, depending on physician's preference.

NOTE. Arterial blood gases should be checked before removal, during period of cuff deflation and following removal of the tube. Supplemental oxygen through face mask may be required until patient can maintain adequate blood gases while breathing room air.

EXTUBATION OF TRACHEOSTOMY TUBE

Equipment
Sterile gloves

Sterile 4 × 4s (without cotton batting)

Suction

Sterile suction catheters

Tape

Scissors

Procedure
1. Explain procedure to patient.
2. Put patient in semi-Fowler's position.
3. Suction tracheostomy tube and oropharynx and deflate cuff prior to removal of tube.
4. Assist physician in the following manner as he removes tube.
   • Cut ties
   • Instruct patient to cough as tube is removed.
   • Cover stoma with 4 × 4 (without cotton batting) and secure with tape.
5. Monitor patient's respirations closely following procedure.
6. Keep sterile tracheostomy equipment readily available in case tube replacement is indicated.
7. Change dressing as necessary.

EMERGENCY AIRWAYS

ESOPHAGEAL OBTURATOR
General Information
An esophageal obturator is a temporary airway only.

Cuffed tube is passed into the esophagus.

The upper portion of the tube contains holes to permit air passage; the part in the esophagus is occluded.

If continued airway assistance is necessary, an endotracheal tube is inserted prior to removal of esophageal obturator.

Equipment
Esophageal obturator (attached mask)

Suction source

Suction catheters

Ambu bag and mask

50-ml syringe

Lubricant (water soluble)

Preliminary Actions
1. Assess need for therapy. Use esophageal obturator only if endotracheal intubation is not possible.
2. The patient should be positioned on his back with head and neck in normal body alignment. The neck should not be hyperextended (would facilitate entry into the trachea).

Procedure
1. Suction or manually remove any foreign material in the mouth.
2. Open the patient's mouth and grasp the tongue and jaw lifting them forward.
3. Insert the lubricated tube into the mouth, and pass it into esophagus.
4. At this point, the mask should closely fit the patient's face.
5. Check for placement by attaching Ambu bag to adapter on mask (or placing mouth on adapter), and ventilate.
   • Check breath sounds.
   • Watch for bilateral chest excursions.
6. After ascertaining that the tube has been properly positioned, inflate the balloon with 30 ml of air.
7. Begin ventilations.
8. To extubate, be sure the balloon has been deflated before removal.

Contraindications
Children

Severe head or face injuries

Conscious patients

Esophageal trauma

CRICOTHYROID STAB (CRICOTHYROTOMY)
General Information
Cricothyroid membrane is opened horizontally with any sharp instrument or object (as performed in field situation).

Cricothyroid stab is performed when the airway is totally occluded, endotracheal intubation is impossible, and there is not sufficient time to perform a tracheotomy.

Serious bleeding will not occur with this procedure because this is not a very vascular area.

Hollow object must be inserted into opening to maintain airway.

This method is replaced by endotracheal or tracheal intubation as soon as possible.

ENDOTRACHEAL SUCTIONING THROUGH ENDOTRACHEAL OR TRACHEOSTOMY TUBE

Equipment
Sterile gloves

Sterile suction catheters (should have intermittent suction control port)

Suction set-up

Sterile normal saline

Sterile basin or cup

Preliminary Actions
1. Explain the procedure to the patient.
2. Preoxygenate patient with 100% oxygen by way of Ambu bag.
3. Prepare equipment, using the following aseptic technique.
   - Wash hands.
   - Pour sterile saline into sterile basin or cup.
   - Open catheter package at suction attachment end. (Catheter should not exceed one third the diameter of the airway.)
   - Turn on suction.
4. Put on gloves (Dominant hand should be considered sterile and nondominant hand clean.)

Procedure
1. Attach catheter to connecting tubing.
2. Lubricate catheter by placing in basin or cup with sterile normal saline.
3. Disconnect ventilator, keeping end of tubing clean.
4. Using dominant hand, insert catheter into tube.
5. Feed catheter into tube without applying suction as far as possible.
6. When proper level is reached, apply intermittent suction as catheter is withdrawn, using a rotating motion.
7. Clean tubing and catheter by flushing with sterile saline.
8. Administer 100% oxygen for several minutes by Ambu bag.
9. Check patient for effectiveness of suctioning.
10. Repeat suctioning, using fresh sterile catheter and gloves as necessary.

Special Considerations

Do not suction for more than 10 seconds at a time; patient's lungs should be hyperinflated with Ambu bag before and after each suctioning.

Suction catheters should be used only once and then discarded.

Sterile saline may be instilled in tube to loosen secretions. (This is usually a standing order in the unit.)
- 3 ml to 5 ml are instilled (less in pediatric patients).
- Needle should be removed from syringe before instillation.
- Hyperinflate the lungs following instillation and prior to suction with Ambu bag.

Positioning of patient's head determines location of the catheter.
- Head turned to right—left bronchus is suctioned.
- Head turned to left—right bronchus is suctioned.

Never suction the mouth and the nose, and then the trachea.

Suction only when necessary.

Maintain strict aseptic technique.

Closely monitor heart rate and rhythm. If heart rate drops or arrhythmias develop suddenly, stop suctioning immediately and administer oxygen. Continue to monitor.

Generally, oxygenate patient with 10 breaths before suctioning, five breaths between suctionings, and 10 breaths after the procedure.

Problems

Hypoxia

Bradycardia (and other arrhythmias)

Atelectasis

Infection

Mucosal trauma

ENDOTRACHEAL SUCTIONING WITHOUT ENDOTRACHEAL OR TRACHEOSTOMY TUBE

Procedure

Follow procedure for endotracheal suctioning with tube, with the following exceptions
- Lubricate the catheter with a water-soluble jelly.
- Following preoxygenation, insert tube through nose and feed into pharynx.
- Have patient take a deep breath, and advance catheter into trachea.
- Encourage patient to breathe slowly and deeply as catheter is advanced as far as possible. (Do not force if resistance is met.)
- Apply suction as catheter is removed.
- Hyperinflate lungs with oxygen following the procedure.

Special Consideration

If bronchospasm occurs, preventing removal of suction catheter, try the following approaches to aid in catheter removal until bronchospasm subsides:

- Convert suction catheter to a temporary airway by disconnecting from suction tubing.
- Administer oxygen through suction catheter.

NOTE. Do not force catheter removal. Remove suction catheter immediately after bronchospasm subsides.

Closely monitor heart rate and rhythm. If heart rate drops or arrhythmias develop suddenly, stop suctioning immediately and administer oxygen. Continue to monitor.

15
Mechanical Ventilation

Mechanical ventilation is frequently used to treat respiratory failure in the critical care unit. The types and basic functions of mechanical ventilators, nursing considerations, adverse effects, and weaning techniques are presented in this chapter.

TYPES OF MECHANICAL VENTILATION

The various modes of operation of ventilators are summarized in Table 15-1.

PRESSURE-CYCLED VENTILATOR

Delivers gas with the desired concentration of oxygen at a preset pressure

Used for assisted and controlled ventilation

Powered by gas (air or oxygen)

Generally, not used for long-term therapy; used primarily for IPPB

Examples
  Monaghan 225
  Bird Mark 7

VOLUME-CYCLED VENTILATOR

Delivers gas with the desired concentration of oxygen at a preset volume

Used for controlled and assist-contol ventilators

Powered by electricity

Generally used for long-term therapy.

Examples
  Bennet MA-1
  Bennet MA-2
  Monaghan 225

TIME-CYCLED VENTILATOR

Delivers gas with the desired concentration of oxygen for a preset period of time, after which inspiration ends and expiration begins

Variable volume and pressure, depending on lung compliance and airway resistance, necessitating constant monitoring of volume to be certain that adequate ventilation is occuring.

Examples
  Air Shields
  Babybird
  Monaghan 225

TABLE 15-1. **Modes of Operation of Ventilators**

Mode	Patient's Ability	Ventilator Response
Assisted ventilation	Breathing on his own but ventilation is inadequate	Triggered by patient's own inspiration to ensure an adequate depth of inspiration and concentration of oxygen
Controlled ventilation	No spontaneous respirations or ineffective respirations	Assumes total control of respirations, delivering an adequate concentration of oxygen at a preset rate and volume, regardless of the patient's efforts
Assist control	Respiratory drive is irregular	Acts as an assist-type ventilator if spontaneous respiratory rate remains above a preset rate, and functions as a control-type ventilator if spontaneous respirations fall below the preset rate
Intermittent mandatory ventilation (IMV)	Breathes spontaneously	Intermittently forces the patient to take a deeper breath at a preset rate; useful in weaning a patient from a respirator (preset to deliver a breath at certain intervals; over a period of time, these intervals are gradually lengthened, according to the patient's tolerance, until the patient is able to breathe on his own)
Synchronized intermittent mandatory ventilation (SIMV), or intermittent demand ventilation (IDV)	Breathes spontaneously	Operates as an assist-type mechanism, allows the patient to breathe spontaneously and at the same time provides mechanical hyperinflation of the lungs at a preset rate; synchronized to deliver a control breath when the patient initiates the next inspiration (this prevents the ventilator from cycling during a patient's spontaneous respiratory cycle); useful in weaning patient from respirator

VENTILATOR ASSISTANCE DURING THE EXPIRATORY PHASE

Many mechanical ventilators have the ability to maintain positive pressure throughout expiration (which prevents alveolar collapse). The alveoli stay open longer, causing an increase in functional residual capacity and a decrease in shunting, resulting in increased alveolar oxygenation.

PEEP (Positive End Expiratory Pressure)

Continuous positive pressure is applied to airway throughout expiration.

PEEP may cause pneumothorax or hypotension.

CPAP (Continuous Positive Airway Pressure)

Positive pressure is applied to the airway throughout the respiratory cycle.

CPAP may be used in patients with spontaneous ventilations.

It may cause pneumothorax or a decrease in cardiac output.

NURSING CARE FOR THE PATIENT RECEIVING MECHANICAL VENTILATION

1. Explain the purpose of mechanical ventilation if time and the patient's condition permit. (Usually done by the physician.)
2. Obtain arterial blood sample for baseline blood gas analysis.
3. Obtain the following equipment for mechanical ventilation.
   • Proper type of ventilator and humidifier as ordered by physician
   • Sterile distilled water for humidifier
4. Prepare for endotracheal intubation, including several sizes of endotracheal tubes, laryngoscope with blades of different sizes, suction equipment with sterile catheters and gloves, and an Ambu bag.
5. Intubate the patient with a cuffed endotracheal tube. (This is usually performed by a physician, anesthetist, respiratory therapist, and, in some institutions, an RN in a critical care unit.) See procedure for Endotracheal Intubation, chapter 14.
   • Tape securely in place.
   • Inflate the cuff.
   • Mark a line on the tube so that it can be properly repositioned if the need arises.

NOTE. Tracheotomy may be performed by a physician under strict aseptic conditions.

6. Set up the ventilator according to the manufacturer's guidelines.
   • This is primarily the function of respiratory therapists, with direction from the physician.
   • Procedure for setting up ventilator should be easily accessible for all staff in critical care areas in case they have to perform this task in an emergency.
   • Ventilator settings are highly individualized.

7. Connect the ventilator to the endotracheal tube (or tracheostomy tube).

8. Make sure the patient is being properly ventilated.
   - Auscultate the lungs frequently.
   - Note quantity and quality of respirations. Rate should be checked even if the patient is on a control mode respirator.
   - Both sides of the chest should be auscultated.

9. Monitor the patient closely for his toleration of the procedure.
   - Patient should be under constant observation.
   - Any adverse changes should be reported to the physician immediately.
   - Observe closely for problems due to mechanical ventilation. (See Table 15-2, Adverse Effects of Mechanical Ventilation, immediately following this section of the chapter.)

10. Monitor arterial blood gases closely, beginning 20 to 30 minutes following institution of mechanical ventilation.

11. Closely observe ventilator and equipment.
    - Settings and gauge readings should be documented by the respiratory therapist on a flow sheet to establish a baseline for comparison by the nursing staff.
    - Humidifiers should be filled with sterile distilled water.
    - Tubing should be clear of excess moisture and free of kinks.
    - Make sure alarms are set.
    - Tubing should fit endotracheal or tracheal tubing securely.

12. Maintain airway patency.
    - Suction endotracheal or tracheal tube as needed, using sterile technique; mouth should also be kept clear of secretions.
    - Always preoxygenate patient with 100% oxygen by using an Ambu bag before suctioning and between repeat suctionings.

    ALERT. Do not suction longer than 10 seconds.

    - Prevent internal kinking of tubes by keeping the airway straight.
    - If endotracheal tube was inserted through the mouth, an airway should be placed in the mouth beside it to prevent biting down and possible occlusion of the tube.

13. Positioning
    - The patient should be turned every 1 to 2 hours, including right and left semiprone positions, depending on patient's condition.
    - Perform passive range of motion exercises.
    - Prevent tension on tubing.
    - Elevate head of bed periodically.

14. Perform chest physiotherapy as specified by the physician.

15. Perform ongoing assessment and monitoring.
    - Monitor vital signs, heart rate, and neurological signs.
    - Monitor closely to detect any adverse changes.
    - Frequency depends on patient status.
    - Temperature may be checked every 4 hours unless it is abnormal.
    - Report adverse changes to the physician. *(Text continues on p. 174)*

TABLE 15-2. **Adverse Effects of Mechanical Ventilation**

Adverse Effects	Probable Cause	Action
Breath sounds heard on one side only	Endotracheal tube in one bronchus (may occur following deflation of cuff)	Reposition endotracheal tube.
Breath sounds not heard at all	Tube in esophagus	Remove tube and reintubate the patient.
Airway obstruction	Tubing kinked	Properly position patient and equipment.
	Respiratory secretions	Suction respiratory secretions. Supply adequate humidification of inspired air to help loosen secretions. Instill sterile saline to loosen secretions if necessary. See endotracheal suctioning in chapter 14.
	Biting down on endotracheal tube	Insert airway in mouth beside tube. Airway obstruction may be relieved by suctioning, changing position, and removing inner cannula of tracheostomy tube if occluded. If airway (endotracheal or outer cannula of tracheostomy tube) is totally obstructed and is not relieved by the above methods, immediately deflate the cuff and support respirations with Ambu bag. Notify physician or respiratory therapist immediately. Prepare for tube removal and insertion of a new one.
Tracheal necrosis (can cause fistulas into the innominate artery and esophagus)	High cuff pressure	Use high-volume, low-pressure cuff. Inflate by using minimal air leak technique. Monitor cuff pressure. (Cuff deflation has not been found to significantly reduce complications such as tracheal necrosis.)

TABLE 15-2. **Adverse Effects of Mechanical Ventilation** (Continued)

Adverse Effects	Probable Cause	Action
Pulmonary infection	Poor technique	Use strict aseptic technique.
	Improperly cleaned equipment	Clean equipment properly. (Tubing should be changed every 24 hr.)
Pneumothorax	Adverse effect of PEEP Complication of insertion of CVP line Rupture of a bleb in the lung	See Pneumothorax in chapter 10.
Hypoventilation or hyperventilation	Arterial blood gases not monitored closely enough to correct imbalances	Monitor arterial blood gases closely and correct imbalances as necessary. Increasing mechanical dead space is sometimes used to treat or prevent hyperventilation. (Increasing the length of hose between the endotracheal tube and exhalation port increases the amount of rebreathed carbon dioxide.)
Atelectasis	Constant tidal volume Inappropriate sighing (either mechanical or hand ventilation with Ambu bag if ventilator does not have a sigh mechanism)	Adjust sigh mechanism. If ventilator does not have a sigh mechanism, hand ventilate with Ambu bag 6 to 8 times an hour.
Gastrointestinal bleeding	Exact cause unknown— possibly stress, ulcer, or steroid therapy	Administer antacids prohylactically. Insert nasogastric tube to decompress the stomach if indicated. Avoid steroids. Administer sedative if needed. Check stool and nasogastric drainage daily for guaiac (blood).
Decreased cardiac output (hypotension, decrease in urinary output, cerebral anoxia)	Decrease in venous return to the heart owing to an increase in intrathoracic pressure (especially with PEEP)	Monitor arterial and venous pressures, urine output, heart rate, and neurological signs to quickly detect significant decrease and effect of cardiac output, and report any adverse effects to physician immediately. (Continued)

TABLE 15-2. **Adverse Effects of Mechanical Ventilation** (Continued)

Adverse Effects	Probable Cause	Action
		Most patients can tolerate this decrease. Effects of inaction (no mechanical ventilation) versus effects of action (mechanical ventilation) have to be considered in those patients who do not tolerate a decrease in cardiac output.
	Large tidal volumes in patient with emphysema	Patients with emphysema need to have tidal volumes adjusted specifically to individual needs.
Water imbalances		
Retention (positive water balance)—weight gain, decrease in serum sodium and hematocrit	Exact cause unknown—possibly humidification, increase in antidiuretic hormone (ADH) production due to decreased cardiac output, or reduced flow in pulmonary vessels	Monitor daily weight. Carefully measure intake and output, serum sodium, and hematocrit. Carefully check chest x-ray film. Administer diuretics if needed.
	NOTE. Humidification not only delivers extra moisture but also prevents the normal loss of 500 ml water/day, which is usually eliminated by expiration.	
Dehydration	Inspired air improperly humidified or overheated	Make sure humidifier is filled with sterile distilled water and is working properly. Closely monitor temperature. (Dial should be kept as close to body temperature as possible.)
Fear Panic Disorientation Paranoid delusions	Fear of being unable to control respiratory function Lack of sleep owing to noise (*e.g.*, respirator, alarms, cardiac monitor) and constant activity that may be going on in the unit	Provide emotional support. Explain what is going on at the level of the patient's understanding. Reassure him that he will not be alone, and do not leave him unattended. Organize nursing care so that rest is promoted.

TABLE 15-2. **Adverse Effects of Mechanical Ventilation** *(Continued)*

Adverse Effects	Probable Cause	Action
	Cerebral hypoxia	Cut down on excessive noise. Dim the lights in the patient's cubicle or room. Provide sedation as ordered. Provide security information—date, day, time. Provide means of communication. Have experienced personnel primarily in charge of his care. Reassure patient that mechanical assistance is a temporary treatment. Encourage patient to help with his care as much as possible to maintain independence, a sense of worth, and a feeling of having some control over the situation. Closely monitor arterial blood gases to prevent or detect hypoxia and institute treatment.
Subcutaneous emphysema (patient is being ventilated by way of a tracheostomy tube)	Too small a tube Improperly inflated cuff	Insert larger tube. Inflate cuff properly.
Oxygen toxicity Early Phase (Exudative phase) Alveolar edema Pulmonary congestion Intra-alveolar hemorrhage Formation of hyaline membrane Late Phase (Proliferative phase) Hyperplasia of alveolar cells Increased alveolar edema Fibrosis	FIO_2 above 50% for more than 24 hr	Prevent oxygen toxicity by keeping FIO_2 below 50% or do not administer high concentrations longer than 24 hours. Treat condition with PEEP, chest physiotherapy, and diuretics.

- Hemodynamic monitoring may be indicated to monitor the effect on cardiac output.
- Monitor intake and output.
  - Check intake and output carefully at least every hour until the patient is stable.
  - Daily weights are indicated.

16. Administer sedatives or muscle relaxants (curare) as ordered.
    - Patient must be monitored continuously following the administration of these types of drugs as they may completely eliminate spontaneous breathing, making the patient totally dependent on the respirator. (These medications are administered to patients who override or "fight" the respirator.)
    - Vital signs and heart rate should also be monitored, paying particular attention to the adverse effects these drugs may have on them.

17. An Ambu bag, sterile suction equipment, and emergency drugs should be kept readily accessible at all times.

18. Maintain adequate nutrition.
    - Intravenous fluids are usually administered to the critically ill patient receiving mechanical ventilation.
    - Nasogastric or gastrostomy feedings may be instituted.
    - If a cuffed tracheostomy tube is in place, oral feedings may be permitted.

19. Use high volume low-pressure cuff to prevent complications such as tracheal necrosis.
    - Inflate cuff, using minimal air leak technique.
      - Attach 10-ml syringe to port of cuff tubing.
      - Place stethoscope over trachea or to one side of it.
      - On inspiration, or cycling the ventilator, inflate cuff until no breath sounds are heard.
      - Slightly deflate the cuff until a small air leak is heard.
      - Check air volume on ventilator. May need to be adjusted to compensate for leak.
    - If no-air-leak technique is required (danger of aspiration), following above procedure, slowly inject air until no-air leak is detected.
    - Check cuff pressure every 2 hours by using either the commercial manometer if available or the sphygmomanometer technique as follows:
      - Deflate cuff.
      - Insert one end of a stopcock into the port of the cuff tubing.
      - Attach a 10-ml syringe to opposite end of stopcock.
      - Attach end of rubber tubing connected to pressure gauge of sphygmomanometer to remaining port of stopcock. Stopcock lever should be turned towards pressure gauge (off position).
      - Inflate cuff.
      - Turn stopcock lever towards syringe.
      - Observe dial on pressure gauge and document pressure reading.
      - Cuff pressure should be less than 25 cm H_2O or 15 mm Hg.

20. Deflate cuff as ordered by physician or according to hospital procedure.
    - Explain procedure to patient.
    - Suction endotracheal or tracheostomy tube if necessary, using sterile technique.
    - Suction mouth, oropharynx, and nose before deflation.

    NOTE. *Never* suction the mouth and nose, and then the trachea.

    - Deflate cuff by withdrawing air with the syringe from cuff inflation tubing.
    - Notify physician if the tube cannot be inflated or deflated.
    - Check breath sounds after deflation and reinflation to check position of the tube because it may slip out of place following deflation.
    - Check for effects that cuff deflation may have on ventilators.
        - Pressure-cycled—may not cycle (ventilate) unless flow rate is increased
        - Volume-cycled—will continue to cycle (It may be necessary to increase volume.)

NOTE. Cuff deflation is a controversial issue; opponents claim that it does not appear to significantly prevent tracheal ischemia or necrosis. Check with physician concerning his particular preferences and, also, the manufacturer's guidelines. Many cuffs do not require deflation.

21. Provide some means of communication for patient since he will be unable to speak.
    - Provide slate board or pen and paper.
    - If he is unable to write, communicate with hand signals or by pointing to pictures of objects on a poster board. (This is easily handmade to include basic equipment, common questions and answers, and feelings, and should be standard equipment in the unit.)
    - If patient is unconscious, continue to talk to him in a calm and confident manner, explaining function of equipment. (He may very well be able to hear you.)
22. Ambulation will be instituted as soon as the patient's condition warrants.
    - Patient may still be receiving mechanical ventilation.
    - Nurse should be in constant attendance.

GENERAL GUIDELINES FOR WEANING FROM THE VENTILATOR

1. Patient should meet criteria for weaning.
2. Weaning should be done during the waking hours.
3. Vital signs and ECG should be monitored before, during (every 5–10 min), and after the process until they remain stable.
4. Arterial blood gases are monitored before, during, and after the process.
5. Proper position for weaning is an upright or sitting position.

6. Weaning is stopped immediately if adverse effects occur (resulting from hypoxia or alveolar hypoventilation).
7. Do not leave patient unattended during weaning.
8. An Ambu bag with oxygen tubing connected should be readily accessible during the procedure.
9. Resuscitative equipment and drugs should be readily accessible.
10. Ventilator connector should be kept sterile during the procedure.

Conditions in which weaning may be contraindicated are summarized in the summary chart below.

CONDITIONS THAT MAY PREVENT WEANING

Malnutrition

Arrhythmias

Pain

Hypovolemia

Hypervolemia

Anemia

Metabolic acidosis

Metabolic alkalosis

Fatigue

Elevated temperature

Decrease in level of consciousness

NOTE. Conditions should be corrected or brought within normal limits prior to weaning.

WEANING FROM MECHANICAL VENTILATION

USE OF IMV

1. Check vital signs, ECG, and arterial blood gases to establish a baseline.
2. Ventilator is adjusted to either the IMV or SIMV.
3. IMV (or SIMV) is gradually reduced over a period of time, as tolerated by the patient.
4. Arterial blood gases, vital signs, and ECG should be monitored closely throughout the process.
5. Generally, mechanical ventilation is discontinued when the IMV is reduced to 2 to 3 breaths/min.

USE OF T-TUBE (T-PIECE)

1. Check vital signs, ECG, and arterial blood gases to establish a baseline.

2. The patient is removed from mechanical ventilation and the T-tube is connected to endotracheal or tracheostomy tube for 5 to 10 minutes an hour as tolerated by the patient. Oxygen and humidity are delivered through the T-piece instead of the ventilator.

3. Vital signs and ECG should be monitored throughout the process.

4. Arterial blood gases may be monitored during the procedure.

5. Following the allotted time, the T-tube is removed and the patient reconnected to the mechanical ventilator.

6. Arterial blood gases are checked following the procedure.

NOTE. Time for T-tube connection is gradually increased as the patient tolerates it and according to physician's orders.

Adverse effects associated with weaning are summarized below.

ADVERSE EFFECTS THAT MAY OCCUR DURING WEANING

Arrhythmias

Dyspnea

Rapid, shallow respirations

Behavior changes (agitation, fear)

Cyanosis

Pulse and blood pressure changes (elevation or decrease)

NOTE. Weaning should be stopped immediately if adverse effects occur.

Renal Nursing

16
Renal Failure

Acute renal failure receives the primary emphasis in this chapter because it is most commonly seen in the critical care unit. Chronic renal failure is discussed briefly.

CHRONIC RENAL FAILURE

Chronic renal failure is an insidious disorder involving progressive renal deterioration which may not become evident for months or years.

Causes

Collagen diseases

Congenital anomalies of the kidney

Acute and chronic glomerulonephritis

Obstruction of the urinary tract and infection

Hypertension

Metabolic disorders

Clinical Manifestations

Anorexia

Nausea

Vomiting

Change in level of consciousness (from lassitude to unconsciousness)

Convulsions

Edema

Hypertension

Anemia

Breath smells like acetone

Pruritus

Discoloration of skin

Uremic frost may be present on face (late change)

Gradual physical deterioration in general

Treatment

There is no cure.

Treat the underlying cause.

Utilize hemodialysis or peritoneal dialysis to rid body of waste products.

The patient may be maintained in this manner until a kidney transplant can be made.

If untreated, or if treatment is ineffective, the condition will progress to uremia, resulting in death.

ACUTE RENAL FAILURE

Causes

Acute glomerulonephritis

Occlusion of renal vessels by thrombus or embolus

Severe dehydration

Circulatory failure

Hemorrhage

Kidney stones

Following vascular surgery in which the aorta or renal arteries are clamped

Toxemia of pregnancy

Hypersensitivity reaction

Acute tubular necrosis which may be caused by the following:
• Transfusion reactions
• Crush injuries
• Major shock
• Major burns
• Septicemia
• Complications of pregnancy including the following:
  • Septic abortion
  • Hemorrhage (concealed)
  • Abruptio placentae
  • Preeclampsia
• Nephrotoxic agents including the following:
  • Antibiotics (*e.g.*, kanamycin, gentamicin, colistin, cephaloridine)
  • Organic solvents (*e.g.*, carbon tetrachloride)
  • Pesticides (*e.g.*, DDT)
  • Heavy metals (*e.g.*, lead, mercury, bismuth, arsenic)
  • Phenacetin
  • Salicylate poisoning
  • Carbon monoxide
• Mushroom poisoning

Clinical Manifestations

Sudden onset

Usually oliguria (less than 400 ml/24 hr)

Total anuria (rare)

Confusion, disorientation

Nausea

Vomiting

Diarrhea

Headache

Irritability

Lethargy

Convulsions

Dehydration (accompanied by dry skin and mucous membranes)

Halitosis (may be suggestive of urine)

Body odor (suggestive of urine)

NOTE. Clinical manifestations increase as retention of the products of metabolism increases.

NOTE. In nonoliguric or high output failure, normal or increased urinary output may occur even though renal function has decreased and nitrogen retention has increased. This condition is seen predominantly with trauma, severe burns, or drug toxicity.

PHASES OF ACUTE RENAL FAILURE

PERIOD OF OLIGURIA

General Information

Oliguria lasts from several days up to 2 weeks or more. (Generally lasts 10–12 da)

Clinical Manifestations

Nausea

Lethargy

Urinary output less than 400 ml/24 hr (may be bloody)

Significant Laboratory Values

Elevated levels of elements that are usually excreted by the kidneys (*e.g.*, potassium, magnesium, creatinine, urea, uric acid)

Complications

Overhydration from sodium and water retention leading to pulmonary edema and cardiac failure

Hyperkalemia

Acidosis

Uremia

Death

PERIOD OF DIURESIS

General Information
Urinary output begins to increase gradually, perhaps to normal levels.

Output depends on degree of fluid overload present from oliguric phase when this stage is entered.

Diuresis usually lasts a week

Complications
Marked sodium wasting due to excessive urinary output

Dehydration

Hypovolemia

NOTE. Remember that actual renal function is not normal at this time.

PERIOD OF RECOVERY (CONVALESCENCE)

General Information
Renal function is gradually restored, although it may never return to prefailure levels; for example, ability to acidify or concentrate urine may be decreased.

It takes several months to a year for restoration of renal function.

Treatment and Nursing Considerations
1. Closely monitor vital signs and ECG.
   - Electrolyte disturbances (specifically hyperkalemia) may result in cardiac arrhythmias and cardiac failure.
   - Severe hypertension may be present. (See electrolyte disturbances, Chap. 31.)
   - Heart and lung sounds should be auscultated frequently to detect the presence of pulmonary edema or heart failure.
   - Notify the physician immediately of significant abnormalities.
   - Keep emergency drugs and equipment readily available.
2. Check neurological signs frequently. Mental changes are common and may be unpredictable.
3. Monitor serum electrolytes frequently and correct imbalances. (See Fluid and Electrolyte Imbalances, Chap. 31.)
4. Monitor fluid level closely.
   - Weigh daily.
   - Closely monitor input and output.
   - CVP monitoring may be indicated.
   - Correct imbalances as indicated.
5. Treat and correct the underlying cause and complications if possible.
   - Shock
   - Burns
   - Transfusion reactions

- Hypertension
- Arrhythmias

6. Start an IV with a large bore needle in a large vein.
   - Administer fluids as ordered.
   - Fluid replacement during oliguric phase is usually limited to 400 ml–500 ml/24 hr, plus measurable fluid loss.

7. Keep strict intake and output records.
   - Record all measurable sources of fluid losses.
   - Watch the patient closely during IV therapy to determine adverse effects (pulmonary edema, heart failure).
   - Measure the urine specific gravity frequently.

8. Administer potent diuretics (*i.e.*, furosemide, ethacrynate sodium, or mannitol) as ordered during the oliguric phase.
   - These drugs may help maintain urinary output.
   - Keep in mind that the fluid and electrolytes must be replaced.

9. Promote proper nutrition.
   - Promote a high calorie diet.
   - Restrict protein intake to prevent elevations in blood urea nitrogen.
   - Administer multivitamin supplements.
   - Restrict foods and fluids that contain large amounts of potassium and phosphorus.
   - Administer total parenteral nutrition if needed.

10. Protect from infection.
    - Resistance to infection is impaired.
    - Avoid indwelling urinary catheter if at all possible.
    - Use strict aseptic technique during insertion and care of IV and CVP.
    - Use strict aseptic technique during wound care.
    - Notify physician immediately if infection is suspected anywhere.

11. Prevent pulmonary complications.
    - Keep the airway patent.
    - Suction secretions if the patient is unable to remove them effectively.
    - Change position at least every 2 hours.
    - Encourage coughing and deep breathing at regular intervals.
    - Incentive spirometry may be indicated.
    - Closely monitor intake and output.

12. Protect integrity of the skin.
    - Change position frequently.
    - Keep off pressure areas as much as possible.
    - Utilize special devices to prevent undue skin pressure (*e.g.*, foam-rubber pads, sheepskin pads, alternating pressure mattress).
    - Alleviate pruritus by applying topical ointments as ordered and bathing with a weakened vinegar and water solution.

13. Administer medications with extreme caution because of reduction of kidney function.
    - Digitalis dosages should be reduced (digitalis levels should be monitored).

- Antacids containing magnesium are contraindicated.
- Antibiotic dosages are frequently reduced.

NOTE. Any drug that is excreted by the kidney or may have adverse effects on the kidney, or that affects electrolyte balance should be used with extreme caution if used at all.

14. Provide protective measures.
    - Electrolyte, water imbalances, and elevated BUN will adversely affect the level of consciousness. The patient may be unconscious or combative.
    - Utilize protective measures. (Keep siderails up if patient is lethargic, stuporous, or unconscious; do not leave on back to prevent aspiration; do not leave unattended if disoriented, confused, or dizzy; a body restraint and padding the sides of the bed may be necessary if the patient becomes combative.)
    - Keep padded tongue blade at the bedside for use if convulsions occur.

15. Promote rest.
    - Bed rest is indicated during acute failure to lower metabolic needs.

16. Support the patient emotionally.
    - This is a very frightening condition.
    - The underlying cause (*e.g.*, trauma) may be just as devastating.
    - Spend time with patient and the family.
    - Allow venting of feelings.

17. Begin dialysis if needed.
    - Peritoneal dialysis
    - Hemodialysis

NOTE. If patient fails to recover from acute renal failure, chronic renal failure may result.

17
Dialysis

DIALYSIS

The procedure for peritoneal dialysis is discussed in depth in this chapter. The procedure for hemodialysis is complex and depends on the particular dialyzer used as well as on institutional practices; therefore, only a general overview in presented here.

HEMODIALYSIS

Purpose

Hemodialysis is used to remove the end products of metabolism and excess water.

Principle

1. Blood flows into dialyzer.
   - On either side of the blood compartment there are dialysate compartments.
   - Separating the two is a semipermeable membrane of cellophane.
2. Small pores in the membrane permit the passage of water, uric acid, creatinine, urea, and other metabolites from the blood into the dialysate solution. They prevent the passage of blood cells, plasma proteins, and bacteria generally because these cells are larger.
3. The dialysate is composed of electrolytes. Electrolyte levels are adjusted according to the individual patient's needs.
4. Following dialysis, the "cleansed" fluid is routed back to the patient. The time required for dialysis depends on the type of dialyzer used (usually 6–10 hr).
5. Results of dialysis are as follows: removal of the end products of metabolism, correction of electrolyte and fluid imbalances, correction of imbalances of the buffer system, and removal of excess water.

Common Means of Access to the Circulation

Arteriovenous fistula—this is a surgical procedure in which an artery (usually the radial) is anastomosed to a vein in a side-to-side manner, creating a fistula. Blood leaking from the higher pressure artery into the vein will distend it, facilitating entry for the repeated venipunctures that are necessary for hemodialysis.

Arteriovenous shunt (external)—this is a surgical procedure in which an artery and a vein, usually in the nondominant arm, are cannulated separately. The cannulas are connected by a Teflon bridge or connector. During dialysis, the bridge is removed and the cannulas are connected appropriately to the dialysis machine.

Femoral artery cannulation—this procedure is used when immediate access is necessary or the other methods (fistula or shunt) are not functioning properly.

Types of Dialyzers

Parallel plate or flow

Coil

Hollow-fiber

Major Components of the System

Dialyzer

Dialysate

Blood pump

Heparin and Protamine infusion pumps

Monitoring devices (air in system, blood leak, system pressure, dialysate temperature, and dialysate concentration)

Complications

Hepatitis

Emboli

Disequilibrium syndrome (neurological symptoms of varying severity—from headache, nausea, and vomiting to confusion, twitching, and convulsions)

Infection (local and systemic)

Hemorrhage

NOTE. Complications depend on method used for circulatory access.

PERITONEAL DIALYSIS (MANUAL METHOD)

General Information

End products of metabolism, excess fluid, and toxic substances are removed by the process of osmosis and diffusion by using the peritoneum as a semipermeable membrane.

The procedure may be performed by either of the following methods:
• Manual method using bottles—dialysate is prepared and is then infused and removed by gravity. The manual method will be discussed.
• Automated peritoneal dialysis method—this method mixes the dialysate and, at timed intervals, automatically infuses and removes the solution (more commonly used for chronic dialysis).

Peritoneal dialysis is contraindicated in the following situations:
• Peritonitis
• Abdominal adhesions
• Abdominal surgery

Equipment

Peritoneal dialysis catheter

Peritoneal dialysis administration set

Trocar set

Sterile dialysate as ordered (prewarmed to body temperature or perhaps slightly higher)

IV pole

Local anesthetic (Lidocaine)

Heparin

Supplemental drugs may be ordered (potassium, antibiotics)

Sterile gown and gloves

Cap and mask

Povidone-iodine solution

Sterile drapes
• 4 large towels
• 1 fenestrated towel

Sterile instruments
• 4 towel clips
• Hemostats
• Curved Kelly
• Needle holder
• Suture scissors
• #15 scalpel blade
• #11 blade handle
• Forceps with teeth
• Sponge forceps
• Suture material (check with physician)
• Syringes (5 ml, 10 ml)
• Needles (25-gauge, 20-gauge 1½ in long)
• Sterile 2 × 2s and 4 × 4s
• Tape
• Prep kit

Preliminary Actions

1. Explain the procedure to the patient. Obtain signed consent form from patient.

2. Instruct the patient to empty his bladder to prevent accidental puncture during the procedure.

3. Place in the supine position.

4. Prep the abdomen (shave from xyphoid process to symphysis pubis).

5. At this point, everyone in the room will don a mask and the physician will put on surgical garb.

6. Set up the equipment. Prime the tubing. Be sure excess water has been dried off the bottle prior to inverting it to prevent contamination of the solution.

7. Perform surgical scrub using povidone-iodine solution. Start at umbilicus and prep in a circular motion to the outside edge.

Procedure

The physician will perform the insertion procedure.

1. The abdomen is draped appropriately and a small incision is made midline (3–5 cm) below the umbilicus.

2. The trocar is inserted into the peritoneum through the incision.

3. Following removal of the obturator, the catheter is inserted, the trocar removed, and the catheter sutured in place.

4. A sterile dressing is applied to the site around the catheter and is taped in place.

5. Connect the primed tubing of the dialysate administration set to the connector of the catheter.

6. Allow the dialysate to flow into the peritoneum (inflow usually lasts 5–10 min).

7. Clamp the tubing following infusion.

8. Leave the dialysate in the peritoneum for 15 minutes to 30 minutes (diffusion phase).

9. Unclamp the tubing to the drainage bottle (outflow tubing) positioned on the floor and permit the solution to drain by gravity. Outflow usually takes about 10 minutes.

NOTE. If the solution bottle is also being used for drainage, simply lower to floor, unclamp, and allow fluid to drain as above.

10. Clamp the outflow tubing when no more drainage is noted.

11. The next exchange is infused as above.

12. The process is continued (usually from 12–36 hr) until the blood chemistry levels are brought to the desired level.

Special Considerations

Prior to beginning, inform the patient that there will be some discomfort during catheter insertion and positioning so that he will not be surprised and startle health team members with sudden movement.

After the trocar is inserted, instruct the patient to lift his head to tighten abdominal muscles. This will facilitate further introduction of the trocar and lessen the chances of trauma to organs.

The dialysate may be allowed to flow through the catheter during positioning to prevent its adherence to the omentum.

If the dialysate does not flow in quickly, catheter repositioning is indicated. Notify the physician immediately.

If the dialysate does not flow out well, turn the patient from side to side and elevate the head of the bed. If these measures are not successful, catheter repositioning is indicated. (Notify physician immediately.)

Monitor the vital signs and ECG closely throughout the procedure.
• Prior to beginning the procedure, check vital signs and ECG to establish baseline.
• Check patient every 15 minutes during the first exchange.
• If patient is stable, check at least every hour.
• Emergency drugs and equipment should be readily available.

Keep an accurate account of intake and output.
• The outflow should equal or exceed the inflow. If it is less, it should only be a slight reduction.
• Notify the physician immediately if there is a significant difference in the exchange volumes.

Protect the insertion site from infection.
• Using aseptic technique (and wearing a mask), clean the site with povidone-iodine solution (going from in to out).
• Be sure to remove any dried blood. (Hydrogen peroxide will accomplish this.)
• Cover with a sterile dressing fitted around catheter, and tape edges in place.
• A sterile plastic drape may be indicated to keep the area dry and free of contamination.

Weight and abdominal girth should be checked prior to and following the procedure.

The color of the outflow should be inspected frequently.
• Normal—straw colored
• Peritonitis—cloudy

Blood chemistries are checked prior to and during the procedure.

Heparin is added to the dialysate to prevent clot formation in the catheter.

Antibiotics may be added to prevent infection.

Xylocaine may be added to lessen abdominal discomfort.

Potassium chloride may be added to the solution if the patient is not hyperkalemic.

Solutions containing large percentages of dextrose may result in hypotension due to the excessive amounts of fluid removed.

See Table 17-1 for specific problems with peritoneal dialysis.

TABLE 17-1. **Specific Problems of Peritoneal Dialysis**

Problems	Actions
Respiratory difficulty	Slow the inflow. Elevate the head of bed. Check tubing for air. Do not introduce air into peritoneum.
Respiratory distress	Stop the inflow. Open the outflow and drain the solution immediately. Notify the physician immediately. Support respiratory function as necessary.
Hypotension	Notify the physician immediately. Frequent vital sign checks should detect this in the early stages so that the problem (*e.g.,* excessive fluid loss) can be corrected before shock ensues.
Hypertension	If measures for increasing fluid return are not successful, notify the physician immediately. (Condition may indicate fluid overload resulting from inadequate return of fluid.) Notify the physician immediately if the increase in blood pressure is significant. If inflow and outflow are equal and there are no other symptoms to suggest other complications, the rise in pressure may be caused by apprehension or discomfort.
Congestive heart failure and arrhythmias	Notify the physician immediately. Treat accordingly. (Condition may indicate fluid overload resulting from inadequate return of fluid.)
Bleeding around insertion site	Notify the physician. If catheter is sutured in place, slight bleeding should be controlled. Perform site care to keep the area free of dried blood, a perfect medium for bacteria. Small amount of bleeding may be noted with first few exchanges. If bleeding is excessive, notify the physician immediately. This is abnormal.
Mild abdominal pain	Elevate the head of the bed 45° to lessen this normal discomfort. Change position frequently. Mild analgesics may be administered as prescribed. Offer food and fluids in small amounts during outflow.
Severe abdominal pain	Severe pain is abnormal and may indicate infection (peritonitis) or paralytic ileus. Notify the physician immediately.

IV

Neurological Nursing

18
Common Neurological Problems

Neurological problems commonly seen in the critical care setting are presented in this chapter—increased intracranial pressure, subdural hematoma, epidural hematoma, subarachnoid hemorrhage, cerebrovascular accident (CVA), and spinal cord injury. Specific nursing considerations are included. For general treatment and nursing considerations for the patient with neurological problems, see chapter 19.

INCREASED INTRACRANIAL PRESSURE

Causes

Trauma

Cerebral edema (resulting from trauma and occurring postoperatively)

Brain tumor

Brain abscess

Hemorrhage

Meningitis

Clinical Manifestations

Headache

Vital sign changes
- Increased respirations (early); change in pattern (late)
- Increased blood pressure (next change to occur)
  - Elevation of systolic pressure
  - Widened pulse pressure
  - Decreased pulse (last change to occur)
    - Rapid and shallow pulse in terminal stage
  - Moderate rise in temperature (terminal stage)

Vomiting (may be projectile and of long duration)

Decline in level of consciousness (restlessness, confusion, agitation progressing to obtunded, stuporous, and finally comatose states)

NOTE. Level of consciousness is the single most important indicator of neurological function.

Pupil changes
• Fixed; unilaterally dilated (initially)
• May progress to fixed and bilaterally dilated.
• Other possible changes are as follows:
  • Slow reactions
  • Unequal pupils
Bulging of operative site following surgery
Bulging of fontanels in infant or small child
Aphasia
Hemiparesis
Hemiplegia
Abnormal posturing (decorticate or decerebrate)

Nursing Considerations

Closely monitor level of consciousness.
• If patient is sleeping, wake him up and check response at specified time intervals to make certain that he is indeed sleeping rather than unconscious.
• Notify physician immediately of any changes.

Try to prevent anything that causes an increase in intracranial pressure.
• Vomiting or retching
• Coughing
• Straining at stool; straining against restraints
• Head in a dependent position
• Excessive movement
• Fluid overload
• Emotional displays (either excessively happy or sad)

Closely monitor pupillary reactions, size, and shape. Notify physician immediately of any change.

Remember that restlessness may represent a deteriorating condition as well as distended bowel and bladder and pain. (See Treatment and Nursing Considerations for the Patient with a Neurological Disorder, chapter 19.)

Elevate the head of the bed slightly unless contraindicated.

If patient is in shock, do not place in Trendelenburg position.

SUBDURAL HEMATOMA

Subdural hematoma is located between the dura mater and the arachnoid.

Causes

Trauma

May occur during a complicated delivery

Clinical Manifestations

May be acute, subacute, or chronic (Latent period can last days, weeks, or months.)

Headache

Unequal pupils (Pupil on side of hematoma may be dilated and nonreactive.)

Weakness or paralysis on opposite side from hematoma

Change in level of consciousness (irritability, confusion, unconsciousness)

Seizures (may be focal)

Nausea and vomiting

Signs of increased intracranial pressure

Positive Babinski reflex

Bloody or yellow tinged (xanthochromic) cerebrospinal fluid

Increase in cerebrospinal fluid pressure

Infants and small children—in addition to exhibiting the other signs of increased intracranial pressure, may also present with any of the following:

Bulging fontanels

Enlargement of head

Retinal hemorrhage

Significant lowering of hematocrit in infants due to blood loss

Nursing Considerations

Subdural hematoma is treated by surgical interventaion.

Remember the time interval involved between the injury and the onset of symptoms.

- Chronic—symptoms may not be evident for several weeks or months following the injury. Patient may not have any memory of trauma due to the length of time involved.
- Subacute—symptoms are usually evident within several days to 2 or 3 weeks.
- Acute—symptoms are evident shortly following trauma. Surgery should be performed without delay.

The intoxicated patient who is unconscious or has received trauma to the head (perhaps by a fall) should be checked for the presence of subdural hematoma. Remember that the clinical manifestations may be obscured by intoxication.

Monitor closely for signs of increased intracranial pressure. Report any changes to physician immediately.

Lumbar puncture is contraindicated.

EPIDURAL HEMATOMA

Epidural hematoma is located between the skull and dura.

Cause

Trauma

Clinical Manifestations

Loss of consciousness immediately following the injury may occur (If consciousness is lost, it may be regained for several hours ["lucid interval"] followed by a progressive deterioration in the patient's condition [both level of consciousness and vital signs] however, the patient may not regain consciousness.)

Unequal pupils (Pupil on side of hematoma may be dilated and nonreactive.)

Paralysis on side opposite hematoma

Nursing Considerations

Epidural hematoma is treated by surgical intervention.

This is the most serious and life threatening of the intracranial hemorrhages because it usually involves arterial bleeding. (Usually, the middle meningeal artery is lacerated following fracture of the temporal bone.)

Progression of this condition is rapid.

A large amount of blood is required for replacement because of arterial bleeding

Monitor closely for signs of increased intracranial pressure. Report any changes to physician immediately.

SUBARACHNOID HEMORRHAGE

Causes

Trauma

Rupture of an aneurysm

Blood dyscrasia

Angiomas

Clinical Manifestations

Sudden onset of headache (explosive quality) followed by mental confusion

Nuchal rigidity (stiff neck; may be extreme—when head is lifted, the trunk also raises due to the rigid neck)

Grossly bloody cerebrospinal fluid

Increase in cerebrospinal fluid pressure

Hemiparesis or hemiplegia

Cranial nerve involvement (visual disturbances, facial pain)

Speech difficulties

Unconsciousness

Dilated pupil on affected side

NOTE. Temporary spasm of the artery may occur following the hemorrhage. Clinical manifestations are transient.

Nursing Considerations

Make sure that patient has strict bed rest to lessen the chance of rebleeding. Avoid anything that may cause increased intracranial pressure.

Elevate the head of the bed slightly.

Closely monitor for signs of increased intracranial pressure. Notify physician immediately of any changes.

Closely monitor vital signs.

• Patient may be severely hypertensive, which caused the aneurysm to rupture.

• Hypotensive agents may be needed to lower the pressure.

Lumbar puncture is indicated to confirm the diagnosis.

Surgical intervention may be indicated to clip the aneurysm, but this is dependent of the patient's condition and stability.

CEREBROVASCULAR ACCIDENT (CVA)

Causes

Embolus

Thrombus

Intracerebral hemorrhage

Hypotension

NOTE. Hemorrhage may be caused by trauma, hypertension, or blood dyscrasia.

NOTE. Embolism may be caused by heart disease or following valve surgery.

NOTE. Hypotension may be caused by acute blood loss, drug therapy, or myocardial infarction.

NOTE. Thrombus is caused by atherosclerosis. It is usually preceded by little strokes or transient ischemic attacks (TIA).

Clinical Manifestations

Headache

Visual disturbances (double vision, loss of vision)

Aphasia

Change in level of consciousness (confusion, drowsiness, comatose)

Dizziness

Loss of memory

Difficulty in swallowing

Paresthesia

Paralysis (partial or complete)

Weakness

Incoordination

Convulsions

Signs of increased intracranial pressure

Bloody cerebrospinal fluid (with hemorrhage)

Hypotension

Hypertension (associated with intracerebral hemorrhage)

Nursing Considerations

Remember the time interval that is involved.
- Hemorrhage—onset is sudden.
- Thrombus—onset is slow and progressive (may take hours or days).
- Embolus—onset is sudden and acute. It is associated with heart disease and is common following valve surgery.

Monitor vital signs and ECG closely.
- Myocardial infarction may be an underlying cause
- A change in vital signs may indicate increasing intracranial hemorrhage.

Do not administer narcotics.

Keep the patient on complete bed rest.

Raise the head of the bed slightly to decrease intracranial pressure.

Monitor closely for signs of increased intracranial pressure. Notify physician immediately.

Monitor pupillary changes. Notify physician of changes immediately.

Administer hypotensive agents if indicated when hypertension is present.

Prepare for surgical intervention if indicated.

SPINAL CORD INJURY

Causes

Trauma

Difficult delivery

Clinical Manifestations

Total sensory loss and motor paralysis below injury level (permanent if complete transection; some return expected if incomplete transection)

Priapism (persistent erection of penis, especially seen in children)

Loss of bowel and bladder control (fecal incontinence and abdominal distention; urinary retention and bladder distention)

Initially, loss of sweating below injury level

Spinal shock (See shock, chap. 21)

Nursing Considerations

Remember the possible effects of the different levels of injury.

- Cervical—quadriplegia; respiratory failure
- Thoracic—paraplegia
- Lumbar—paralysis of lower extremities

Immobilize the patient

- Keep the back straight and flat.
- Keep the head, neck, and spine in normal body alignment.
- Place sandbags on either side of head and neck to prevent turning. If none are available, the nurse or rescuer should place her hands on either side of the head and gently support, preventing any movement, until more definitive methods can be instituted.

Prepare for insertion of Crutchfield tongs (skeletal traction).

Closely monitor vital signs and ECG. Be alert for symptoms of spinal shock. Notify physician immediately of occurence.

Closely monitor neurological signs. Be alert for symptoms of increased intracranial pressure. Notify physician immediately of occurrence.

An indwelling urinary catheter should be inserted and connected to a drainage bag.

A Levin tube should be inserted to treat or prevent abdominal distention.

Oxygen therapy with mechanical ventilation may be indicated.

Start an IV.

Closely monitor intake and output.

Administer Decadron as ordered.

Prepare for surgery if indicated. (See spinal shock chap. 21)

19

General Treatment and Nursing Considerations for the Patient with a Neurological Disorder

The treatment and nursing care of the patient with a neurological problem are discussed in this chapter. Nursing actions and accompanying rationale that are essential in providing quality care are also included.

GENERAL TREATMENT AND NURSING CONSIDERATIONS

1. Closely monitor vital signs and ECG.
   - Note quality and quantity, especially respirations.
   - Watch for widening pulse pressure.
   - Report significant changes to physician immediately; changes may indicate a further increase in pressure.

2. Promote respiratory function.
   - Keep airway open.
   - Suction as necessary.

   NOTE. Nasal suctioning is contraindicated in patient with head injury or postoperative neurosurgical patient.

   - Encourage removal of secretions.
   - Keep the airway straight.
   - Perform chest physiotherapy.
   - Change positions frequently unless contraindicated.
   - Oxygen therapy may be indicated, including entubation and mechanical ventilation in the unconscious patient if respirations are inadequate.
   - Check arterial blood gases to establish a baseline, and then monitor closely throughout the acute and subacute stages.

NOTE. Coughing, suctioning, and other procedures related to respiratory care may increase intracranial pressure.

3. Closely monitor and document neurological status.
   - Assess the following:
     - Level of consciousness (assess frequently) and response to commands. (See insert, Levels of Consciousness.)

LEVELS OF CONSCIOUSNESS

Full consciousness—fully aware of surroundings

Drowsiness—inactive; responds slowly to stimuli

Stupor—responds to painful stimulus only

Coma—response to intense stimuli is reflex

- Spontaneous movement of extremities (purposeful)
- Pupil reaction, size, shape, and movement
- Extremities for strength
- Facial movement (ability to perform the following commands: grimace, show teeth, stick tongue out, open and close eyes, and wrinkle forehead)
- Speech
- Vision
- Breathing pattern
- Posture (position)
- Babinski reflex
- Monitor intracranial pressure
  - Observe waveform and readings closely and document at least every 15 minutes in an unstable patient.

NOTE. Decompensation may occur in 30 minutes or less.

- Notify physician immediately if significant changes (plateaus) or trends occur.
- Observe for presence of the following:
  - Vomiting (retching)
  - Convulsions (describe)
  - Twitching
  - Tremors
  - Restlessness
  - Abnormal posture (See Abnormal Posture chart.)
  - Abnormal muscle tone
    - Flaccid (no muscle tone or response; limp body)
    - Spastic (involuntary muscle spasms or movements)

ABNORMAL POSTURE

- *Decorticate*

  Arms are flexed rigidly on chest; hands are rotated internally; wrists and fingers are flexed; legs are stiffly extended; feet are plantar flexed. If head is turned to left, left arm may relax and the right arm will flex. If the head is turned to the right, the opposite occurs. The legs remain hyperextended in both.

  Significance. Damage is above the brainstem, near the brain cortex or high midbrain.

- *Decerebrate*

  Jaws are clenched; all extremities are rigidly extended; arms are hyperpronated; fingers and wrists are flexed; feet are plantar flexed.

  Significance. Damage is in the upper brainstem.

- Combination of the above postures may occur.

- *Opisthotonic*

  Back is arched forward; head is hyperextended; rigidity of arms and legs in an extended or straight position.

  Significance. There is meningeal irritation.

---

4. Mechanically hyperventilate the patient if necessary to decrease high intracranial pressure.
   - Begin hyperventilation at once if an increase is noted.
   - Use an Ambu bag or volume-controlled ventilator.
   - Notify the physician immediately.
   - Keep in mind that this is a temporary measure.

NOTE. CO_2 is a potent cerebral vasodilator. Hyperventilating the patient reduces the level of CO_2, resulting in cerebral vasoconstriction and a decrease in edema and pressure.

This is sometimes done in an emergency when reducing the pressure is critical to prevent further cerebral damage from the increased pressure and herniation of the brain through the foramen magnum. The patient may survive until more definitive therapy may be instituted.

5. Administer medications as prescribed.
   - Osmitrol (Mannitol)
     - Osmitrol is an osmotic diuretic.
     - This drug lowers intracranial pressure (ICP) by dehydrating the brain.
     - Indwelling urinary catheter should be inserted to remove extra urine volume.
   - Dexamethasone (Decadron)
     - Dexamethasone is a steroid (anti-inflammatory).

- This drug reduces cerebral edema.
- Decadron does not act as fast as Mannitol and therefore is not the drug of choice for extreme emergencies.
- Furosemide (Lasix)
  - Furosemide is a diuretic.
  - This drug reduces cerebral edema.
  - Lasix is thought by some sources to be as beneficial in action as Mannitol.
- Paraldehyde
  - Paraldehyde is a hypnotic.
  - This drug is used to sedate the severely combative patient.

ALERT. Do not administer sedatives or analgesics because they may mask the underlying condition as well as cloud the observation of level of consciousness.

- Phenytoin (Dilantin)
  - Phenytoin is an anticonvulsant.
  - This drug is used to stop seizures.
- Antibiotics

6. Elevate the head of the bed slightly (30°–45°), unless contraindicated.
   - Elevation promotes cerebral venous return to the heart.

ALERT. Elevation is contraindicated in spinal shock and spinal injuries.

7. Protect the patient from harm.

NOTE. The underlying condition may cause the patient to be aggressive, combative, highly suspicious, or agitated concerning any activities going on around him.

- Keep the environment calm.
- Approach the patient cautiously. Avoid sudden movements or actions that he may perceive as a threat.
- Talk to him in a firm and clear but nonthreatening manner.
- Give him time to respond. Remember, his senses and understanding may be somewhat dull and slow.
- Pad the bed rails to prevent injury if the patient is restless.
- Avoid restraints if at all possible, including both commercially-made restraints and physical restraint (literally restraining patient by holding).
  - Restraints tend to increase restlessness and agitation, and consequently cause an increase in intracranial pressure.
  - If a patient must be restrained, a chest restraint is indicated because it allows movement of the extremities.
- Paraldehyde may be administered if patient is severely combative or in danger of inflicting physical harm on himself.

NOTE. Restlessness may indicate situations other than deterioration of the condition. It may be caused by a distended bowel or bladder, pain, restraints, bandages (including casts) that are too tight, cerebral hypoxia, or some degree of obstruction of the airway. These other causes should be investigated and corrected immediately. Most causes can be prevented or quickly detected and and corrected before extreme restlessness occurs by close nursing observations and actions.

8. Monitor intake and output closely.
   - Restrict intake in the presence of increased intracranial pressure as ordered by physician.
   - Monitor IV infusions carefully to prevent overhydration.
   - Weigh the patient daily.
   - Insert an indwelling urinary catheter if the patient is unconscious, has a spinal cord injury, is receiving diuretic therapy, or is excreting large amounts of urine (diabetes insipidus).
   - Do specific gravity checks as indicated. (Sodium content in urine may be ordered.)
   - Closely monitor and document bowel function.
     - Administer suppositories, mild laxatives, or stool softeners as needed to promote bowel function.
     - Instruct patient not to strain at stool because straining increases intracranial pressure.
9. Promote proper nutrition, and fluid and electrolyte balance.

   NOTE. Unconscious or semiconscious patient should receive nothing by mouth due to danger of aspiration.

   - Provide nasogastric feedings if the patient is unable to swallow.
   - Administer intravenous fluids in the unconscious patient.
   - Monitor serum electrolytes closely.
     - Diuretic therapy lowers potassium level.
     - Diabetes insipidus causes an elevated serum sodium.
   - Replace fluid in the treatment of diabetes insipidus to prevent extreme dehydration.
10. Treat patient who is in shock.
    - If shock is present due to other injuries, manage accordingly. (See Shock, Chap. 21.)

    ALERT. Do not place the patient with a neurological disorder in Trendelenburg position.

11. Check for an elevated and rising temperature. (Hypothermia may be indicated to lower temperature.)
    - Use hypothermia blanket to lower temperature.
    - Sponging is also used to reduce temperature.

12. Position patient properly.
    * Change the patient's position as ordered or at least every 2 hours. Range of motion exercises should also be carried out.
      * Change patient's position to prevent skin breakdown and respiratory problems due to pooling of secretions and poor oxygenation.
      * Keep patient in cervical traction flat unless he can be placed on a CircOlectric bed or Stryker frame which allows him to be turned in one motion with support.
      * Keep patient with head injuries off the injured area.
      * Keep postoperative patient off the operative site.
      * Keep unconscious or comatose patient in the side-lying or semiprone position to lessen the danger of aspiration and to facilitate drainage of the mouth and nose. Never leave flat on his back.
      * Keep the patient with opisthotonic posturing turned at the hips to a side-lying position, with the knees flexed; pillows should support the head, the arms, and the legs. Patient should not be left flat on his back (will increase abnormal muscle tone).

13. Provide eye care.
    * Protect the eyes from corneal irritation.
    * Blinking reflex may be absent or impaired, hence the eyes must be protected.
    * Irrigate eyes with sterile normal saline or prescribed solution. Instill methylcellulose eye drops or sterile mineral oil and cover with sterile eye pads, securing in place with nonallergic or eye tape (tape from inner to outer area). Repeat at least every 4 hours or as ordered.
    * Sometimes suturing of the eyelids in a closed position is performed as a temporary measure.

14. Check nose, ears, and head dressing covering surgical wounds for evidence of leakage of spinal fluid.
    * Check for ear or nose drainage in patient with head injury.
      * For otorrhea—place sterile cotton ball or pad loosely over ear (do not push into ear) and tape in place.
      * For rhinorrhea—place sterile cotton pad under nose and tape in place. Nasal secretions may be tested for glucose. Normal secretions do not contain glucose but cerebrospinal fluid does.

    NOTE. Drainage from the ear or nose may indicate a basilar skull fracture.

    * Check for drainage from surgical wound.
      * Head should be placed on sterile towel to prevent introduction of bacteria into brain.
      * Cerebrospinal fluid will cause a halo effect on dressing or towel—a bloody area surrounded by a light pink area (the cerebrospinal fluid).
      * Mark the boundaries of drainage to keep up with the amount.
    * Physician should be notified immediately.

15. Monitor ventriculostomy tubes for patency and proper drainage of fluid.
    - Tube is inserted by physician to remove cerebrospinal fluid and decrease intracranial pressure. Also inserted in patients with surgery of the posterior fossa.
    - Cerebrospinal fluid should pulsate in tubing if patent.
    - Tubing is connected to a sterile external drainage bag.

16. Attempt to remove dentures and place a padded tongue blade or bite block between the teeth to prevent biting of the tongue if patient is having a seizure.
    - Do not force anything into mouth if jaws are clenched too tightly.
    - Turn patient to side if possible to prevent aspiration of secretions or vomitus.
    - Suction as indicated.
    - Do not restrain. Protect from hitting bed rails or falling.
    - Notify the physician immediately.
    - Be sure to note and record your observations concerning description, length, presence of aura, and recurrence (may indicate status epilepticus).

17. Start rehabilitation as soon as possible.
    - Position properly.
      - Keep hands in functional positon.
      - Use foot board on bed.
    - Put extremities through range of motion.
    - Change position frequently to prevent pressure sores.
    - Do not overlook mental rehabilitation.
      - Stimulate mental activity as tolerated by patient.

20
Special Procedures

Procedures commonly used in the critical care unit for patients with neurological problems are presented in this chapter. Nursing responsibilities are discussed in detail. Lumbar puncture, hypothermia, and intracranial pressure monitoring are also described.

LUMBAR PUNCTURE

Description
A lumbar puncture involves the insertion of a needle into the lumbar subarachnoid space. Strict aseptic technique is required.

Purposes
To check cerebrospinal fluid pressure

To obtain specimen for laboratory examination of cerebrospinal fluid

To reduce cerebrospinal pressure by removing cerebrospinal fluid

To check for presence of blood or pus

To administer anesthetics

To inject radiopaque substances for x-ray studies

Contraindications
Papilledema (indicates a great increase in intracranial pressure)

Intracranial tumor

Subdural hematoma

Infected area at puncture site

Normal Value
- Normal initial cerebrospinal pressure reading is 80 to 180 mm of H_2O or 6 to 13 mm Hg.

Equipment
Sterile lumbar puncture tray

Povidone-iodine swabs

Sterile gloves

Local anesthetic

Band-aid

Preliminary Actions

1. Explain procedure to patient. A signed consent form should be obtained.
2. Position as specified
   - Lying on side—head and neck are flexed with head supported by pillow.
     - Knees are flexed up on abdomen and drawn up toward chin as much as possible. Patient should clasp his knees to provide support.
     - Nurse should support the position by placing her hands on the neck and behind the knees.
   - Sitting—patient straddles a straight-backed chair.
     - He folds his arms on the back of the chair and rests his head on his arms.
     - Nurse should support the position by standing beside the patient and placing her hands on the head or back of the neck to remind the patient to remain still.
3. The vital signs and ECG should be checked prior to the procedure to establish a baseline.
4. Set up equipment, using sterile technique.

Procedure

1. The physician performs the procedure. He inserts the spinal needle between the L3–L4 or L4–L5 interspace.
2. Monitor the pulse and respirations for quality and quantity throughout the procedure. Be alert for signs of increased intracranial pressure and notify physician immediately of their occurrence.
3. Instruct the patient to relax and slowly straighten his legs following introduction of the needle and prior to checking cerebrospinal pressure. Also, encourage him to breathe normally.
4. Properly label test tubes #1, #2, or #3 as physician hands them to you.
   - Be sure requisitions are properly filled out.
   - Protect test tubes from breaking.
5. Assist in performing Queckenstedt test.
   - Nurse compresses jugular vein(s) as directed by physician for 10 seconds; or
   - Places a blood pressure cuff around the patient's neck and inflates it to 20 mm Hg.
   - The physician takes readings of the cerebrospinal pressure at 10 second intervals.
   - Normally, there is a rapid rise of pressure during compression, and a rapid return to normal after release.
   - A slow rise and fall is abnormal and indicates a spinal subarachnoid block.

6. Place a Band-aid over the needle site following the procedure. Check frequently for signs of bleeding or drainage.
7. Instruct the patient to lie flat for 6 to 12 hours.
   • Patient may lie on side, back, or stomach as long as he remains flat.
   • This position helps to prevent or lessen the severe headache that may occur following the procedure.
   • Encourage fluid intake.

NOTE. For cisternal puncture, place patient in the same position as for lumbar puncture. Instruct him to flex his chin onto the chest.

HYPOTHERMIA

Description

In the procedure described, hypothermia (a state of lowered temperature) is induced by means of a cooling blanket. Close monitoring of the patient is essential.

Purposes

To reduce high temperatures

To reduce metabolic demand

NOTE. Each degree of temperature elevation (centigrade) results in increasing metabolism of approximately 7%.

Phases

Cooling

Hypothermia (usually around 32° C, 89.6°F)

Rewarming

Effects of Hypothermia

Vital Signs

Initially, vital signs increase.

All vital signs will decrease in 15 to 20 minutes.

Cardiac

Ventricular irritability occurs with rapid hypothermia.

PVC's result in ventricular tachycardia or fibrillation if temperature goes below 28°C (82.4°F).

All ECG intervals are prolonged.

Sensorium

Sensorium fades at 33°C to 34°C (91.4°F to 93°F). This includes hearing.

Artificial tears should be instilled. The eye is then covered with an eyepad which is secured with tape.

Drug Absorption

Drug absorption is altered significantly.

Medications should be given IV.

Deep IM injection may be given if absolutely necessary.

Ability of the liver to detoxify certain drugs is altered. Watch for cumulative effects.

Urinary Output

Urinary output is decreased.

Specify gravity may decrease.

Blood

Hemoconcentration may develop due to fluid shift.

Acid-base Balance

Acidosis may develop. (Ventilations decrease faster than production of CO_2.)

Complications and Preventive Nursing Actions

Downward drift—after discontinuing hypothermia (*i.e.*, machine turned off) temperature continues to drop (usually 1° but may be more).

Action
• Turn off machine before reaching desired temperature.

NOTE. The obese patient experiences a greater degree of drift.

Skin breakdown or frostbite
Action
• Protect hands, feet, and face by preventing direct contact with the blanket.
• Change position frequently (at least every 2 hr) to avoid pressure areas.
• Protect the skin by applying a light application of lotion followed by talcum powder that is applied sparingly.

Arrhythmias
Action
• Lower the temperature slowly (not more than 1 degree in 15 min).
• Do not lower the temperature below 28°C (82.4°F).

Thrombus or embolus formation
Action
• Turn patient at least every 2 hours.
• Perform passive range of motion exercises frequently.

Shivering (begins in masseter muscles)
Action
• Slow the temperature decline rate.
• Administer medications as ordered.

Rewarming

Natural rewarming is the recommended method.

Artificial rewarming may result in muscles and skin warming before the heart. The heart is unable to meet the metabolic demands in warmer areas.

Shock may occur from rapid rewarming.

Cumulative effects of drugs administered during the procedure may occur during this stage.

Comments

Monitor vital signs every 15 minutes until desired hypothermia is reached and then at least every 30 minutes during the procedure.

Temperature is usually monitored with rectal probe.
- Rectal probe should be taped in place to prevent inadvertent removal.
- Rectal probe should not be inserted in feces.
- The patient's temperature should be periodically checked throughout the procedure with a glass rectal thermometer to check accuracy of rectal probe.

Be sure hypothermia machine has been properly set to turn off automatically when the desired temperature range is reached.

Monitor ECG constantly.

INTRACRANIAL PRESSURE MONITORING

Description

Intracranial pressure monitoring is a means of measuring intracranial pressure continuously with a greater degree of accuracy.

Types of Intracranial Pressure Monitoring Systems

Intraventricular—ventricular catheter is attached, using a stopcock and pressure tubing, to a pressure transducer and connected to the monitor. The system is primed with sterile normal saline or Ringer's lactate solution.

Subarachnoid (subdural)—the screw is attached to the transducer using pressure tubing and connected to the monitor. The system is primed with sterile normal saline or Ringer's lactate solution.

Epidural—monitoring system will depend on the type of epidural device used.

The characteristics of these systems are described in the Characteristics of Intracranial Pressure Monitoring Systems chart.

Normal Value

4 mm to 15 mm Hg or 50 mm to 200 mm H_2O

CHARACTERISTICS OF INTRACRANIAL PRESSURE MONITORING SYSTEMS

Intraventricular Method

LOCATION
- Ventricular catheter is inserted through a burr hole into the anterior (usually) or occipital horn of the lateral ventricle (nondominant side).

ADVANTAGES
- Large amounts of CSF can be drained and sampled.
- CSF pressure is measured directly.
- Contrast medium can be instilled into the ventricles for diagnostic tests.
- Intracranial compliance can be tested.
- Intraventricular method is the most accurate type.

DISADVANTAGES
- The dura is entered, increasing the chance of infection.
- There is difficulty in inserting the catheter in certain conditions (cerebral edema, collapse of ventricle, midline shift).
- Loss of CSF may be excessive. If there is a sudden drop in intracranial pressure, the brain may herniate.
- The catheter may be blocked with blood clots or brain tissue.

Subarachnoid (subdural) Method

LOCATION
- A hollow screw is inserted through a hole made by a twist drill into the subarachnoid space.

ADVANTAGES
- Subarachnoid method is easier to insert.
- CSF can be drained or sampled.
- Brain matter is not entered.
- CSF pressure is measured directly.
- Subarachnoid method is an accurate monitoring method.

DISADVANTAGES
- The dura is entered, increasing the chance of infection.
- The subarachnoid method causes a loss of CSF.
- Contrast media cannot be instilled for diagnostic tests.
- Catheter may be blocked with blood clots or brain tissue.
- Testing for intracranial compliance is not reliable.
- Large amounts of CSF cannot be drained.

Epidural Method

LOCATION
- An intracranial transducer (fiberoptic transducer or intracranial balloon connected to an extracranial transducer) is inserted through a burr hole between the skull and the dura.

(Continued)

ADVANTAGES
- The dura is not entered, decreasing the chance of infection.
- Complications of central nervous system damage and hemorrhage are minimal.
- The system will not become occluded with blood clots or brain tissue.

DISADVANTAGES
- CSF cannot be drained or sampled.
- The intracranial transducer cannot be recalibrated.
- Intracranial compliance cannot be tested.
- Reflection of CSF pressure is questionable.

INTRACRANIAL PRESSURE WAVES (Fig. 20-1)

"A" WAVE

"A" waves are generally called "plateau waves."

Pressure is elevated to 50 mm-100 mm Hg, lasting 5 to 20 minutes, and then drops sharply.

"A" waves occur when the mean intracranial pressure is 20 mm Hg.

"A" waves are a significant abnormality, indicating decompensation.

"B" WAVE

"B" waves have a sharp, rhythmic saw-tooth appearance.

The pressure is elevated up to 50 mm Hg.

They occur every 30 seconds to 2 minutes.

Change is related to respirations.

The significance of "B" waves is unclear.

They may precede "A" waves.

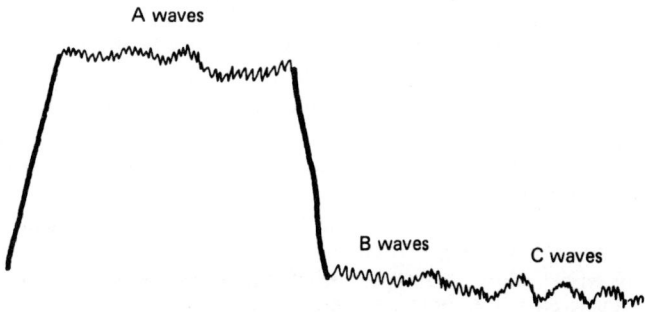

FIG. 20-1. *Intracranial pressure waves.*

"C" WAVE

"C" waves are smaller, rapid and more rhythmic waves.

The pressure is elevated up to 20 mm Hg.

They occur every 4 minutes to 8 minutes.

"C" waves correspond to arterial blood pressure changes.

They are not clinically significant.

Equipment

Sterile tray for ventriculostomy

Monitoring device (catheter, subarachnoid screw, or epidural)

Sterile twist drill

Scalpel

Sutures

Local anesthetic (syringe and needle)

Povidone-iodine solution

Sterile dressing (occlusive) 2 x 2s, 4 x 4s, Kerlex

Sterile gloves

Monitor

Transducer

Sterile normal saline solution (without preservatives)

High-pressure tubing

3-way stopcocks (3)

IV pole

IV tubing

Skin prep tray or razor

Syringes for system (20 ml and tuberculin)

Preliminary Actions

1. Explain procedure to patient. Obtain signed consent form.
2. Set up equipment as follows.
   - Set up flush or irrigation solution on IV pole.
   - Remove 20 ml and 1 ml in appropriate syringes from this system.
     - Flush or irrigation solution may be removed directly from bag.
     - IV tubing and 3-way stopcock may be attached; fluid is removed by stopcock.
   - Do not connect flush line to monitoring system of ventricular catheter or subarachnoid screw.
     - Danger of accidentally infusing large amounts of the flush solution into the subarachnoid space or ventricle is great.
   - Using strict aseptic technique, prime the monitoring system using the 20 ml syringe.

- Balance and calibrate the monitor according to manufacturer's instructions.
- Be sure all air bubbles are removed from the system.
- The transducer should be level with the point of reference as specified by the physician (usually level of the lateral ventricles).

3. Position the patient properly.
   - Elevate head slightly (30°–45°).
   - The patient's head should be held firmly during the procedure.

Procedure

1. The physician will prepare the area and perform the procedure, using strict sterile technique.
2. Assist physician as necessary.
   - Following insertion of device, the skin will be sutured and a sterile occlusive dressing applied.
   - Observe the waveform. The physician may want the line flushed (damped waveform).
   - To flush the line, attach the prefilled tuberculin syringe to the 3-way stopcock connected directly to the monitoring device. Turn the stopcock to the syringe and monitoring device.
   - Monitor waveform.
   - Slowly inject the amount ordered by the physician (usually 0.25 ml)

   ALERT. Do not aspirate prior to flush. (Brain tissue might be aspirated into line.)

   - Monitor waveform again following the flush.
   - Turn the stopcock back to the transducer and the monitoring device.
3. Perform the following if the physician orders CSF to be drained.
   - Drain a 500 ml sterile solution bag of normal saline, maintaining sterility.
   - Attach macrodrip tubing. Clamp should be closed.
   - Attach drainage system to 3-way stopcock attached to monitoring device. Open clamp. Turn stopcock to monitoring device and drainage bag.
   - Keep drainage bag at level of ventricles.
   - Drain amount ordered by physician.
   - Monitor patient closely for signs of adverse effects. Herniation of the brain can result if an excessive amount of CSF is removed.
   - When the desired amount is removed, turn the stopcock back to the transducer and the monitoring device.
   - Disconnect the drainage system.
   - Attach a sterile cap to the middle port of the stopcock.
4. Test compliance by doing the following.
   - Introduce a small amount of sterile fluid (ordered by the physician) into the ventricular monitoring system.
   - Note the resulting pressure.
     - Normal intracranial pressure—the fluid instillation results in a slight increase in pressure and amplitude (less than 2 mm Hg)

- Significantly increased intracranial pressure—the fluid instillation results in a greatly increased pressure and amplitude
5. Monitor cerebral perfusion pressure (CPP) as follows.
  - Subtract diastolic blood pressure from systolic pressure (readings from an arterial line are recommended).
  - Take ⅓ of the difference obtained from the first step.
  - Add result to diastolic pressure to get the mean arterial pressure.
  - Subtract intracranial pressure from mean arterial pressure to get CPP.
  - Increased intracranial pressure causes a decrease in CPP. Cerebral hypoxia is the result of a significant decrease in CPP (40 mm Hg or below).
  - Normal CPP is at least 50 mm Hg, up to 90 mm Hg.

Special Considerations

Avoid taking pressure readings during any activity that may increase intracranial pressure temporarily (*e.g.*, coughing, sneezing, moving, laughing, straining, diaphragmatic breathing, turning of head to the side) and give a false high reading.

Take pressure readings as ordered, at least every hour if stable. This depends entirely on the patient's status.

Keep the head of the bed elevated slightly and the transducer at the proper level. These two points should remain constant for all readings.

Recalibrate and balance the monitor according to manufacturer's instructions.

Check system frequently to make sure all connections are secure.

Keep extra pressure tubing and stopcocks at the bedside.
- If system becomes disconnected, cover line from patient with a sterile dressing.
- Prime new pressure tubing and stopcocks as before and attach to system immediately.
- Notify physician.

NOTE. The disconnected line is contaminated and should not be reconnected to the line.

Notify the physician immediately concerning any significant changes in the pressure or waveform.

V

Care of the Patient in Shock

21

Commonly Occurring Forms of Shock

A general overview of the "shock state" and detailed descriptions of the different forms of shock—cardiogenic, hypovolemic, spinal cord, septic, and anaphylactic—are presented in this chapter.

Shock is a general term used to describe those situations in which the circulation or perfusion is inadequate to meet the metabolic demands of the tissues.

Types of Shock

Cardiogenic shock occurs when the pumping ability of the heart fails to produce an adequate cardiac output to maintain proper tissue perfusion. This type of shock may be caused by arrhythmias, acute myocardial infarction, or acute left ventricular failure.

Hypovolemic shock occurs when a significant amount of circulating blood volume is lost (*e.g.*, loss of whole blood, plasma, or extracellular fluid), resulting in a level that is unable to meet metabolic demands. This type of shock may be caused by internal or external hemorrhage (hemorrhagic shock), severe burns (burn shock), excessive loss of fluid from the gastrointestinal tract (from vomiting or diarrhea), and crushing injuries.

Shock occurring from massive vasodilatation in the vascular bed resulting in poor vascular tone may be classified as neurogenic shock when the underlying cause involves nervous control of the vessels, and vasogenic shock when the underlying cause involves vasoactive or humoral substances (*e.g.*, histamine). Neurogenic shock may be caused by spinal cord transection (spinal cord shock), drugs (*e.g.*, anesthesia), head injury, and fainting. Vasogenic shock may be caused by septicemia due to gram-negative and gram-positive organisms (septic shock) and hypersensitivity reactions (anaphylactic shock).

Diagnostic Tests

Electrocardiogram

Laboratory tests—hemoglobin, hematocrit, complete blood cell count, electrolytes, arterial blood gases

X-ray films of chest and abdomen

Cultures of blood or other possible source of infection (*e.g.*, urine, sputum)

Clinical Manifestations

The clinical manifestations depend on the underlying cause. General effects are as follows:

Blood pressure
- In early shock, the blood pressure may remain normal.
- It will eventually fall, and may even be unobtainable except by palpation (a grave sign).
- A narrowed pulse pressure is significant.
- If blood pressure is normal but shock is suspected, check patient for orthostatic hypotension. Vital signs in the sitting position will show an increased pulse and a decreased blood pressure in shock.
- Blood pressure change depends on patient's normal blood pressure. If the patient is normally hypertensive, an unexpected drop of 30 mm Hg below the patient's usual pressure is significant.

Pulse
- Pulse initially increases.
- It will become weak and thready as shock progresses.
- Bradycardia is more common in neurogenic shock due to head or cord injury.

Level of consciousness
- Early changes are apprehension and restlessness.
- As shock ensues and cerebral anoxia increases, the patient may become extremely restless or agitated, progressing eventually to a stuporous state. Coma is an ominous sign and usually appears very late.

NOTE. The elderly patient will show these changes much earlier than the young.

Respirations
- Initially, hyperventilation occurs and progresses to the gasping respirations of air hunger.
- Breathing may be diaphragmatic in spinal shock.

Urine output
- Output below 30 ml/hr is significant.
- Anuria is an ominous sign.

Skin
- The skin is pale, cool, and clammy.
- Cyanosis may occur later or if the condition is severe.

NOTE. In early septic shock, the skin may be pink, warm, and dry.

Mucous membranes
- Mucous membranes become pale and dry.
- Patient complains of thirst.

Nail beds
- Capillary filling is slow in shock.

Body temperature
- Body temperature is lowered.

Pressures
- Central venous pressure is high in heart failure or cardiac tamponade and lower in hypovolemia.
- Pulmonary artery wedge pressure is high in acute left ventricular failure or acute MI and low in hypovolemia.

CARDIOGENIC SHOCK

Clinical Manifestations

Acute onset (usually)

Changes in level of consciousness (initially, apprehension, staring, anxiety, confusion; progresses to unconsciousness if untreated)

Narrowing pulse pressure (a significant sign)

Oliguria or anuria

Pale, cool, clammy skin

Weak, rapid pulse

Cyanosis

Hypotension (systolic pressure less than 80 mm Hg or 30 mm Hg below normal reading)

Treatment and Nursing Actions

1. Monitor vital signs and ECG continuously.
   - Auscultate heart and lung sounds.
     - Rales and gallop rhythm indicate acute left ventricular failure.
   - Check apical-radial pulse.
   - Check for life-threatening arrhythmias which may occur at any time.
   - Report abnormalities immediately. This type of shock can progress extremely rapidly.
   - Keep emergency drugs and crash cart with defibrillator readily available.
   - Check level of consciousness frequently.
2. Support respiratory function.
   - Keep airway patent.
   - Suction as indicated.
   - Administer oxygen therapy.
   - In advanced shock, entubation and mechanical ventilation may be indicated.
   - Monitor arterial blood gases closely.
3. Support cardiac function.
4. Start an IV of 5% dextrose in water if not already in place with a large bore needle.

- A peripheral and central line may be indicated.
- Select a large vessel to facilitate administration of emergency drugs.
- Avoid intravenous saline solutions.
5. Monitor intake and output closely.
   - Watch for symptoms of fluid overload.
   - Insert an indwelling catheter into the bladder and monitor output continuously.
6. Perform hemodynamic monitoring.
   - Prepare for and assist physician with insertion of central venous pressure line, arterial line, and Swan–Ganz catheter.
   - Obtain readings initially to establish baseline and frequently thereafter to assess degree of shock or success of therapy.

NOTE. In cardiogenic shock, central venous pressure is usually elevated, pulmonary artery pressure is significantly elevated, and pulmonary artery wedge pressure is significantly elevated.

7. Administer medications as ordered.
   - Inotropic drugs are given to support the failing myocardium (*e.g.*, digitalis, Levophed, Isuprel, dopamine, glucagon).
   - Sodium bicarbonate is administered to correct acidosis.
   - Vasodilators may be administered to improve cardiac output by decreasing peripheral vasoconstriction of shock. They should only be used if the systolic pressure is above 100 mm Hg (*e.g.*, Nipride, regitine).
   - Vasopressors may be administerd to raise the blood pressure (*e.g.*, Aramine).
   - Arrhythmias are treated as indicated.
   - Pain medication (morphine) may be administered to relieve chest pain resulting from myocardial ischemia. Pain medication should be given in small doses and with caution.
   - Dopamine may be administered simultaneously with Nipride.
     - Dopamine increases myocardial end-diastolic fiber length (length of myocardium at end of filling period—diastole or preload), which results in improving the contractability of the myocardium.
     - Nipride decreases the resistance to ventricular ejection (afterload), which results in an increase in cardiac output.
   - Administer diuretics as ordered (*e.g.*, Lasix, Mannitol)
   - Steroids may be administered (*e.g.*, Solu-medrol, Decadron)

NOTE. Medications should be administered intravenously.

8. Perform a fluid challenge for the patient in cardiogenic shock that is thought to be the result of hypovolemia. (The CVP and pulmonary artery pressures are not elevated.)
   - Take initial CVP and pulmonary artery pressure readings.
   - Rapidly infuse 200 ml of fluid, usually 5% dextrose in water over a ten-minute period.

- Response should be an increase in pressure readings, urine output, and blood pressure if the patient is hypovolemic.
- Replace volume as ordered. Whole blood, blood products, or blood expanders may be necessary to correct the imbalance.
- If the pressure readings increase, but blood pressure and urine output do not, heart failure is most likely the underlying cause. Excessive fluid volume in this situation would increase heart failure and result in pulmonary edema.

NOTE. Cardiogenic shock occurring secondary to hypovolemia has a better prognosis than that occuring as a result of heart failure.

9. Keep the patient in the supine position.
   - Change position hourly if the situation permits.
   - Trendelenburg position is contraindicated in this situation.
   - The head may be elevated slightly.
10. Promote complete bed rest.
11. Closely monitor the patient's response.
    - The patient may sense an impending catastrophe.
    - Explain procedures to patient in an easy to understand manner.
    - Encourage an air of calm and assurance among all staff members no matter how serious the situation. If the patient senses your uneasiness, resulting fear on his part may cause progression of shock.
    - Do not leave the patient unattended.
12. Counterpulsation may be employed, either external (MAST suit) or internal (intra-aortic balloon pump).
    - Blood flow to coronary arteries is increased.
    - Ventricular work load is decreased.
13. Prepare for emergency surgery as indicated.

HYPOVOLEMIC SHOCK

NOTE. Suspect hypovolemic shock with acute blood loss, burns, protracted vomiting, or diarrhea.

Clinical Manifestations

Apprehension

Hypotension

Thirst (significant)

Oliguria, anuria

Pale, cold, clammy skin

Cyanosis (late)

Weak, rapid pulse

Rapid respirations

Impairment of sensory perception (advanced shock)

Treatment and Nursing Actions

1. Monitor vital signs and ECG continuously.
   * Check neurological signs frequently.
   * Auscultate heart and lung sounds.
   * Report any abnormalities to physician immediately.

2. Support respiratory function.
   * Keep airway patent.
   * Suction as indicated.
   * Administer oxygen therapy.
   * Entubation and mechanical ventilation may be indicated.
   * Monitor arterial blood gases closely.

3. Support cardiac function.

4. Stop obvious bleeding if possible.

5. Begin hemodynamic monitoring (arterial line, central venous pressure line, possibly pulmonary artery catheter).

6. Start an IV with a large bore needle.
   * A peripheral and a central line may be indicated.
   * Type of fluid administered depends on situation (initially, 5% dextrose in saline or Ringer's lactate).
   * Colloids (whole blood, plasma, albumin, or dextran) for hemorrhage or burns
   * Crystalloids (Ringer's lactate or normal saline)—for volume replacement
   * If an abdominal injury is present, start IV in upper extremities.
   * Fluid should be rapidly infused to raise CVP level 5 cm H_2O above initial reading and keep systolic blood pressure at 80 mm to 90 mm Hg.

7. Monitor strict intake and output.
   * Watch patient closely for symptoms of fluid overload.
   * Insert an indwelling urinary catheter in the bladder and monitor urine output closely.

8. Type and crossmatch blood.

9. Administer medications as ordered to treat the symptoms.
   * Vasopressors (Levophed, Aramine)
   * Vasodilators (see Cardiogenic Shock)
   * Steroids
   * Inotropic drugs (digitalis, Levophed)
   * Sodium bicarbonate (if the patient is in acidosis)
   * Pain relievers if necessary (Pain may intensify shock.)

10. Monitor the patient's response.
    * Patient may sense an impending catastrophe.
    * Do not leave patient unattended.

11. Position patient on back with legs straight and slightly elevated.
    * Head should be level with chest or slightly higher.
    * Do not place in severe head-down position.
    * This position is contraindicated with head injuries.

12. Maintain the body temperature.

13. Provide external counterpulsation (MAST suit) if indicated.

14. Prepare for emergency surgery as indicated.

SEPTIC SHOCK

Septic shock is usually caused by a gram-negative organism.

Clinical Manifestations

Elevated temperature (may occur intermittently, with "spikes")

Chills, shaking

Rapid, weak pulse

Initially, warm, dry skin (progresses to cold and clammy)

Changes in level of consciousness (dullness, inappropriate behavior; listlessness, progresses to delirium and coma)

Purpuric or petechial skin eruptions

Rapid pulse

Hypotension

Oliguria

Cyanosis

Rapid respirations

General vascular collapse

Treatment and Nursing Actions

1. Monitor vital signs and ECG continuously.
   - Check levels of consciousness frequently.
   - Auscultate heart and lung sounds.
   - Report abnormalities to physician immediately.

2. Support respiratory function.
   - Keep airway patent.
   - Suction as indicated.
   - Administer oxygen therapy.
   - In advanced shock, entubation and mechanical ventilation may be indicated.
   - Monitor arterial blood gases closely.

3. Support cardiac function.

4. Start an IV with a large bore needle.
   - Use peripheral and central line if indicated.
   - Select a large vessel to facilitate administration of emergency drugs and irritating antibiotics.
   - Administer normal saline, whole blood, plasma, or blood expanders if indicated.

5. Type and crossmatch blood.

6. Monitor intake and output closely.
   - Report decrease in output (below 30 ml/hr) to physician immediately.

- Monitor closely for signs of fluid overload.
- Measure central venous pressure to determine if fluid replacement therapy is needed.

7. Administer medications as ordered.
   - Administer Cephalosporins, Gentamicin, and Tobramycin (drugs of choice) as ordered by the physician to control the infection.
   - Administer antipyretics to reduce high temperature elevations.
   - Administer specific medications as ordered for complications (digitalis may be given to support ventricular function; sodium bicarbonate for acidosis).

8. Obtain laboratory studies.
   - Draw a blood sample for culture and sensitivity.
   - Culture other potential sites of infection (*e.g.*, wounds, urine, sputum)
   - Culture suspect equipment (*e.g.*, angiocath, urinary catheter)

9. Monitor patient's response.
   - Patient may sense an impending catastrophe.
   - Do not leave patient unattended.

10. Prepare for immediate surgery as indicated (Abscess may be drained).

SPINAL CORD SHOCK (NEUROGENIC SHOCK)

Clinical Manifestations

Complete loss of motor, sensory, reflex and autonomic nervous system function below the level of injury

Hypotension

Loss of bowel and bladder control (fecal incontinence and abdominal distention; urinary retention, and bladder distention)

Complete paralysis below the level of injury

Slow pulse

NOTE. Cervical injuries result in minimal to absent function of intercostal muscles and diaphragm.

Treatment and Nursing Actions

1. Monitor vital signs and ECG continuously.
   - Watch for cardiac or respiratory arrest which may occur at any time.
   - Look for respiratory complications with cervical cord injury.
   - Auscultate heart and lung sounds.
   - Notify physician immediately of any adverse changes.

2. Closely monitor neurological signs. Report increasing deficits to physician immediately.

3. Support respiratory function.
   - Keep the airway patent.
   - Suction as necessary.
   - Begin mechanical ventilation, control or assist, if necessary, especially if C3, C4, or C5 are involved.
   - Administer oxygen therapy as ordered.
   - Monitor arterial blood gases.

4. Support cardiac function.

5. Keep the patient flat. Cardiac or respiratory arrest may follow elevation of the head of the bed even at a slight incline.

6. Start an IV with a large bore needle in an upper extremity vein.

7. Support circulating volume.
   - Blood transfusions may be indicated if hemorrhage has accompanied this injury.
   - Monitor central venous pressure if indicated.
   - Monitor intake closely.
   - Watch for symptoms of circulatory overload.

8. Completely immobilize the patient.
   - Keep the spine in proper alignment, with special attention to the head and neck, especially if cervical injury is suspected.
   - Place sandbags on either side of the head and neck to prevent turning. If none are available, the nurse should place her hands on either side of the head and gently support it, preventing any movement until more definitive methods can be instituted.
   - Failure to properly immobilize the patient can cause further damage, progression of shock, or death.
   - Prepare for type of immobilization as ordered by physician (*e.g.,* Crutchfield tongs).
   - Prepare frame (*e.g.,* Stryker frame) or bed (*e.g.,* CircOlectric bed) as ordered by physician.

9. Insert an indwelling catheter into the urinary bladder to relieve urinary distention.
   - Monitor urinary output closely.

10. Support gastrointestinal function.
    - Insert a nasogastric tube to relieve abdominal distention.
    - Connect nasogastric tube to low intermittent suction.

11. Administer Decadron as ordered.

12. Keep NPO.

13. Auscultate bowel sounds.

14. Prepare for surgical intervention as indicated.

NOTE. The higher the level of injury, the greater the degree of shock. This type of shock is usually temporary (several days) but may last weeks or even months.

ANAPHYLACTIC SHOCK

Clinical Manifestations

Sudden anxiety	Restlessness
Irritability	Dyspnea

Feeling of choking or suffocating (shortness of breath)

Chest pain or feeling of tightness

Headache (throbbing)

Coughing, wheezing, bronchial asthma

Difficulty in swallowing

General vasodilation (erythema, warm feeling)

Hives (massive facial swelling may indicate upper respiratory edema)

May be incontinent of stool and urine

Nausea, vomiting

Severe abdominal cramping

Profound vascular collapse in periphery (absence of pulse, cyanosis)

Circulatory and respiratory failure

Convulsions

Coma

Death (unless treatment is begun promptly)

Treatment and Nursing Actions

1. Monitor vital signs and ECG continuously.
   - Respiratory and circulatory collapse is imminent.
   - Upper airway may be occluded by swelling.
   - Auscultate heart and lung sounds.
   - Notify physician immediately of abnormalities.

2. Support respiratory function.
   - Keep airway patent.
   - Suction as necessary.
   - Begin entubation with mechanical ventilation if needed.

3. Support cardiac function.
   - Perform CPR if necessary.
   - Keep emergency drugs and crash cart readily available.

4. Administer medications intravenously as prescribed.
   - Epinephrine
   - Antihistamines (usually Benadryl)
   - Vasopressors for hypotension (Levophed)
   - Steroids (Solu-Cortef)
   - Aminophyllin or theophylline to relieve bronchospasm and asthma
   - Valium for convulsions

5. Start an IV with 5% dextrose in water in a large vessel to facilitate an emergency drug route. Replace volume as indicated.

6. Monitor patient's reaction.
   - Patient may sense impending doom.
   - Do not leave unattended.

7. Continue to monitor patient for several hours following the successful treatment of shock in order to quickly detect its recurrence.

22
Special Treatment Devices

The antishock suit (MAST), external counterpulsation pressure device, and the intra-aortic ballon pump (for internal counterpulsation) described in this chapter are special devices used in the treatment of shock.

ANTISHOCK SUIT

Description and Purpose

Antishock suit is also referred to as Military Anti-Shock Trousers (MAST).

It is a device needed in the treatment of shock due to hypovolemia and hypotension.

The antishock suit consists of a one-piece wrap-around trouser suit that is secured with Velcro fasteners. There are three inflatable compartments (one for each leg and the abdomen). It is inflated with a foot pump. A pressure relief valve is attached to prevent excess pressure.

The device is inflated until the blood pressure approaches the normal limit. Vital signs, especially blood pressure, must be closely monitored during this time.

It may be left in place for 24 hours to 48 hours or until the patient's condition stabilizes.

Contraindications

Advanced pregnancy

Congestive heart failure

Pulmonary edema

Severe head wounds

Chest injuries and resulting respiratory difficulty

Severe bleeding for any reason above the MAST suit

Treatment and Nursing Actions

1. Treatment of underlying cause of shock should be started immediately.
2. Fractures should be immobilized with splints prior to application.

3. Sterile dressings should be applied to wounds prior to application.

4. When discontinuing the procedure following stabilization of the patient's condition, observe the following guidelines:
   - Release pressure gradually.
   - Monitor vital signs closely during this time. If an adverse change occurs, immediately reinflate.
   - After all the pressure has been released, leave the suit in place for a while and observe patient response.
   - If any adverse effects occur, reinflate immediately.

COUNTERPULSATION DEVICES

Description and Purpose

Counterpulsation devices are used to augment or strengthen the heart during diastole.

The purpose of these devices is to improve coronary and systemic perfusion.

There are two methods available.
   - External counterpulsation pressure (noninvasive technique) and the intra-aortic balloon pump (an invasive technique)

Monitoring

The patient should have continuous ECG monitoring during the procedure.

Hemodynamic monitoring is indicated.

Renal function should be monitored closely. An indwelling urinary catheter is indicated.

Contraindication

Counterpulsation is contraindicated if an aneurysm of the descending thoracic aorta is present or with an incompetent aortic valve.

EXTERNAL COUNTERPULSATION PRESSURE
Procedure

1. The patient's legs are encased in two rigid support forms shaped in a V and lined with inflatable bags.

2. The bags, which encircle the legs from ankle to thigh, are filled with water to completely avoid any free space inside the device.

   NOTE. The feet are not included.

3. The hydraulic pumping unit, which is positioned between the ankles, is connected to the system by hoses.

4. The pump functions to alter the bag pressure synchronously. The following sequence occurs:
   - During diastole, water is pumped into the bags.

- This pressure causes squeezing of the patient's legs.
- The squeezing motion forces blood from the arteries and veins back to the heart.
- Diastolic pressure is strengthened and central venous return is increased.
- Bag pressure is released immediately before systole.
- The arteries and veins fill with blood.
- This results in a lowered systolic pressure.

5. The process is repeated.

Effects

Cardiac function improves for the following reasons:
- Increased diastolic pressure results in increased coronary artery blood flow.
- Increased venous return to the heart increases cardiac output.
- Workload of left ventricle is reduced.

INTRA-AORTIC BALLOON PUMP

1. The intra-aortic balloon pump is inserted through the femoral artery and is positioned in the descending thoracic aorta just distal to the left subclavian artery.
2. Timed in sequence with the QRS complex, the balloon pump is inflated shortly after the T wave occurs and deflated when the QRS occurs.
3. The balloon pump is powered by either helium or carbon dioxide.
4. The balloon is connected to a bedside console with the following features: controls that activate the alarms, balloon function synchronized with cardiac action, and pneumatic controls for balloon inflation and deflation.

Effects

Cardiac function improves for the following reasons:
- Increased diastolic pressure results in increased coronary artery blood flow.
- Oxygen requirements of myocardium are reduced.
- Arterial resistance to emptying of ventricle is decreased, resulting in increased cardiac output and decreased workload of heart.
- In addition, the device continues to support systemic perfusion.

23
Hemodynamic Monitoring

This chapter describes in detail the many types of hemodynamic monitoring and associated nursing considerations. It discusses indwelling arterial line, central venous pressure, pulmonary artery catheter, cardiac output, cardiac index, arteriovenous oxygen difference, and left arterial pressure monitoring.

ARTERIAL LINE (INDWELLING)

Description and Purpose

An indwelling arterial catheter, cannula, is used for continous monitoring of arterial blood pressure. This invasive form of monitoring is more accurate than cuff measurement.

The arterial line facilitates monitoring of sustained hypertension or hypotension, and the administration and effects of hypotensive or hypertensive medication as well as hypovolemia. It is also used when frequent samples for blood gas analysis are required.

Prerequisites

Adequate arterial circulation must be present in the area for insertion. Check by performing Allen's Test which is described in Chapter 30.

Systolic, diastolic, and mean pressure readings may need to be taken.
- Systolic—indicates injection of blood into the aorta
- Diastolic—indicates coronary circulation
- Mean—indicates renal and cerebral circulation
- Normal pressure readings:
  - Systolic—below 140 mm Hg
  - Diastolic—below 90 mm Hg
  - Mean—70–90 mm Hg

Equipment

1 16–18 gauge (2 in) Longdwell

Sterile transducer and dome

Sorensor Intraflo with arterial pressure tubing

3 sterile stopcocks

500 ml normal saline with 500–1000 U heparin

Pressure pump (inflate to 300 mm Hg)

IV pole

IV administration set (microdrip and pressure tubing)

Local anesthetic (usually lidocaine 1%)

Povidone–iodine solution

Sterile 4 x 4s and 2 x 2s

Tape

Arm board

4–0 suture

Preliminary Actions

1. Explain procedure to patient.
2. Set up equipment. Make sure all air is removed from tubing.
3. Calibrate the monitor.
4. Make sure that the transducer is level with the right atrium.
5. Perform the Allen test to check for circulatory efficiency.

Procedure

1. The physician performs the procedure, using strict sterile technique.
2. After proper placement, connect patient to primed arterial pressure monitoring system.
3. Close the 2-way stopcock of the transducer to room air.
4. Close the 3-way stopcock to the IV solution.
5. Take the desired reading (depress systolic, diastolic, or mean buttons).
   - Pressure will appear on digital readout.
   - Dicrotic notch must be visible.
6. To display waveform (Fig. 23-1) on monitor, switch dial from ECG to BP.
7. Set the alarms appropriately and activate by depressing the ready button.
8. Apply small sterile dressing to site.

Comments

1. The system should be flushed as necessary by pulling the valve stem quickly in the following situations:
   - After all blood samples
   - If the waveform damps out
   - If blood backs up into the line
2. Continue to monitor the extremity for temperature, color, and sensation. It is very important that the extremity be left exposed (except for the small area covered by the dressing) so that frequent checks can be made.
3. The arm should be immobilized on an arm board.

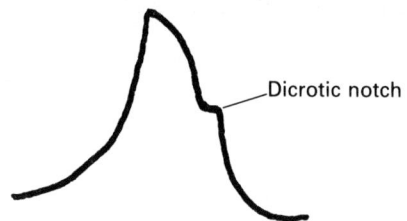

FIG. 23-1. *Arterial blood pressure waveform.*

4. Recalibrate the monitor every 8 hours.

5. Remember that the monitor reading is usually 20 mm Hg greater than the cuff reading.

6. Chart the total amount of blood aspirated for blood samples on output and include the discarded blood.

7. Chart the amount of heparinized saline (3 ml) infused every hour to flush the line.

8. Be sure to chart arterial pressure (both monitored and cuff readings) on graphic sheet.

Nursing Considerations

1. Check all connections. Hemorrhage and death could occur if the system is disconnected.

2. If a line clots, try to free it by gentle aspiration with a tuberculin syringe. Never manually irrigate the line.

ALERT. Never administer medications through the arterial line because this could result in arterial spasm and possible necrosis. *Exception*—heparinized solution is used to continually flush with the intraflow.

3. Always check cuff pressure to correlate reading, especially if the arterial pressure is suspected to be inaccurate.

4. Do not allow bag to run dry. Change it when the level gets low.

5. See Table 23-1 for problems associated with arterial lines and appropriate actions.

TABLE 23-1. **Problems Associated with Arterial Lines**

Problem	Cause	Action
Damped pressure tracing	Clot	Try to gently aspirate. If unsuccessful, notify physician. Do not manually irrigate.
	Catheter position (against vessel wall)	Gently reposition catheter while observing waveform.
	Air bubbles	Flush, being careful to prevent entry of bubbles into artery.
		NOTE. If above attempts are unsuccessful, notify physician.

TABLE 23-1. **Problems Associated with Arterial Lines** *(Continued)*

Problem	Cause	Action
Damped pressure tracing *(continued)*	Hypotension	Check blood pressure with cuff. Notify physician if reading is significant.
No waveform attainable	Incorrect setup of equipment	Check system, including settings on monitor and stopcock opening the transducer to the catheter. If everything is in order and there is still no waveform, notify physician.
Waveform ragged and erratic in appearance	Movement of catheter tip	Attempt to stop by stabilizing the catheter (2×2s, tape, and placing extremity on arm board) If unsuccessful, notify physician.
Waveform is slightly rounded; systolic height consistently varies	Mechanical ventilation with PEEP or Pulsus paradoxus	Check systolic pressure regularly. If the difference between the highest and lowest is greater than 10 mm Hg, pulses paradoxus may be the underlying condition. Notify physician.
Absent or weak pulse below insertion site (waveform may be straight or damped)	Thrombosis of artery	Do not flush. Notify the physician immediately. Depending on the situation, he may discontinue the line or attempt to remove the clot by arteriotomy and Fogarty catheterization.
Absent or intermittent pulse below insertion site (waveform will be irregular)	Spasm of artery	Notify physician immediately. Prepare for lidocaine injection at site and in catheter by physician.
Sudden appearance of symptoms of air embolism (waveform damped) **NOTE.** Symptoms depend on location of embolus and its effects (see Thromboembolic Events Chap. 2 and Pulmonary Embolus, Chap. 10)	Air bubbles from system entering artery	Position patient on his left side and in Trendelenburg position to try to keep bubbles in right side of heart where they will be absorbed by the pulmonary artery. Notify the physician immediately. Administer oxygen therapy as ordered. Have resuscitative equipment available. Check line to make sure all connections are tight. Do not leave patient unattended.

Care of the Insertion Site

1. The dressing should be removed and the site observed every 48 hours.
2. Tubing and fluid should be changed every 48 hours.
3. Using a sterile technique, clean the site with povidone-iodine swabs.
4. Apply sterile 2 × 2s and tape securely.
5. Note date and time of dressing change on nurse's notes and tape over dressing.

CENTRAL VENOUS PRESSURE MONITORING

Description and Purpose

Central venous pressure monitoring (CVP) is a method used for continuous monitoring of right atrial pressure to reflect the pressure and function of the right ventricle.

It indicates the function and pumping ability of the right side of the heart.

It is not a reliable indicator of the function and pumping ability of the left side of the heart or rapid changes in the cardiovascular status. It may be the last parameter to change in these situations.

It determines fluid status (whether to replace fluid or restrict fluid intake), and it determines the ability of the cardiac pump to handle blood volume (circulatory dynamics).

CVP may be monitored continuously by connecting to a monitoring system or intermittently by connecting to a water manometer.

Catheter is inserted into superior vena cava in close proximity to the right atrium or in the right atrium.

Normal Reading

Normal CVP reading is 5 cm H_2O to 15 cm H_2O.

Continuous central venous pressure measurement may be obtained by attaching the proximal lumen of the pulmonary artery catheter to the transducer and monitor (see Pulmonary Artery Catheter Setup on p 242). Normal right atrial mean pressure is 1 mm Hg to 6 mm Hg.

To convert pressure readings from mm Hg (used with pressure monitoring) to cm H_2O (used with manometer), if the systems are converted, use the following formulas:
- mm Hg × 1.36 = cm H_2O
- cm H_2O ÷ 1.36 = mm Hg

Equipment

Central venous pressure tray

Deseret catheter—large bore (used for percutaneous insertion); or cutdown tray with long intracatheter or feeding tube as ordered by physician

CVP manometer with tubing

Sterile 3–way stopcock

IV pole

IV solution as ordered by physician

Buretrol

Povidone-iodine swabs and ointment

Sterile 4 × 4s

Tape

Sterile gloves

Preliminary Actions

1. Explain the procedure to the patient.
2. Place the patient in slight Trendelenburg position to allow for better filling of the vein and lessen the chances of an air embolus if insertion is performed through the internal or external jugular or subclavian vein. The patient should also be instructed to bear down as the physician inserts the catheter into the vein—another measure used to lessen the chances of air embolus.
3. If the catheter is inserted in a large vein in the arm, the arm may have to be straightened or rotated to facilitate catheter passage at the shoulder area.
4. Set up the equipment.

Procedure

1. The physician inserts the catheter either percutaneously or by cutdown using sterile technique.
2. Following insertion, the catheter is connected to the primed IV setup.
3. Catheter patency is tested by lowering the IV solution which normally should have a free backflow of blood.
4. The catheter should be sutured into place and taped to secure its position.
5. Povidone-iodine ointment is applied to the site and a sterile dressing is applied and taped in place.
6. A chest x-ray film is used to confirm the proper positioning of the catheter and to detect the presence of a pneumothorax (a complication of insertion when the subclavian approach is used).

Monitoring CVP Pressure

1. Position the patient flat on his back without a pillow under his head if possible.
   - If the patient is unable to tolerate this position select the most comfortable position and use it for all subsequent readings. Semi-Fowler's position is usually well tolerated.
   - The legs should never dangle, even with the modified position, because this would give a false low reading.
   - The position should be recorded on the nurse's notes and used for all subsequent readings.

2. Position the manometer correctly.
   - Manometer should be level with the right atrium.
   - Point where reading is taken should be marked on chest with a felt-tip pen.
   - Readings should always be taken at this point.
3. Respirator should be disconnected if possible while the reading is being taken.
   - If patient is unable to be off respirator, take reading and document in nurse's notes that the patient was on a respirator.
   - Subsequent readings should be taken this way as necessary.
4. Flush line with IV fluid to assure patency (stopcock should be in "keep open" position).
5. Close stopcock to patient and allow fluid to fill the manometer above the estimated CVP level.
   - Do not overfill.
   - Fluid spillover could contaminate the system.
6. Close stopcock to IV fluid.
7. Observe manometer at eye level.
8. Take reading when fluid ceases to fall in the manometer.
   - The level will fluctuate slightly with respiration (falling on inspiration and rising with expiration) when the CVP is reached.
   - The reading is taken when the fluid level stops falling.

   NOTE. Reading is taken from base of meniscus of fluid.

9. Close stopcock to manometer after the reading is taken and open to IV fluid.
10. Flush the line.
11. Adjust the flow rate to that specified by physician.
12. Document reading in nurse's notes.
13. Reconnect the respirator.
14. Assist the patient to a comfortable position.

Comments

Take readings as specified by the physician or as follows: every hour for 24 hours; every 2 hours for 24 hours and then every 4 hours if stable.

Check system frequently to make sure all connections are secure.

Do not infuse the following solutions through the system without a physician's order: potassium (administered hourly through buretrol), blood, plasma, or albumin.

Never leave the system open to air (negative pressure produced in the central venous pressure on inspiration facilitates the entry of an air embolus).

Take blood samples from catheter by using the following procedure:
- Place the patient in slight Trendelenberg or flat position.
- Instruct patient to take a deep breath and hold it while samples are being removed.
- Attach sterile syringe to 3-way stopcock (stopcock should be turned to syringe and catheter).
- Aspirate 5 ml of blood to clear the fluid from the tubing (amount depends on length of tubing).
- Turn stopcock to halfway position. (This closes all ports to air.)
- Remove syringe and discard.
- Attach another sterile syringe. (turn stopcock back to syringe and catheter.)
- Aspirate desired amount of blood.
- Turn stopcock to halfway position and remove syringe.
- Turn the stopcock back to IV and catheter to clear the line.
- After the line is cleared, readjust the flow rate to that ordered.
- Cover the exposed port with a sterile protective cap.

See Table 23-2 for problems associated with CVP monitoring and appropriate actions.

TABLE 23-2. **Problems with CVP Monitoring**

Problem	Cause	Action
Fluid level in manometer rising on inspiration and falling on expiration	On positive pressure breathing	Normal
	Catheter that perforates vessel when femoral approach is used	Notify physician immediately.
Sluggish infusion of IV fluid	Clot	Try to aspirate with syringe. If unsuccessful, notify physician.
	Kinked tubing	Remove dressing and check for kinked tubing. Reposition, apply sterile dressing, and tape in place.
High pressure; active fluctuation with heartbeat	Cathether that has migrated into right ventricle	Notify physician. Chest x-ray film confirms the position. Physician repositions the catheter
Sudden appearance of PVC s in the absence of underlying cardiac disease symptoms or drugs	Catheter that has migrated into right ventricle, causing PVCs	Notify physician immediately. Catheter needs to be repositioned immediately.

Care of the Insertion Site

1. Remove the dressing and check the site every 24 hours.
2. Change the IV setup (including buretrol and stopcock) and fluid daily. Use the following procedure to change the IV set up and fluid:
   • Place the patient in slight Trendelenburg position if it can be tolerated.
   • Instruct the patient to hold his breath and bear down (unless contraindicated).
3. Using sterile technique, cleanse the site with povidone-iodine swabs.
4. Apply povidone-iodine ointment at insertion site and cover with a sterile dressing. Secure with tape.

PULMONARY ARTERY CATHETER (Fig. 23-2)

The pulmonary artery catheter is usually referred to as the Swan–Ganz catheter. (Swan–Ganz is a trade name for a flow-directed pulmonary artery catheter; however, the two terms are used interchangeably.)

Description and Purpose

The pulmonary artery catheter is an indirect means of measuring the pressure and function or pumping ability of the left ventricle.

The wedge position actually reflects left atrial pressure, which in the presence of normal function of the left ventricle and mitral valve is closely related to the filling pressure of the left ventricle (i.e., left ventricular end-diastolic pressure).

It is used to determine optimal fluid replacement therapy, to determine alterations in left ventricular function (as may be seen with heart failure), and to indicate the quality and quantity of systemic perfusion.

General clinical situations that utilize this type of monitoring are heart failure, MI, shock (hypovolemia, cardiogenic), unexplained tachycardia, pulmonary disease or conditions (pulmonary edema), and left ventricular failure.

General Information

The pulmonary artery catheter may be positioned with or without the use of fluoroscopy, the position being monitored by the pressure tracing on the monitor.

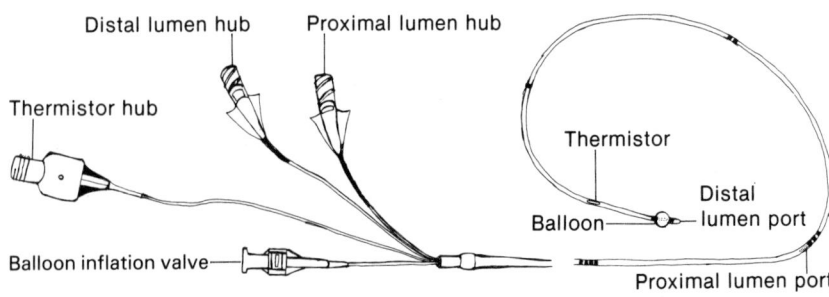

FIG. 23-2. *Pulmonary artery catheter (Swan-Ganz).*

The catheter is inserted into any large vein by cutdown of the antecubital, internal jugular, femoral, or subclavian vein. It may be inserted percutaneously by using special venous introducers.

The balloon is not inflated following insertion until it reaches the superior vena cava. The inflated balloon prevents irritation from the catheter as it passes through the valves and chambers of the heart.

The inflated balloon moves easily with the blood flow through the right side of the heart and into the pulmonary artery and a smaller branch where it wedges.

The length is 110 cm with markings placed every 10 cm (Measurements are given for Swan–Ganz catheter.)

The balloon is usually inflated with air, although carbon dioxide is recommended.

ALERT. Never use air to inflate the balloon if there is a chance the air could enter arterial circulation following balloon rupture (i.e., any type of shunt within the heart or pulmonary artery where venous and arterial blood might mix).

NOTE. Never inflate the balloon with any type of solution because it causes incomplete balloon deflation and decreases the catheter sensitivity.

The catheter is connected to a transducer that translates pressure waves into electrical impulses on a monitor.

Normal Pressures

Commonly used pulmonary artery pressures are abbreviated as follows:
- PAD—pulmonary artery diastolic pressure
- PAWP—pulmonary artery wedge pressure, or PCWP—pulmonary capillary wedge pressure

Normal pulmonary artery pressures are as follows:
- Systolic—20 mm Hg to 30 mm Hg
- Diastolic—5 mm Hg to 15 mm Hg
- Mean—below 20 mm Hg

Normal pulmonary artery wedge pressure:
- Mean—4 mm Hg to 12 mm Hg

ALERT. PAD should always be slightly higher than PCWP. A PAD that is more than 6 mm higher than the PCWP is significant and should be reported to the physician. It indicates an increase in pulmonary resistance associated with conditions such as primary pulmonary hypertension or pulmonary embolus.

TYPES

Double-lumen catheter
- One lumen (located one mm from catheter tip) is for balloon inflation

(shorter tubing); the other lumen (located at catheter tip) is for monitoring pressures (distal lumen port).

- It monitors pulmonary artery pressure and pulmonary artery wedge pressure and samples mixed venous blood (to determine O_2 concentrations).
- Intravenous solutions may be infused through second lumen.

Triple-lumen catheter
- Triple-lumen catheter has a lumen for balloon inflation and one to monitor pulmonary artery pressure.
- It has an additional lumen (proximal lumen) that lies in the right atrium (20 or 30 cm from the tip).
- Proximal lumen may be used to monitor central venous pressure or infuse intravenous solutions.

Thermodilution catheter
- The thermodilution catheter has the same features as the triple-lumen catheter.
- It also has a thermistor tip which measures changes in blood temperature. These changes are used to compute the cardiac output.

Equipment for Insertion

Sterile Swan–Ganz catheter set

Sterile cutdown tray

Introducer (one size larger than catheter)

Sterile transducer and dome

Transducer holder

Sorensor Intraflo (or other brand) with arterial tubing

IV pole

500 ml normal saline with 1000 U heparin

IV administration set (microdrip, pressure tubing)

Pressure bag (inflate to 300 mm Hg)

Oscilloscope and monitor

Local anesthetic (1% Xylocaine)

Povidone-iodine solution and ointment

Sterile 2 × 2s, 4 × 4s

Tape

Sterile towels

Sterile drape

Sterile solution bowl with sterile normal saline

Sterile gloves, masks, gowns

Caps

Syringes (10 ml and tuberculin)

Needles (25-gauge and 21-gauge)

Suture 3–0 or 4–0 silk

Defibrillator

Lidocaine bolus

Peripheral IV if not already in place

Scalpel with #11 blade

Sterile water to prime dome

Fluoroscope

Sterile 3-way stopcocks (2 for each intraflow and one for administration of medications or blood samples)

Preliminary Actions

1. Explain procedure to patient. Obtain signed consent form.
2. Set up equipment.
   - Assemble heparinized saline solution (flush solution) and equipment.
   - Set up transducer and flush with heparinized saline. Stopcocks should be opened and solution attached to flush out all air bubbles. At this point, close the stopcocks.
   - Calibrate monitor according to manufacturer's instructions.
   - Prepare cutdown tray.
     - Open tray.
     - Add povidone-iodine.
     - Assist physician in drawing up local anesthetic in syringe.
     - Open package containing catheter.
   - Position transducer level with the patient's right atrium.
   - Test the balloon for leaks by inflating it in a basin of sterile saline, maintaining sterility of the catheter.
3. Position the patient appropriately.
   - Patient is usually placed in the supine position.
   - Place in slight Trendelenburg position (rolled towels placed under shoulders) if the internal or external jugular approach is utilized.
4. Connect monitoring system that has been primed and calibrated to distal lumen and proximal lumen ports.
5. Prime distal and proximal lumens.
6. Monitor vital signs and ECG prior to and during the procedure.

Procedure

1. The physician performs the procedure, using strict sterile technique.
   - Assist physician as necessary.
   - Obtain printout of waveforms during insertion.
2. Monitor progress of catheter insertion on the scope (Fig. 23-3). (Fluoroscopy may be used.)
3. When the catheter is properly placed, the physician secures it in place with a suture.
4. Obtain desired pressure readings. Make sure transducer is level with the right atrium.

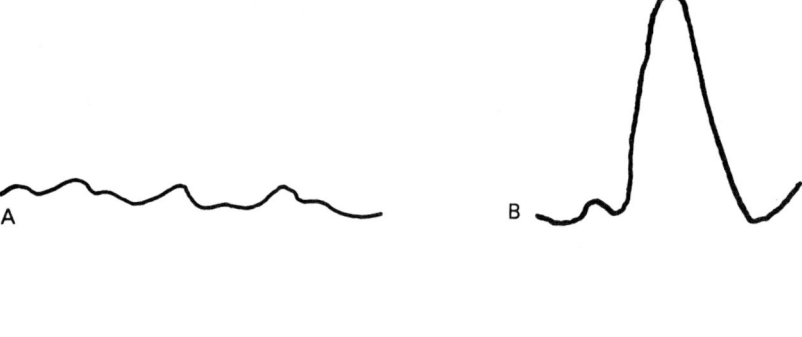

A   B

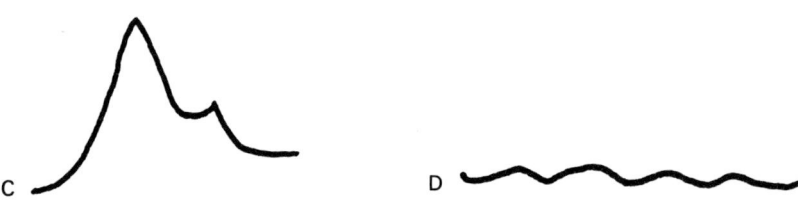

C   D

FIG. 23-3. *Waveforms observed as the pulmonary artery catheter passes through the chambers of the heart and reaches the desired position in the pulmonary artery. (A.) Right atrial pressure. (B.) Right ventricular pressure. (C.) Pulmonary artery pressure. (D.) Pulmonary artery wedge pressure.*

5. Take chest x-ray to check catheter position.
6. Set high and low alarms and activate by depressing the "Ready" button.
7. Continue to monitor vital signs and ECG.

Monitoring Pressures
1. Position the patient flat in bed if possible.

   NOTE. If patient cannot tolerate this position, leave in semi-Fowler's position for pressure reading. Document this position change in nurse's notes, and continue to take subsequent readings in this position.

2. Disconnect respirator during reading if possible.

   NOTE. If patient cannot tolerate being disconnected from respirator, take pressure reading and document the use of respirator in nurse's notes.

3. If excessive respirations are adversely affecting the waveform, instruct the patient to take a deep breath, exhale, and hold his breath during the reading.

4. Check the monitor to be sure the pulmonary artery (PA) waveform is present.
5. Make sure the transducer is level with the right atrium.
6. Flush the line by pulling pigtail on intraflow a couple of times.
7. Turn the machine on for printed readout (should be set at 25 mm paper speed).
8. Make sure the machine is properly calibrated.
9. Close the 2-way stopcock of the transducer to room air.
10. Close the 3-way stopcock to the IV solution.
11. Take the desired readings—systolic, diastolic, mean. Record readings.
12. Remove tuberculin syrige from balloon port to be sure all air has been removed.
13. Reattach syringe.
14. Inflate balloon with just enough air to change pulmonary artery (PA) waveform to PCWP waveform.
    • A slight resistance should be felt during balloon inflation.
    • Overinflation can cause rupture of the balloon.
15. Take the desired reading.
16. Deflate the balloon by removing the syringe immediately.
17. Close the 3-way stopcock to the transducer.
18. Open the 2-way stopcock to room air.
19. Flush the line and return to the continuous irrigation system.
20. Make sure the PA waveform has returned on the oscilloscope.

Comments

Make sure the balloon is completely deflated following pressure reading. If left inflated, pulmonary infarction could result.

Do not infuse any medications, except heparin or Xylocaine drips, through the pulmonary artery (PA) line.

Do not infuse IV solutions through the distal lumen unless absolutely necessary so that the pulmonary artery (PA) waveform will remain unaffected. IV solutions or medications may be infused through the proximal lumen.

Cover all ports on stopcocks with a sterile cover to maintain sterility of the system.

Check system frequently to make sure no air bubbles are in the line.

Check waveforms at least every hour.

Flush the system every 1 to 2 hours.

Check to make sure all connections are secure.

Check readings every 2 hours or as ordered by the physician.

If occlusion of the system is suspected, gently aspirate with a syringe attached to the stopcock closest to patient to see if the clot can be removed.

If this procedure is not successful, inform the physician immediately. Never manually irrigate the catheter.

See Table 23-3 for problems associated with the pulmonary artery catheter and appropriate actions.

TABLE 23-3. **Problems Associated with the Pulmonary Artery Catheter**

Problem	Cause	Action
Damped pressure waveform (Fig. 23-4)	Clot in the system	Try to aspirate blood gently. If successful, continue to do so until a readable pressure waveform appears. If unable to aspirate blood, notify physician immediately. Do not irrigate.
	Malposition of the catheter (tip against arterial wall)	Instruct patient to cough, which may reposition catheter correctly. If unsuccessful, raise patient's arm at a 90° angle to his body and flush the catheter gently. If this is unsuccessful, notify the physician immediately.
	Air in system	Check system for bubbles. Flush until bubbles are removed, being careful to prevent entry of same into the venous system.
	Blood backed up in tubing and is on transducer	Attempt to flush until blood is removed (may be possible if blood is fresh). If unsuccessful, replace with sterile dome.
No PCWP obtainable	Balloon rupture	Notify physician immediately. Prepare for removal of catheter.
	Insufficient balloon inflation	Disconnect tuberculin syringe to allow the balloon to deflate and then repeat.
	Improper position of catheter	Notify physician. (Catheter may have slipped back into right ventricle.) An x-ray film may be ordered to confirm position. Physician may reposition.
PCWP waveform remains after balloon deflation	Balloon not fully deflated	Disconnect tuberculin syringe. If the balloon deflates fully, the PA waveform should return. If unsuccessful, notify physician immediately.

(Continued)

TABLE 23-3. **Problems Associated with the Pulmonary Artery Catheter**
(Continued)

Problem	Cause	Action
PCWP waveform remains after balloon deflation (*continued*)	Tip of catheter has wedged in a small pulmonary capillary	Instruct the patient to cough. If this is not successful in removing the catheter, notify the physician immediately.
Drifting waveform	Insufficient time allowed for monitoring system to warm up	System should be allowed 30 minutes to warm up.
Sudden change of waveform configuration	Improper calibration of transducer	Recalibrate.
	Transducer not level with right atrium	Reposition correctly. Recalibrate.
	Catheter that has drifted out of proper position	Try to wedge the catheter by inflating the balloon. If unsuccessful (the PCWP not obtained), notify the physician.
	Loose connections	Check all connections, especially catheter attachment to transducer. Secure any that are loose.

Care of the Insertion Site

1. Remove the dressing and observe the site daily.
2. Change tubing and fluid daily.
3. Using sterile technique, clean the site with povidone-iodine swabs.
4. Apply povidone-iodine ointment to the catheter site.
5. Apply sterile 4 × 4s and tape securely.
6. Note date and time of dressing change on nurse's notes and tape over dressing.

CARDIAC OUTPUT

Description and Purpose

Cardiac output is the amount of blood ejected by the heart (stroke volume) times the heart rate.

The cardiac output for the right and left ventricles should be the same except in the presence of an intracardiac shunt.

Cardiac output is used to assess left ventricular performance and cardiac status.

FIG. 23-4. *Damped pressure waveform.*

Normal Cardiac Output

Normal cardiac output is 4 to 8 liters/min (resting).

Equipment

Small basin or container filled with ice and water

Sterile 10-ml syringes with needles (at least 5 per reading)

500 ml 5% dextrose in water

Preliminary Actions

1. Fill each syringe with the dextrose solution by inserting the needle through medication port on bag.
2. Cap each needle and place the syringes in ice-slush solution.
3. Monitor the temperature of the solution in the container with the computer probe or remove the plunger from a syringe and insert a glass thermometer to periodically measure the temperature. Temperature should be 0°C.
4. Attach the cable from the machine to the thermistor tip on the catheter.
5. Pretest thermistor tip and calibrate the computer according to manufacturer's instructions. Allow system to warm up as recommended.
6. Check the digital display on the screen (reflects the patient's temperature) and be sure it corresponds closely with predetermined temperature.
7. Check the patient's temperature. Dial results into computer.

Procedure

1. Remove syringe from solution and quickly check to make sure all air bubbles are removed and that it contains 10 ml of solution.
2. Immediately attach to proximal lumen.
   - Do not touch plunger or hold in hand for any length of time as these actions will change the solution temperature.
   - Press the start button and immediately inject the solution as quickly and steadily as possible.
3. Watch the computer for the cardiac output display and record.
4. Turn recorder back to standby.
5. Repeat the above procedure for at least two more injections. If the reading is within a 0.5 liter/min range, take an average for the cardiac output.
6. Discard readings that are obviously inaccurate (in comparison with the others) and repeat the procedure.

CARDIAC INDEX

Description

The cardiac output may be used to determine the cardiac index, a more specific measurement of cardiac function.

The cardiac index is the cardiac output per square meter of body surface area.

This reading is obtained as follows:

- Determine the body surface area according to a height-weight formula. (See Appendix)
- Divide the cardiac output by the body surface area (calculated in square meters).

Normal Index

Normal resting cardiac index is 2.5 to 4 liters/min (m²).

ARTERIOVENOUS OXYGEN SATURATION DIFFERENCE

Description

The arteriovenous oxygen saturation difference (AVO_2 difference) determines the amount of oxygen being extracted from the blood by the tissues.

It varies inversely with the cardiac output. (These relationships are shown in Table 23-4.)

Normal Arteriovenous Oxygen Difference

Normal AVO_2 difference is 3 to 5.5 vol.% (oxygen saturation per 100 ml of blood).

Procedure for Finding AVO_2 Saturation Difference

1. Hemoglobin (gm/100 ml) × 1.34 (O_2 carrying capacity) × O_2 saturation (arterial) = vol. % O_2 content of arterial blood.

2. Repeat step 1 using venous O_2 saturation to find vol. % O_2 content of venous blood.

3. Arterial vol. % O_2 content − venous vol. % O_2 content = AVO_2 difference.

LEFT ATRIAL PRESSURE

Description and Purpose

Left atrial pressure (LAP) is a method of monitoring the pressure in the left atrium. It is used to determine left ventricular function.

Mean left atrial pressure is a reliable indicator of left ventricular end-diastolic pressure in patients with normal mitral valve and left ventricular function.

TABLE 23-4. **Arteriovenous Oxygen Differences**

Cardiac Output	Effect in Tissues	Indication
Greater blood flow	Less O_2 removed; AVO_2—small difference	Normal to high cardiac output
Decreased blood flow	More O_2 removed; AVO_2—large difference	Low cardiac output

The catheter is inserted directly into the atrium during cardiac surgery and is connected to a transducer and monitor.

Normal Pressure

Normal mean left atrial pressure is below 12 mm Hg.

Equipment

Monitor

Sterile transducer and dome

Sorensor Intraflo (or other brand) with arterial tubing

500 ml of 5% dextrose in water with 1000 U of heparin

IV pole

IV administration set (microdrip, pressure tubing)

Air filter

Pressure bag (inflate to 300 mm Hg)

3-way stopcocks (2)

Procedure

1. Set up the monitoring system and prime.
   - Attach an air filter to the system to lessen the chance of introducing an air embolus directly into the left atrium.
   - Check entire system, including tranducer, to make sure all air bubbles are removed.
   - Make sure transducer is level with the right atrium.
2. Attach a 3-way stopcock to the tubing of the air filter.
   - Flush until all air bubbles are removed.
   - Cap middle port with sterile cap.
3. Close stopcock to air filter.
4. Open lateral port on stopcock connected to left atrial (LA) line and allow fluid or blood to drip slowly.
5. Open lateral port on stopcock connected to air filter and allow fluid to drip slowly.
6. Connect the two stopcocks immediately. (Introduction of air embolus is prevented by allowing the fluid to flow from both systems during the connection.)
7. Flush the line until all blood is removed.
8. Rebalance and recalibrate monitor according to manufacturer's instructions.

Monitoring Pressures

1. Depress "mean" button on monitor.
   - Systolic and diastolic pressures are not significant.
   - LA pressures are always taken on "mean."
2. Check waveform (Fig. 23-5) and digital readout.
3. Document findings in nurse's notes.

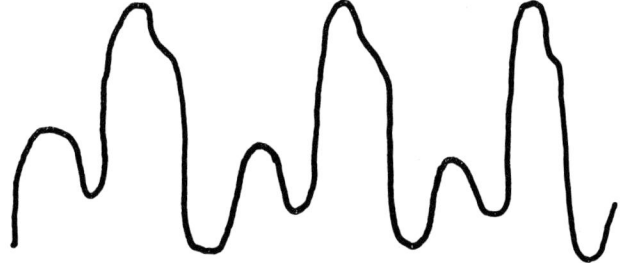

FIG. 23-5. *Left atrial pressure (LAP) waveform.*

Comments

Take LA pressure readings at the end of exhalation.

Do not infuse any other IV solutions or medications through the line.

Take pressure readings when vital signs and other hemodynamic monitoring is performed to correctly assess the patient's status. Heart sounds should be monitored closely.

Take readings every hour or as ordered by physician.

Notify physician of any significant changes (2 mm Hg)

The monitoring system should be calibrated and balanced at least every 8 hours.

Never irrigate or flush the line manually.

Check all connections frequently to assure security of the system.

See Table 23-5 for LAP monitoring problems and appropriate actions.

Care of the Insertion Site

1. Remove the dressing and check the site daily.

2. Using sterile technique, cleanse the area with povidone-iodine swabs.

3. Apply a sterile dressing and tape securely.

4. Change monitoring system setup every 24 hours.

TABLE 23-5. **Left Atrial Pressure Monitoring Problems**

Problem	Cause	Action
Blood clot	Inadequate flow of solution	Notify physician immediately. Do not attempt to flush or aspirate the catheter.
Waveform is of poor quality or unobtainable	Loose connection in system	Quickly check system for proper connections.
	Blood clot on catheter tip	Notify physician immediately.
	Improper position of catheter	Do not attempt to flush or aspirate the catheter.

VI

Care of the Patient with an Acute Abdomen

24

The Acute Abdomen

Acute abdomen is a general term used to describe many conditions. The ones most commonly seen in the critical care unit are presented in this chapter. They are abdominal injuries, acute intestinal obstruction, rupture of the esophagus, ruptured abdominal aneurysm, and acute gastrointestinal bleeding.

ABDOMINAL INJURIES

Cause
Trauma (blunt or penetrating)

Clinical Manifestations
Liver

Pain in right upper quadrant of abdomen with spasm and rigidity

Pain may radiate to shoulder

Shock

Elevated white blood cell count

Decreased red blood cell count

Spleen

Pain and tenderness in left upper quadrant of abdomen

Referred pain in left shoulder (Kehr's sigh) owing to blood under the diaphragm

Shock

Hemorrhage
- May be delayed for 48 hours or longer
- Patient will exhibit symptoms of progressive peritoneal irritation
- Leukocytosis
- Should be suspected with fractures of the lower left ribs or trauma to the lower left ribs

NOTE. Spleen may rupture with no history of trauma.

Pancreas

Epigastric pain that decreases soon after injury and then increases several hours later

Involuntary muscle spasm

Absence of bowel sounds

Elevation of serum and urine amylase may be present (test should be repeated several hours later)

Elevated white blood cell count

Stomach and Duodenum

Epigastric tenderness

Abdominal rigidity, with or without spasm

Blood in gastric secretions (If sufficient time has passed following injury, melena may be present.)

Small Bowel, Colon, and Rectum

Abdominal rigidity with spasm

Peritoneal irritation

Positive test for four-quadrant tap or peritoneal lavage

Blood in rectum

NOTE. Major vascular injuries (laceration of abdominal aorta, inferior vena cava, portal vein) may accompany these injuries, resulting in shock. Bluish discoloration in the flanks indicates a profound hemorrhage located in the retroperitoneal region as a result of major vessel trauma.

Diagnostic Tests

Abdominal x-ray film

Chest x-ray film

Four-quadrant tap

Peritoneal lavage

Laboratory tests:
• Complete blood cell count
• Hemoglobin
• Hematocrit
• Electrolytes
• BUN
• Serum amylase
• Urinalysis

Insertion of nasogastric tube to detect blood in gastric secretions

Treatment and Nursing Care

NOTE. Special considerations for penetrating trauma and suspected abdominal injury are presented in a summary chart following this section.

Monitor vital signs and ECG continuously.
• Neurologic signs should be checked.
• Pulses should be monitored carefully. Absence of pulse may indicate trauma to a major blood vessel.

Treat shock if present.

Auscultate bowel sounds frequently.

Start an IV with a large bore needle.
• Start in upper extremity vessel. DO NOT start in lower extremities, due to possibility of major vessel trauma associated with this type of injury.
• Infuse Ringer's lactate until blood transfusion is ready.

Type and crossmatch blood.
• Administer blood replacement therapy as ordered.
• Be sure that you administer the right blood to the right patient.

Obtain laboratory studies (complete blood cell count, hematocrit, hemoglobin, etc.).

Monitor intake and ouput closely.

Assess the patient's response.
• He may sense an impending catastrophe (shock).
• Fear and apprehension can compound the problem.
• Do not leave patient unattended.

Measure the abdominal girth to establish a baseline for comparison, and then check frequently for increase.

Prepare for emergency surgery as indicated.

SPECIAL NURSING CONSIDERATIONS

PATIENT WITH OBVIOUS PENETRATING TRAUMA
   Do not move the patient until he has been stabilized.

   Assess respiratory and cardiac function and support as indicated.

   Inspect the patient for wounds (front and back).

   For gunshot victims, look for entrance and exit wounds.

   If source of trauma is obvious (knife handle protruding from abdomen), do not remove.

      Secure with sterile dressing and tape.

      Prevent movement.

(*Continued*)

SPECIAL NURSING CONSIDERATIONS (*Continued*)

NOTE. Removal of object is physician's responsibility and will be done in surgery.

Apply direct pressure to wound for external bleeding. Cover with sterile pressure dressing if necessary.

If the bowel is protruding:

Have the patient flex his knees to prevent tension and further protrusion.

Cover the bowel with sterile saline dressings and keep wet to prevent drying of the bowel.

Keep the patient NPO to prevent an increase in peristalsis and possible contamination of the peritoneum if the bowel is lacerated.

Central venous pressure monitoring is indicated.

Insert an indwelling urinary catheter to closely monitor output.

Insert a nasogastric tube.

Attach to low intermittent suction.

Irrigate frequently to keep patent.

Administer antibiotics as ordered to prevent possible infection from bacterial contamination.

Prepare for emergency surgery as indicated.

Administer tetanus therapy as specified.

PATIENT WITH SUSPECTED ABDOMINAL INJURY

Assess respiratory and cardiac functions and support.

Do not move the patient until his condition has been assessed and stabilized.

Assist physician as he performs diagnostic tests and examinations (*e.g.*, four quadrant tap, peritoneal lavage, insertion of levin tube).

Keep patient NPO.

Monitor vital signs every 15 minutes. Vital sign changes or instability may be only indication of an abdominal injury.

Auscultate bowel sounds frequently.

ACUTE INTESTINAL OBSTRUCTION

Causes
Vascular

Infarction of a segment of the bowel owing to thrombosis or embolus of a splanchnic artery or vein

Mechanical (may be inside or outside the intestinal wall)

Malignancy

Intussusception

Volvulus

Adhesions

Strictures

Neurogenic (adynamic or paralytic ileus)

Postoperative complication (especially abdominal)

Peritonitis

Pneumonia (or other severe disease)

Extreme pain

Wound dehiscence

Spinal cord injuries

Clinical Manifestations

(depend on degree of obstruction, location, and cause)

General

Pain, spasmodic

Elevated white blood cell count

Toxicity

Shock

Elevated temperature

Peritonitis

NOTE. The higher the obstruction, the more severe the clinical manifestations.

High Small Intestine

Intense pain

Shock

Severe vomiting occurring soon after obstruction (with pain initially)

Minimal distention of the abdomen in epigastric area (occurs late)

Oliguria (due to loss of fluid and electrolytes)

Low Small Intestine

Symptoms are not as severe and generally appear later.

Vomitus may contain fecal material.

Oliguria does not usually occur at this level.

Conspicuous abdominal distention.

Colon

Symptoms are not as severe as those of obstruction of low small intestine and occur later; may have insidious onset. Vomitus contains fecal material. Constipation may or may not be present.

Vascular

Sudden onset of severe, cramping abdominal pain

Paralytic ileus

Shock

Peritonitis

(See general symptoms.)

Diagnostic Tests

Abdominal x-ray film

White blood cell count

Treatment and Nursing Actions

Monitor vital signs and ECG continuously.
- If shock is present, treat accordingly.
- Fluid and electrolyte disturbances may cause ECG changes.
- Neurologic signs should be monitored. Decreasing level of consciousness may indicate increasing electrolyte imbalance.

Prepare patient for insertion of a gastrointestinal tube to relieve distention. (See Gastrointestinal Tubes, Chap. 25.)

Start an IV.
- Infuse 5% dextrose in saline initially, followed by dextrose in water.
- Obtain serum electrolyte readings as soon as possible to correct any imbalances and to aid in determining fluid therapy.
- Administer saline solutions with caution in cardiac patients.

Administer antibiotics as ordered to prevent peritonitis.

Keep the patient NPO.

Closely monitor the patient's response for possible detection of complications. Do not leave unattended.

Monitor intake and output closely.
- Oliguria may indicate shock. Indwelling catheter may be indicated in acutely ill patients.
- Note quality and quantity of stool. (Test for guaiac.)
- Watch patient for symptoms of fluid overload (pulmonary edema, congestive heart failure).

Obtain routine lab studies (urinalysis, hemoglobin, hematocrit, complete blood cell count).

Prepare patient for emergency surgery (usually indicated with acute obstruction).

RUPTURE OF THE ESOPHAGUS

Causes

Trauma from:
- Automobile accidents
- Gunshot wound
- Swallowed foreign body
- Endoscopy
- Traumatic insertion of a stiff tube (nasogastric, etc.)
- Ingestion of corrosive chemicals

Spontaneous rupture—severe vomiting

Clinical Manifestations

Mild to severe chest pain (usually substernal)

Hematemesis

Temperature elevation (within 24 hours)

Abdominal pain and tenderness may be present

Back pain may be present

Subcutaneous emphysema and crepitus, including chest wall, neck, and face

Shock

Spontaneous rupture
- Cyanosis
- Dyspnea (may be extreme)
- Hamman's sign (crushing sound in the precordium)
- Sudden onset of severe pain in chest or upper abdomen
- Subcutaneous emphysema
- Rigid abdomen

Diagnostic Tests

Chest x-ray film—air in mediastinum will be visible.

Esophagoscopy—confirms the diagnosis.

Treatment and Nursing Actions

Closely monitor vital signs and ECG.

If patients is in shock, treat accordingly.

Insert nasogastric tube.
- Should be performed by a physician.
- Keep patient NPO.

Prepare patient for emergency surgery, as indicated (*i.e.,* perforation from spontaneous rupture, arterial bleeding, etc.).

If due to chemicals, neutralize as soon as possible.

If due to foreign body, prepare patient for endoscopy.

If due to presence of Sengstaken–Blakemore tube, notify physician immediately and prepare for removal.

Start an IV with a large bore needle. (See Acute Gastrointestinal Bleeding in this chapter.)

- Blood replacement therapy may be indicated.
- Nutrition will have to be supplied parenterally until surgical repair is accomplished or spontaneous healing occurs.

Administer antibiotics as ordered to prevent or control possible complication (*i.e.*, pneumonitis or peritonitis).

Obtain hemoglobin and hematocrit.

Type and crossmatch blood if blood replacement or surgery is indicated.

Monitor intake and output closely.

RUPTURED ABDOMINAL ANEURYSM

Cause
Arteriosclerosis

Clinical Manifestations
Sudden onset of excruciating pain (located in abdomen, lumbosacral area, groin, or rectum)

Sudden onset of syncope (results from extravasation of blood into the retroperitoneal cavity)

Hypovolemic shock owing to loss of circulating blood volume

Palpable, pulsating mass, tender to touch, located to left of midline in umbilical area

Pulses:
- Femoral pulses—present
- Popliteal, pedal, posterior tibial pulses—may be weak or absent

Blood pressure—may be undetectable or normal, or may exhibit varying degrees of hypotension

NOTE. Usually seen in men over 60 years of age. The aneurysm may develop without the patient's experiencing any symptoms. When rupture occurs, the patient becomes acutely ill.

Diagnostic Tests
Abdominal x-ray film—reveals calcified mass

Aortogram—confirms the diagnosis

Treatment
Immediate surgical resection and grafting

Nursing Actions
Prepare patient for immediate surgery.

Monitor vital signs, arterial pulses, ECG, and neurologic signs continuously.

Type and crossmatch blood.

NOTE. Patient may require up to 12 units of blood during surgery alone.

Insert intravenous line.
• Use large-bore needle to facilitate blood transfusions.
• Peripheral and central lines may be indicated.

Treat patient for hypovolemic shock. (See Shock, Chap. 21.)

Monitor intake and output closely.
• Indwelling catheter should be inserted in bladder, due to significant decrease in output.
• Fluid volume replacement with Ringer's lactate solution should be started.

Obtain routine preoperative laboratory studies (hematocrit, urinalysis, etc.).

Monitor arterial blood gases.

Hemodynamic monitoring may be indicated. Prepare patient for insertion and monitoring of arterial line, central venous pressure line, and Swan–Ganz catheter.

Provide emotional support.
• Patient may sense an impending catastrophe.
• Explain what is being done.
• Answer any questions.

Administer premedication as ordered.

Do not leave patient unattended at any time. (Nurse should accompany patient when x-ray film is obtained.)

Obtain signed surgical consent form.

Transfer patient to surgery as soon as possible.

ACUTE GASTROINTESTINAL BLEEDING

Cause

Upper Gastrointestinal Bleeding

Malignancy (resulting in erosion of major blood vessels)

Bleeding esophageal or gastric varices (suspect if patient is an alcoholic or shows signs of chronic liver disease)

Perforated peptic ulcer (located in esophagus, stomach, or duodenum)—most common cause

Gastritis

Trauma

Lower Gastrointestinal Bleeding
Diverticulosis (most common)
Ulcerative colitis
Cancer
Colonic ulcers

Clinical Manifestations

Sudden onset of severe, sharp pain in upper abdomen that remains constant and increases with movement

Tachypnea

Rigidity (boardlike) of abdomen

Diminished or absent peristalsis

Hematemesis

Tarry or bright-red stools

Thirst

Poor skin turgor

Shock

Massive bleeding (with esophageal or gastric varices)

Significance of Color of Blood

(See summary chart on the following page.)

NOTE. Occult blood is non-specific. Source of bleeding may be any location in the GI tract, or bleeding may originate in the respiratory system or mouth (blood coughed up and swallowed, severe nosebleed, etc.)

Diagnostic Tests

X-ray film of the chest

X-ray film of the abdomen

Endoscopy (upper GI bleeding)

Abdominal arteriograms

Proctosigmoidoscopy (lower GI bleeding)

Anoscopy (lower GI bleeding)

Barium contrast studies (It is not uncommon for bleeding caused by diverticula to stop following barium enema.)

12-lead ECG (to rule out cardiac complication of acute hemorrhage—MI)

Treatment and Nursing Actions

Monitor vital signs and ECG continuously.
- Hypotension may indicate shock.
- Myocardial ischemia (resulting from massive hemorrhage and a significant drop in oxygen-carrying hemoglobin) may progress to myocardial infarction.

ACUTE GASTROINTESTINAL BLEEDING: SIGNIFICANCE OF COLOR OF BLOOD

Color	Significance
Bright red blood	Fresh blood; massive bleeding
Bright red vomitus	Fresh blood from duodenum or stomach
Dark-red or coffee-ground vomitus	Old blood—perhaps several hours; from duodenum or stomach

NOTE. *Gastric acid turns bright-red blood (red hemoglobin) to dark-red (brown hematin). The brighter the blood, generally, the shorter the time spent in contact with gastric acid.*

Tarry stools	Only 60 ml of blood in the GI tract is necessary to cause this symptom—usually from duodenal rather than gastric ulcers. Most commonly associated with upper GI bleeding, although can occur in lower GI bleeding.
With diarrhea	Bleeding is above the duodenojejunal junction (ligament of Treitz)
Without diarrhea	Bleeding is above the midtransverse colon
Passing of bright red blood which may coat surface of stool	Seen with lower GI bleeding—that is, lower sigmoid and rectum
Maroon-colored blood with diarrhea	Bleeding is located above midtransverse colon
Bright red blood with stool	Bleeding is located below midtransverse colon
Blood and pus with stool	Inflammatory disease (ulcerative colitis)
Dark-red or currant-jelly color	Bleeding is located at Meckel's diverticulum

- Oxygen therapy may be necessary.
- Neurologic signs should be monitored. Decreasing level of consciousness may indicate inadequate cerebral oxygenation.

Treat patient for shock, if present. Place in Trendelenburg position (see Shock, Chapter 21).

Bowel sounds should be auscultated frequently. (A moderate amount of blood may produce a churning sound.)

Start an IV with a large-bore needle.
- Peripheral and central lines may be indicated.
- 5% dextrose in normal saline, or lactated Ringer's solution may be administered until the blood transfusion is ready.

Type and crossmatch for blood replacement therapy.

Administer blood as ordered.
- Be sure that you are administering the right blood to the right person.
- Closely monitor the patient for any transfusion reactions.

Obtain blood studies (complete blood cell count, hemoglobin, hematocrit, coagulation studies, liver and renal function tests).

Arterial blood gases should be checked to establish a baseline.

Monitor intake and output closely.
- Watch patient closely for symptoms of circulatory overload from blood and fluid replacement therapy (*i.e.*, pulmonary edema, congestive heart failure).
- Report decrease in urinary output (below 30 ml/hour) to physician immediately, as this may indicate shock.

NOTE. Urine output of at least 30 ml/hour indicates that blood pressure is sufficient to prevent adverse cardiac or cerebral complications.

- An indwelling catheter is indicated to closely monitor urinary output in the critically ill patient.
- Check specific gravity of urine to assess hydration (should be below 1.030).
- Document quality and quantity of stools or frank rectal bleeding.

Prepare patient for insertion of large-bore nasogastric tube.
- If massive bleeding has occurred, this procedure should be performed by a physician.
- Large-bore tubing should be used to properly evacuate blood clots.
- If aspirate is coffee-ground color or bloody, prepare patient for gastric lavage.

Begin gastric lavage, using either the iced saline or the iced saline with Levophed method, as prescribed. (See summary chart on the following page.)

If hemorrhage is due to esophageal or gastric varices, prepare patient for insertion of the Sengstaken–Blakemore tube by physician. (See Sengstaken–Blakemore tube, Chapter 25.)

Central venous pressure monitoring is indicated to determine the need for and effectiveness of fluid replacement.

Pitressin (Vasopressin) may be infused intravenously or intra-arterially into superior mesenteric artery (after angiography) to control bleeding.
- Generally used for bleeding esophageal varices, but may be used in the treatment of GI bleeding owing to other causes.

GASTRIC LAVAGE FOR PATIENT WITH ACUTE GI BLEEDING

NOTE. *Check for tube placement prior to instilllation of solutions.*

ICED SALINE METHOD
1. Instill 200 ml to 300 ml of iced saline into the stomach, using a continuous infusion system.
2. Clamp the tube to the irrigating solution.
3. Allow the solution to remain in the stomach for 2 to 3 minutes to promote vasoconstriction.
4. Unclamp drainage tube and siphon out solution by manual aspiration, using a 50-ml syringe or gravity drainage into collection bottle.
5. Using a 50-ml irrigating syringe, manually irrigate the tube frequently to dislodge blood clots regardless of the method used for solution drainage.
6. Repeat the above procedure as specified by the physician until the returns are clear or faint pink.

NOTES.
• *Do not use iced water as the irrigating solution because this may cause electrolyte depletion.*
• *Iced saline may cause an increase in circulating volume in susceptible patients due to absorption of sodium chloride. Monitor patient closely for signs of pulmonary edema and congestive heart failure.*

ICED SALINE WITH LEVOPHED METHOD
1. Add 2 ampules to 4 ampules of Levophed (levarterenol) to 1000 ml of normal saline (irrigating solution).
   • Levophed causes vasoconstriction. Systemic effects are prevented by its absorption from the stomach into the portal system and subsequent transport to the liver, where drug metabolism occurs.
2. Follow procedure for irrigating with iced saline.

• Causes general arterial vasoconstriction and decreased portal blood flow and resulting pressure.
• Should not be used in patients with coronary artery disease due to arterial vasoconstriction.

Vitamin K (AquaMephyton) may be administered intravenously or intramuscularly if clotting disorders are present.
• Monitor patient closely for hypersensitivity reaction if administered IV; anaphylaxis may occur.
• IM route preferred.

Cimetidine (Tagamet) therapy may be instituted, initially administered IV and, after bleeding has stopped, orally.

Prepare patient for more definitive diagnostic studies (upper GI series, gastroscopy, proctosigmoidoscopy, etc.) as soon as his condition stabilizes.

Prepare patient for emergency surgery as indicated. (Decision for surgical intervention depends on underlying cause, effect [*i.e.*, perforation], and the patient's response to medical therapy.)

Monitor the patient's response continuously.
- Is he becoming apprehensive?
- Does he complain of thirst?
- Both of the above may indicate continued bleeding and impending shock.
- Is he experiencing respiratory difficulty (from fluid overload)?
- Do not leave the patient unattended.

When bleeding stops, a milk–antacid regimen is started if the patient is not vomiting.
- Milk and antacids are given on an alternating basis around the clock every 1 to 2 hours.
- Include milk with intake monitoring. (Antacids are not absorbed and are not included in intake report.)
- If the patient has an underlying cardiac condition, be sure to use a low-sodium antacid.

Vital signs should continue to be monitored closely (every 15 minutes) until stable, and then every 1 to 2 hours for several hours. If the condition remains stable, advance to every 4 hours.

Continue to monitor gastric aspirate for fresh bleeding.

If not obviously bloody, check fecal material for occult blood.

Continue to monitor the patient for signs of recurring hemorrhage and resulting shock.

Administer a cathartic, as prescribed, to remove old blood. (Blood is an irritant and should be removed as soon as possible.)

25
Special Diagnostic and Therapeutic Procedures

Special procedures used in the diagnosis and treatment of acute conditions of the abdomen are described in this chapter. They include four-quadrant tap, peritoneal lavage, the various gastrointestinal tubes encountered in the critical care unit (Levin, Salem–Sump, Cantor, Miller–Abbot, Sengstaken–Blakemore), and total parenteral nutrition (TPN).

FOUR-QUADRANT TAP

Description and Purpose
Four-quadrant tap is a diagnostic procedure which involves aseptic needle puncture of the four quadrants of the abdomen for the purpose of aspirating fluid. Blood or bloody fluid is considered a positive test.

Equipment
5 10-ml syringes

4 18-gauge spinal needles (short-bevel)

25-gauge needle

Local anesthetic

Povidone-iodine solution

Sterile 4 × 4s

Collection tubes

Tape

Procedure
1. Have the patient empty his bladder, or catheterize.
2. The physician prepares the site and then injects a local anesthetic at each site.
3. Each quadrant is tapped lateral to the rectus sheath and gently aspirated.
4. Aspiration of blood or bloody fluid is considered a positive test.

NOTE. Intraperitoneal blood will not clot. If the aspirate contains blood from a blood vessel accidentally punctured, the blood will clot.

5. If the results are negative but injury is still suspected, peritoneal lavage may be performed.

NOTE. Aspirated fluid may be sent to a lab for analysis (*e.g.*, amylase, etc.).

PERITONEAL LAVAGE

Description and Purpose

Solution is introduced into the peritoneum for the purpose of evaluating the effects of trauma to the abdomen.

Contraindications

This procedure is contraindicated in the following situations:
Pregnancy
Multiple abdominal scars

Equipment

Peritoneal dialysis tray with administration set
Peritoneal dialysis catheter (with stylet and connector)
Povidone-iodine solution
1000 ml. Ringer's lactate or normal saline
Local anesthetic
IV pole
4-0 silk suture
Needle holder
#11 scalpel blade
#3 scalpel handle
Sterile 4 × 4s and 2 × 2s
Sterile gloves
Syringes—5-ml and 10-ml
Needles—22-gauge and 25-gauge
Collection bottle or bag
Razor
Tape

Preliminary Actions

1. Explain the procedure to the patient. Obtain a signed consent form.
2. Have the patient empty his bladder, or catheterize.
3. Prep the area as ordered, usually midline below the umbilicus.
   • Shave the insertion site and surrounding area.
   • Scrub the area with povidone-iodine solution.

4. Attach the cap from the administeration set to the solution bottle and prime, removing all air bubbles from tubing. Clamp. Hang the solution bottle on the IV pole.

Procedure

1. At this point, the physician puts on sterile gloves and begins the procedure.
2. Sterile drapes are placed appropriately.
3. Local anesthetic is injected.
4. A small incision (2 cm–3 cm) is made in the abdomen, and the peritoneal dialysis catheter is inserted.
5. The 10-ml syringe is attached to the catheter, and aspiration is attempted.
6. If no blood is aspirated, the physician will remove the syringe and attach the catheter to the prepared administration tubing.
7. The drainage tube is clamped.
8. The administration tubing is unclamped, allowing 1000 ml of the irrigating solution to infuse into the peritoneal cavity. (For children, use 10–20 ml/kg of body weight.)
9. Following infusion, clamp the administration tubing and turn the patient from side to side to facilitate the passage of the solution to all areas of the abdomen (unless contraindicated).
10. Unclamp the drainage tubing.
11. Bloody fluid indicates the need for emergency surgery. The physician should be made aware of this at once.

   NOTE. Drainage may be sent to the lab for analysis.

12. Following the drainage of the fluid, the physician will remove the tube and suture the incision.
13. The site is cleansed with povidone–iodine solution, and a sterile dressing (4 × 4) is applied.
14. Continue to monitor the patient for complications (perforation of viscera, general deterioration of condition).
15. Significance of the color of the blood is as follows:
    • Straw-colored—weakly positive
    • Grossly bloody—strongly positive

Comments

The absence of fluid return should be reported to the physician immediately.

The infusion should be stopped immediately and the physician notified if the following occur:
• Abdominal cramps—indicates possible perforation of bowel
• Diarrhea of abrupt onset—indicates possible perforation of bowel
• Urgent need to void—indicates possible perforation of bladder

The irrigating solution may be warmed prior to instillation by placing the solution container in a basin filled with warm water (45° C or 110° F).

If nonclotting blood is aspirated following insertion of the catheter, the test is positive, and the patient should be prepared for emergency surgery.

Intravenous tubing may be used for administration tubing. Following instillation, the empty solution bottle is placed on the floor, and the fluid is siphoned from the peritoneal cavity.

GASTROINTESTINAL TUBES

Description

Several types of gastrointestinal tubes are encountered in the critical care unit. Tubes may be inserted through the mouth or the nose, and may be used for diagnosis or treatment. The insertion of specific gastrointestinal tubes and the nursing care associated with their use are described.

LEVIN TUBE

Type

One lumen

Use

Decompression of stomach or upper intestine

Gastric lavage

Administering feedings or medications

Obtaining specimen for analysis

Size

10 Fr to 18 Fr (smaller size used for children)

16 Fr to 18 Fr (used most commonly for adults)

Equipment

Levin tube

Asepto syringe

Adapter

Water-soluble lubricating jelly

Tape

Towel

Emesis basin

Glass of water

Straw

Intermittent suction source

Suction and suction catheters

Stethoscope

Inserted by

Nurse or physician

Procedure

1. Explain the procedure to the patient.
2. Raise the head of the bed slightly (30°–40°).
3. Place the patient on his back, with his head in normal alignment. Do not hyperextend neck.
4. Place towel across patient's chest to protect clothing.
5. Keep emesis basin close at hand.
6. Measure tube as follows:
   • Adult patient
     • Measure tube from ear lobe to bridge of nose, to bottom of xiphoid process, to approximate the distance necessary to reach the stomach. Mark the length with a piece of tape.
   • Pediatric patient
     • Newborn (premature and full-term)—measure tube from bridge of nose to just beyond tip of sternum.
     • Child—measure tube from tip of nose, past the ear, to tip of sternum.
7. Lubricate 3 inches to 4 inches of tubing with a water-soluble jelly.
8. Insert through the nose if no nasal deformity is present.
9. After reaching the pharynx, have the patient swallow sips of water.
10. As he does so, advance the tube 2 inches to 3 inches with each swallow.
11. Continue to advance the tube in this manner until the second or third mark from the end is even with the nose.
12. Check for proper tube position by using one of the following methods:
    • Attach the aseptic syringe to the tubing and aspirate the gastric contents.
    • Place a stethoscope over the epigastrium and inject a small (5 ml) amount of air through the tube. A gurgling or whooshing sound is heard if the tube is in the stomach.
    • Place the end of tube in water. Bubbling indicates tube is in trachea. Remove tube at once if this occurs.
13. Secure the tube to the nose with tape.
14. Connect to low, intermittent suction for continuous drainage.

Special Considerations

Do not force tube if resistance is met. Switch to other nostril.

If used for feedings (gavage) or administration of medications, tube should be clamped following instillation.

Tube should be irrigated every 2 hours, or as ordered, and following feedings or medication instillation with a small amount (15 ml–30 ml) of water. Include amount used on intake record.

Administer frequent mouth care.

Apply cream to nose and lips.

Keep the head of the bed elevated slightly to prevent reflux of gastric contents into the esophagus.

ALERT. Use extreme caution with insertion in the semiconscious or unconscious patient because of the danger of aspiration.

A cuffed, endotracheal tube must be inserted prior to lavage in the unconscious patient.

- This patient should be kept in head-down position for insertion and lavage. (See gastric lavage.)

Keep suction and catheters readily available at all times.

SALEM-SUMP TUBE

Type

Two-lumen—second lumen serves as air vent to prevent blockage of the suction lumen

Use

See Levin tube.

Size

See Levin tube.

Equipment

Salem–Sump tube

(See Levin tube.)

Inserted by

Nurse or physician

Procedure

See Levin-tube insertion.

Special Considerations

See Levin tube, p 275.

CANTOR TUBE

Type

Single-lumen with balloon attached to tip

Marked at specific intervals: S = stomach
P = pylorus
D = duodenum

Contains perforations for aspiration of intestinal contents

Use

Intestinal decompression

Size

12 Fr (pediatric)

16 Fr (adult)

Equipment

Cantor tube

5-ml syringe

21-gauge needle

10 ml of mercury

Asepto syringe

Adaptor

Glass of water

Straw

Water-soluble lubricating jelly

Intermittent suction source

Topical anesthetic (may be used)

Towel

NOTE. Test the balloon for patiency and adherence to tubing prior to beginning.

Inserted by

Physician

Procedure

1. The mercury (approximately 5 ml) is injected into the bag prior to insertion.
2. After insertion, the tube is slowly passed, through the esophagus and stomach, into the duodenum.
3. The tube is then connected to low, intermittent suction.

Special Considerations

The patient should lie on his right side to facilitate entry into the duodenum.

The tube is advanced 2 inches every 30 minutes to 60 minutes by the nurse.

Tube position is checked 2 hours following insertion by abdominal x-ray film.

Do not tape the tubing to the patient's nose. It must be free to travel by gravity and peristalsis.

Protect the tube from being inadvertently removed or pulled from position.

MILLER–ABBOTT TUBE

Type

Double-lumen with balloon attached

Use

Intestinal decompression

Size

18 Fr

Equipment

Miller–Abbott tube
20-ml syringe
3 ml mercury
Water-soluble lubricating jelly
Topical anesthetic
Glass of water
Straw
Intermittent suction source
Towel

NOTE. Check the balloon for leaks by injecting air. Inflate thoroughly prior to insertion.

Inserted by

Physician

Procedure

1. After insertion, the tube is passed through the esophagus and into the stomach.
2. Approximately 1 ml of mercury will then be injected into the balloon to facilitate entry into the duodenum.
3. After passage into the duodenum, the physician will inject 20 ml of air into the bag (depends on pretested volume).
4. The tube is then connected to low, intermittent suction.

Special Considerations

The patient should lie on his right side to facilitate entry into the duodenum.

The tube is advanced 2 inches every 30 minutes to 60 minutes as ordered.

Tube position is checked 2 hours following insertion by abdominal x-ray film.

Do not tape the tubing to the patient's nose. It must be free to travel by gravity and peristalsis.

Protect the tube from being inadvertently removed or pulled from position.

SENGSTAKEN–BLAKEMORE TUBE

Type

Triple-lumen—for aspiration of gastric contents and inflation of two balloons

Proximal balloon—will be positioned in distal esophagus

Distal balloon—will be positioned in cardio-esophageal junction

Use

Control of bleeding caused by esophageal and gastric varices

Size

Standard size

Equipment

2 Sengstaken–Blakemore tubes

Sphygmomanometer (with 2½ feet of rubber tubing)

50-ml syringe

Lidocaine jelly

2 suction sources

Cube of sponge rubber

Y-connector

Adhesive tape

Topical anesthetic (lidocaine)

4 hemostats (rubber-tipped)

Scissors

Glass of water

Straw

NOTE. Both balloons should be checked for leaks prior to insertion by inflating with air and holding under water. Thoroughly deflate both balloons after check.

Inserted by

Physician

Procedure

1. After insertion, the tube is gently passed into the esophagus and the stomach. Proper positioning is essential to prevent inflation of the gastric balloon in the esophagus.

2. At this point, the physician will inject 150 ml to 200 ml of air into the gastric balloon and then double-clamp the air-intake valve.

3. Traction is then applied to pull the inflated balloon snugly against the cardia of the stomach, indicated by meeting resistance.

4. Maintaining this traction, a foam sponge is placed around the tube at its point of exit from the nose and is taped in place. (Tube may be attached to a football helmet with mouthguard.)

5. The esophageal balloon is then inflated with a sphygmomanometer to 40 mm Hg and is double clamped.

6. Using an asepto syringe, gastric contents are aspirated through the third outlet, and then the tube is attached to intermittent suction.

Special Considerations

A nasogastric tube is sometimes inserted through the opposite nostril to a position beside the Sengstaken–Blakemore tube in the upper esophagus to prevent the danger of aspiration and to remove secretions.

The patient is kept NPO. Remember: The esophagus is totally occluded.

Monitor the balloon pressures every 30 minutes to 60 minutes.

Lavage the stomach every 30 minutes to 60 minutes to remove blood clots and to prevent occlusion of the tube.

Keep the head of the bed elevated.

Keep a pair of scissors at the bedside at all times. Rupture of the gastric balloon may result in complete airway obstruction due to the rising of the tube into the nasopharynx. The tube should be cut immediately and then removed.

Provide frequent mouth care and suction as necessary.

Continuously monitor patient for symptoms of esophageal rupture. Report to physician immediately.

The esophageal balloon may remain inflated for up to 72 hours. Periodically, the nurse may lower the pressure according to the degree ordered by the physician.

The gastric balloon may remain inflated for up to 24 hours. It is the physician's responsibility to deflate this balloon.

Generally, the balloon is deflated following cessation of bleeding for 24 hours. If bleeding does not recur, the tube is cut and removed.

An extra tube should be kept at the bedside in case balloon rupture occurs, necessitating insertion of a new one.

TOTAL PARENTERAL NUTRITION (TPN)

Description and Purpose

Total parenteral nutrition, also known as parenteral hyperalimentation, is indicated in any condition in which the gastrointestinal tract is unable to function adequately. The catheter is inserted under strict, aseptic conditions.

General Information

Solutions contain hypertonic glucose, electrolytes, amino acids, vitamins, minerals, and other trace elements.

The catheter is placed in regions of high blood flow because the solution is hypertonic and would cause thrombosis at the catheter tip very quickly.

Ideally, the TPN solution should be prepared in the pharmacy under a laminar air-flow unit.

The solution must be refrigerated until used.

The solution expires in 24 hours from the time of preparation.

Nothing else should be infused via the TPN line.

If albumin is included in the solution, a final filter should not be used because the albumin will not pass through it.

Blood volume should be normal to ensure adequate venous pressure, which facilitates venipuncture.

The catheter is usually inserted into the subclavian vein and is passed into the superior vena cava.

Equipment

Subclavian catheter—16-gauge, 20-cm (8-in)

Cutdown tray

5% dextrose in water, 500 ml, for IV infusion (with macrodrip and extension tubing without stopcock)

TPN solution

Face masks

Sterile gowns

Sterile gloves

2 3-ml syringes with 25-gauge needles

Local anesthesia (Xylocaine 1%)

Povidone-iodine solution and ointment

Alcohol or alcohol wipes

3-0 silk suture

Dressing—2 × 2s, 4 × 4s

Tincture of benzoin spray

Tape (1 in)

IV pole

IVAC or Holter pump

Prep tray (if necessary)

Rolled towel

One bottle of acetone or ether

Sterile adhesive-backed drape or dressing

NOTE. All equipment (including tape and solutions) should be fresh.

Preliminary Actions

1. Explain the procedure to the patient.
2. Wash hands thoroughly, using surgical scrub technique, before setting up any equipment.
3. If excessive body hair is present, shave a large area around the insertion site.
4. Set up IV with 5% dextrose in water.
   - Prime the tubing.
   - Make sure all air is expelled.
5. Place patient in a supine position with the head turned opposite to the insertion site.
6. Place in Trendelenberg position (45°) to prevent an air embolus during insertion and to facilitate catheter entry by dilating vessels in the shoulder and neck.
7. A rolled towel may be placed vertically along the spinal column to hyperextend the shoulder.
8. At this point, everyone in the room should be masked and the physician will gown and glove.
9. Open the sterile tray. Pour solution into containers (acetone, povidone–iodine, or tincture of iodine and alcohol).

Procedure

(Assist the physician.)

1. The area is initially cleaned with acetone to remove oil on the skin.
2. Then, povidone–iodine or tincture of iodine is applied, and the area is thoroughly cleaned, going in a circular motion from inside to out. It is allowed to dry 5 minutes to achieve maximum effects.
3. The tincture of iodine is then removed with alcohol to prevent skin irritation.

NOTE. Povidone–iodine should not be removed.

4. The area is then draped with sterile towels or drapes, and the physician begins the procedure. Using a large needle attached to a syringe, the physician begins the procedure.

5. After the needle is inserted and after the position in the vein is confirmed by aspiration of blood, the patient is instructed to perform the Valsalva maneuver (bear down), before the syringe is removed, to prevent the introduction of an air embolus during introduction of the catheter.

6. The syringe is removed and the catheter is advanced into place.

7. The primed IV system is connected to the catheter and is maintained at a keep-open rate. (The TPN solution should not be hung until x-ray films confirming the position have been taken.)

8. The physician will suture the catheter in place. Be sure to note and document the number of sutures applied.

9. The physician will lower the IV solution momentarily to check for proper positioning (determined by venous backflow into the IV tubing).

10. The drapes are removed.

11. The bed is returned to normal position and the patient is made comfortable.

Continuing Care—Dressing

1. Repeat the skin preparation using strict aseptic technique.

2. Place povidone-iodine ointment on sterile dressing (double thickness) and apply to insertion site.

3. Using benzoin spray or Elastoplast spray, spray the area surrounding the site and allow to dry (should be sticky).

4. Create an air-tight dressing by:
   • Covering the dressing with a sterile adhesive-backed drape or dressing.
   • Sealing all borders with adhesive tape.
   • Making sure all edges are firmly sealed, including the area under the catheter hub.

5. Tape all connections of the IV system, including the catheter, to prevent separation.

6. Anchor IV tubing with tape on patient's skin. (If filter is used, system should be anchored here.)

7. Label the dressing: date, time, and initials of person applying it.

8. Prepare patient for follow-up chest x-ray study.

9. After catheter position is confirmed, connect TPN solution to the system.
   • An IVAC pump should be used.
   • When connecting the solution, be sure to place the patient in Trendelenberg position and have him perform the Valsalva maneuver while the tubing is quickly switched from the "keep-open" solution to the TPN solution.
   • Adjust flow rate as ordered.

10. Monitor patient closely for complications (*i.e.*, symptoms of air embolism, pneumotherax, hematoma at insertion site, protein allergy).

Special Considerations

It is imperative that the solution be infused as ordered.
- If the rate gets behind, do not speed up, but recalculate to ordered rate.
- Ideally, an IVAC should be used to keep the flow rate constant.
- A rate that is either too slow or too fast may cause hypoglycemia or hyperglycemia, respectively.
- A rate that is too fast causes hyperosmolar diuresis (an excessive excretion of sugar). If severe, this condition may be fatal.
- The flow rate should be checked every 30 minutes.

Vital signs should be checked every 2 hours or as ordered.
- Any abnormalities, especially temperature changes, should be reported to the physician immediately.
- Sepsis is indicated by:
  - Temperature spikes
  - Low-grade temperatures that may or may not be constant
  - A grossly elevated temperature with signs of sepsis

NOTE. Glucose intolerance is another sign (early) of sepsis.

TPN solution should not be used if cloudy or if precipitates are observed.
- If any precipitation is noted in the system, the line should be discontinued immediately and 10% dextrose in water should be hung.
- Notify the physician and pharmacy (if solution is made there) immediately.

Serum electrolytes should be checked closely to monitor the effects of therapy.

Urine sugar, acetone, and specific gravity should be checked as ordered or every 6 hours.

TPN solution should be changed at least every 12 hours.

Weigh daily.

Monitor intake and output closely.

The IV tubing should be changed every time a new bag of TPN solution is hung.
- Strict aseptic technique must be used.
- New tubing should be primed with TPN solution.
- Exposed tubing on extension line should be thoroughly cleaned with a povidone-iodine swab prior to connection to the new system.
- Place the patient in Trendelenberg position and instruct him to perform a Valsalva maneuver during the tubing change.

The tubing is changed and cultured if infection is considered.
- The catheter may have to be removed.
- This should be cultured, also.

TPN DRESSING CHANGE

Equipment

Povidone-iodine solution and ointment, or tincture of iodine

Acetone or ether

Alcohol or alcohol wipes

Tincture of benzoin spray or Elastoplast spray

Sterile adhesive-backed drape

Adhesive tape

Sterile 2 × 2s, 4 × 4s

3 sterile solution bowls (small)

Sterile suture set

Sterile towel or drape

Sterile gloves—2 pair

Mask

Procedure

1. Explain the procedure to the patient.
2. Put on mask.
3. Set up equipment. Pour solutions into containers (acetone, povidone-iodine, or tincture of iodine and alcohol).
4. Place patient in semi-Fowler's position or supine position.
5. Put on sterile gloves.
6. Remove old dressing entirely.
7. Remove gloves and put on a sterile pair.
8. Use sterile towel for draping the patient.
9. Clean areas as before for insertion of TPN line.
10. Apply dressing as before for insertion of TPN line.
11. Label the dressing with the date, time, and initials of the person applying it. Document in nurse's notes.

VII

Burns

26

Care of the Burn Patient

The assessment, treatment, and nursing care of the burned patient are covered in this chapter. Methods of evaluating the depth and extent of burn injury, phases reflecting systemic changes, specific treatment (fluid replacement, methods of wound care with skin grafting, topical chemotherapy), and general nursing considerations are described.

FACTORS IN THE ASSESSMENT OF BURN INJURIES

Cause of the Burn Injury

Heat
- Dry heat—flame, hot metal, hot grease
- Moist heat—steam, boiling water

Chemicals
- Acids
- Alkalies
- Phosphorus

Electricity
- Lightning
- Electric current source

Radiation
- Ultraviolet rays
- X-rays
- Radioactive substances

Patient's Age and General Health Status

Obtain from history and observation.

These factors affect prognosis and treatment.

Methods Used to Calculate the Extent of Burn Injury

The rule of nines—specific areas of the body are assigned numerical values, all multiples of 9 (Fig. 26-1).

Burn evaluation chart based on the percentage of areas affected by growth (*i.e.,* according to age; Fig. 26-2).

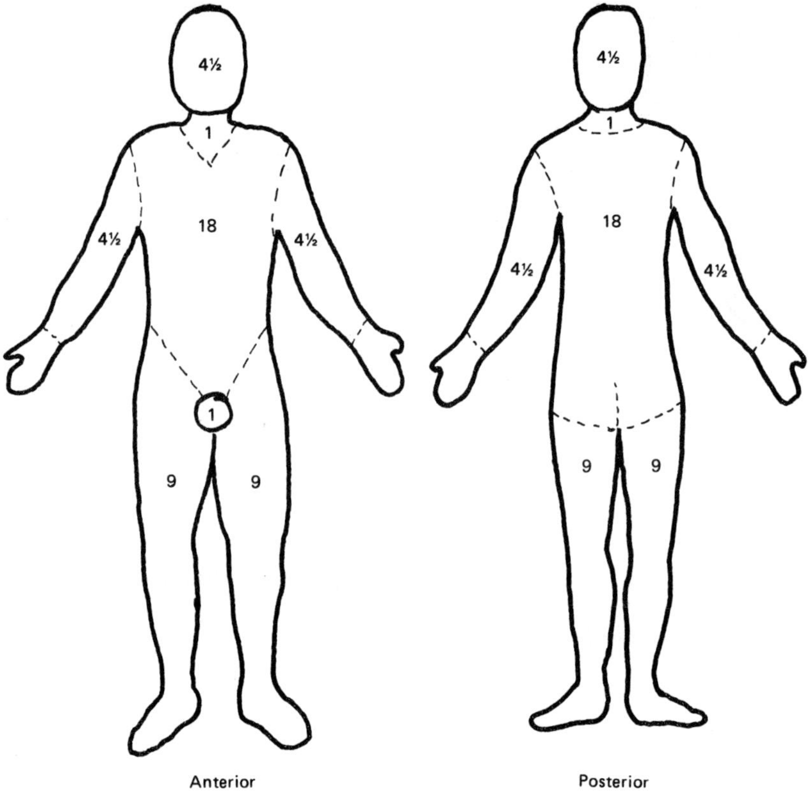

FIG. 26-1. *Burn evaluation chart based on "Rule of Nines."* (Left) *anterior,* (right) *posterior.*

Depth of Burn

Depth of burn may not be clearly visible at first, but a rough estimate can be made. Characteristics of first, second, third, and fourth degree burns are presented in Table 26-1.

First degree burn—partial thickness, involves epidermis

Second degree burn—involves epidermis and part of dermis
- Superficial—partial thickness
- Deep—deep partial thickness

Third degree burn—full thickness; involves epidermis, dermis, and subcutaneous tissue

Fourth degree burn—full thickness; involves epidermis, dermis, subcutaneous tissue, and may include subcutaneous fat, muscles, and bone

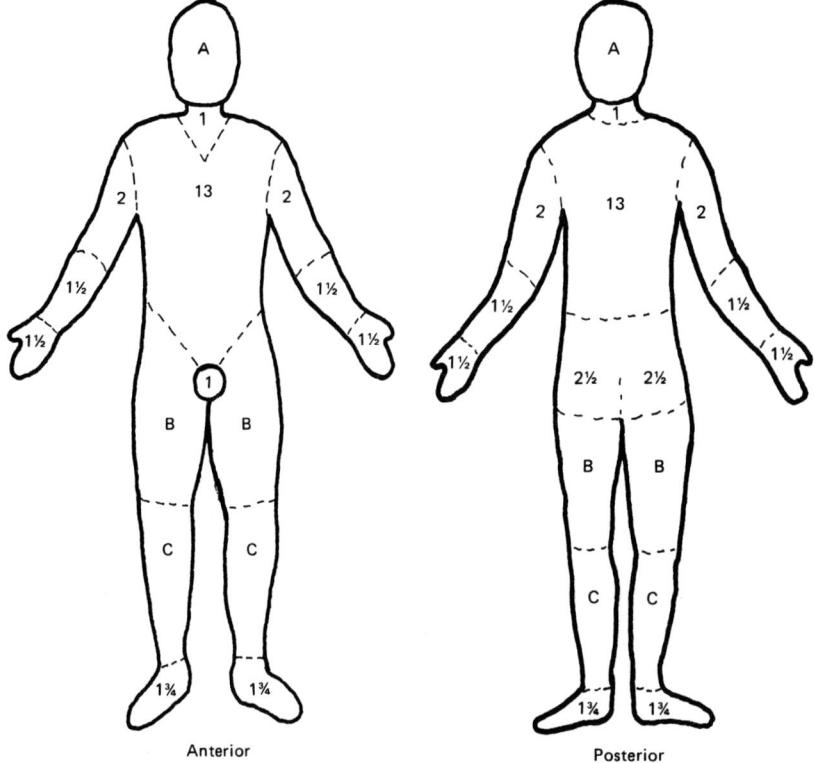

	Age in Years					
	0	1	5	10	15	Adult
A = ½ head	9½	8½	6½	5½	4½	3½
B = ½ one thigh	2¾	3¼	4	4¼	4½	4¾
C = ½ one leg	2½	2½	2¾	3	3¼	3½

FIG. 26-2. *Burn evaluation chart based on percentage of areas affected by growth.* (Left) *anterior,* (right) *posterior. Areas on chart with numerical designations remain fairly constant from birth through adulthood. Areas on chart with letter designations vary according to age.*

Location of Burn

This factor is important because a burn in one area can affect another. For example, burns of the head may affect the respiratory system. Burns of the hands, feet, face, and perineum are associated with severe effects (disease [*e.g.*, infection] and death).

Table 26-1. **Characteristics of First, Second, Third, and Fourth Degree Burns.**

Type	Clinical Manifestations	Healing Period	Scarring
First Degree (partial thickness)	Redness of skin No blister formation	1 wk (skin grafting not necessary)	No
Second Degree			
Superficial (partial thickness)	Redness of skin Blister formation Edema	10 da–2 wk (skin grafting not necessary)	No
Deep (partial thickness)	White blister formation May or may not be sensitive to touch Resembles third degree burn	Several wk–2 mo (skin grafting may be done to speed up healing process but is not necessary)	Yes
Third Degree (full thickness)	Whitened or browned skin Reddened areas do not blanch when pressure is applied No pain Leathery appearance Massive edema	Depends on extent, location, and success of skin grafting	Yes
Fourth Degree (full thickness)	Charred Depressed area May extend down to bone	Depends on extent, location, and success of skin grafting	Yes

PHASES REFLECTING SYSTEMIC CHANGES DUE TO BURN INJURIES

In the hours, days, and weeks following a burn injury, the systemic changes brought about by the burn become evident. Three general phases can be identified—a shock phase (plasma-interstitial fluid shift), a phase of fluid remobilization (state of diuresis) and a recovery phase.

SHOCK PHASE (PLASMA-TO-INTERSTITIAL FLUID SHIFT)
Time Interval Postburn

First 48 hours (especially first 8 hours following the burn)

Significant Laboratory Values

Elevated serum potassium

Decreased serum sodium

Elevated hematocrit

Bicarbonate deficit

Clinical Manifestations

Decreased blood pressure

Decreased cardiac output

Oliguria or anuria

Edema

Dehydration

Elevated pulse

Shock

Metabolic acidosis

FLUID REMOBILIZATION PHASE (STATE OF DIURESIS)

Time Interval Postburn

48 to 72 hours following the burn

Significant Laboratory Values

Decreased hematocrit

Decreased serum sodium

Decreased serum potassium

Bicarbonate deficit

Clinical Manifestations

Increased urine output (tremendous increase)

Pulmonary edema due to circulatory overload

RECOVERY PHASE

Time Interval Postburn

5 days following the burn

Significant Laboratory Values

Decreased serum calcium, serum sodium, and serum potassium

Negative nitrogen balance (may last throughout convalescence)

Clinical Manifestation

Weight loss

TREATMENT

FLUID REPLACEMENT

Fluid replacement is a primary concern in the treatment of the burned patient. Standardized formulas are modified by the physician for the individual patient. The Brooke, Baxter or Parkland, and Evans formulas are presented in the Formulas for Estimating Fluid Replacement chart.

FORMULAS FOR ESTIMATING FLUID REPLACEMENT

NOTE. Colloids include whole blood plasma and plasma expanders. Electrolytes include normal saline, lactated Ringer's solution, and Hartman's solution.

BROOKE FORMULA
First 24 hours
- Colloids 0.5 ml × weight in kilograms × percent of burn (body surface area)
- Electrolytes 1.5 ml × weight in kilograms × percent of burn
- Five percent dextrose in 2000 ml water (proportionately less in children)

NOTE. One half of the above total should be administered during the first 8 hours and the rest over the remaining 16 hours.

Second 24 hours
- One half of the colloids and electrolyte solutions + all of the 5% dextrose in water

BAXTER OR PARKLAND FORMULA
First 24 hours
- 4 ml of lactated Ringer's solution × weight in kilograms × percent of burn.

NOTE. One half of the formula is administered during the first eight hours and the rest over the remaining 16 hours.

Second 24 hours
- Fluids administered by mouth
- No formula used

EVANS FORMULA
First 24 hours
- Colloids 1 ml × weight in kilograms × percent of burn
- Electrolytes 1 ml × weight in kilograms × percent of burn
- Five percent glucose in 2000 ml water (proportionately less in children)

Second 24 hours
- One half of the colloid and one half of the electrolytes + all of the 5% dextrose in water

METHODS OF TREATING BURN WOUNDS
OPEN (EXPOSURE) METHOD

Air dries the exudate forming a hard crust within 3 days, which serves as a protective barrier.

This method is used most commonly to treat burns of the face, neck, perineum, and extensive trunk burns.

Skin regeneration under crusts occurs within 2-3 weeks in a second degree burn.

There is no regeneration under eschar. The eschar of a third degree burn generally separates within 2 to 3 weeks. Grafting is usually indicated.

Temperature and humidity regulation in the room is imperative to prevent loss of body fluids due to overheating or excess expenditure of energy due to shivering.

Reverse isolation is required. All dressings, clothing, or linen should be sterile.

Environment must be kept as clean as possible.

If the wound has adhered to linen or clothing, moisten the area with sterile normal saline, and leave in place for a few minutes until the material can be removed without causing trauma. Special sheeting that is placed over the regular bedding and prevents wound adherence is available commercially.

Occlusive (Pressure) Method

The occlusive method is most commonly used for burns of hands and feet.

Fine mesh gauze with a topical antimicrobial agent impregnated in it is applied next to the wound. It is covered with a dressing and held in place with an elastic bandage or stockinette dressing.

Care must be taken to dress the fingers and toes separately and in positions of function.

This method is useful for holding grafts in place and protecting them.

Bandage must be changed if drainage is noted.

There is a high incidence of infection.

Circulation below the dressing must be checked closely.

Pain during dressing change is a problem

If dressing has adhered to wound, it must be saturated with sterile normal saline and left in place for a few minutes until it can be removed without causing trauma.

OPEN WOUND WITH TOPICAL ANTIMICROBIALS (SEMIOPEN)

The wound is left open.

Topical antimicrobials are applied directly to the site.

Usually, a single-layer dressing is applied and held in place by a net tube dressing (or other single layer bandage).

The wound is cleaned and debrided as usual, with all the medication thoroughly removed. Then, a fresh layer of medication is applied and redressed as discussed.

WET DRESSINGS

The burn wound is covered with a dressing and kept wet with a prescribed solution ($\frac{1}{2}$% silver nitrate, normal saline). It is then covered with a dry sterile towel to prevent excess evaporation.

Dressing must be kept wet.

Sometimes a fine mesh gauze is applied next to the wound to aid in debridement.

GRAFTS (BIOLOGICAL DRESSINGS)

Grafts may be used as a protective cover (homograft or heterograft) or to aid in the formation of granulation tissue (autograft).

Types of Grafts

Autograft—taken from patient; permanent graft

Homograft (allograft)—taken from cadaver

Heterograft (xenograft)—taken from a different species (*e. g.*, pig or porcine skin)

Description of Grafts

Full thickness—includes the epidermis and dermis (all layers)

Split thickness—varies in thickness from thin (0.10 in) to thick (0.35 in); does not include the deeper layers of the dermis

Pinch (Punch)—small piece of graft obtained

Mesh—slits cut in graft, giving it a meshlike apperance; may then be stretched to cover a wider area; this technique provides good drainage, preventing fluid collection under the graft which might prevent it from taking

Free—taken from one site (donor site) and moved to wound

Pedicle—the donor site is separated on three sides only; the fourth side remains in the normal site; the other three sides are grafted to the desired area; blood supply to the graft is maintained

Priority of Locations for Grafting

Hands

Face

Neck

Areas of motion (*e.g.*, joints, axillae)

Method of Application

Grafting may be used in conjunction with the open or occlusive method of treating wounds.

• Open method—the grafted area must be immobilized for 2 to 3 days to prevent motion that would tear or pull the graft from its position. The physician may order sterile saline compresses to be applied at regular intervals for short periods to provide adequate humidity.

• Occlusive method—the dressing immobilizes the graft. Excess motion should be prevented.

It is imperative that the graft be flat against the wound. This is usually accomplished by rolling a sterile cotton applicator or swab gently over the graft to smooth the surface and edges. Remove any air or fluid trapped underneath.

A graft is said to be "taking" when circulation is established connecting the wound and graft and when it is providing nourishment.

Homografts or heterografts are replaced approximately every 3 days.

• They are used to protect the wound, prevent fluid loss, and prevent the introduction of bacteria.

• They are only temporary and are replaced as soon as possible by an autograft.

When changing the dressing over a graft, saturate it with sterile normal saline, leave it in place for a few minutes, and then gently remove it without disturbing the graft.

TOPICAL CHEMOTHERAPY FOR BURNS
SILVER NITRATE SOLUTION

Comments

0.5% solution is used.

• Solutions below 0.5% are ineffective.

• Solutions above 1% cause necrosis of the tissues.

Fine-mesh gauze (without the cotton filler) is applied to the wound and saturated with silver nitrate solution. A stockinette dressing is placed over the gauze to keep it in place.

The entire dressing is kept wet (approximately every 2–4 hr) by using a bulb syringe to saturate it.

The dressing is changed as ordered, which may vary from every 12 hours to several days.

Advantages

Inexpensive

Highly effective

Caps, gowns, and masks not necessary

Can be applied to grafts and donor sites

Disadvantages

Silver nitrate solution does not penetrate the eschar which may allow an infection to occur under it.

It is not effective in the presence of oil or grease on the wound.

It may cause hyponatremia, hypokalemia and hypochloremia.

Serum electrolytes must be checked frequently and imbalances corrected.

Silver nitrate solution stains everything it comes in contact with.

MAFENIDE ACETATE (SULFAMYLON CREAM)

Comments

Mafenide acetate is applied to wound in a thin layer (2–4 mm or 1/16 in) Fine mesh gauze is used to cover the area to keep the cream in place.

The cream is removed and the dressing is changed once or twice a day, preferably by placing the patient in a Hubbard tank.

Advantages

Penetrates the eschar

Effective against a broad range of gram-negative and gram-positive organisms

Disadvantages

Mafenide acetate causes sensitivity reactions.

It is a carbonic anhydrase inhibitor which may cause metabolic acidosis due to disturbance of the acid-base balance. Arterial blood gases and pH should be monitored closely.

It is not recommended for use in the presence of pulmonary disease because of an inability to maintain an adequate acid-base balance.

It causes pain (burning sensation) following application, which is usually temporary. Pain medication may be indicated prior to use.

GENTAMICIN SULFATE 0.1% (GARAMYCIN CREAM)

Comments

Gentamicin sulfate is applied in a similar manner as Mafenide Acetate (Sulfamylon Cream).

Advantages

Effective against a broad range of gram-positive and gram-negative organisms

Easy application

No stain (becomes invisible)

Not painful

Disadvantages

Gentamicin sulfate causes sensitivity reactions.

It may promote the growth of gentamicin-resistant organisms; it is primarily used for the most critically burned patient.

It causes nephrotoxicity. (Creatinine levels must be closely monitored.)

POVIDONE-IODINE

Comments

Povidone-iodine is applied in similar manner as Mafenide Acetate (Sulfamylon Cream)

Advantages

Available in solution, spray, or cream

Effective against a broad range of gram-negative and gram-positive organisms, and fungi, viruses, and yeast

May cause staining but can be removed if washed immediately

Disadvantages

Povidone-iodine causes sensitivity reactions.

It may cause crusting.

It may cause staining.

SILVER SULFADIAZINE 1% (SILVADENE)

Comments

Silver sulfadiazine is a combination of sulfadiazine and silver nitrate.

It is applied directly to wound (2–4 mm or 1/16 in thick) or in impregnated gauze.

The area may be left open.

The wound should be kept covered with the medication at all times.

Advantages

Painless

Does not disturb electrolytes or acid-base balance

No stain

Effective against a wide range of gram-negative and gram-positive organisms, and candida albicans

Disadvantages

Silver sulfadiazine causes sensitivity reactions (usually to sulfa).

It is contraindicated for use in term pregnancy, and premature and newborn infants up to one month because sulfa increases the possibility of kernicterus.

GENERAL NURSING CARE OF THE PATIENT WITH SEVERE BURNS
IMMEDIATE CARE

1. Stop the burn process.
   * Remove burned clothing if possible. It may have to be done in conjunction with hydrotherapy.
   * Cool the burn if necessary.

2. Assess the patient closely for respiratory damage.
   * Check to see if the hairs in his nose are singed.
   * Find out if the burn occurred in an enclosed area.
   * Examine the mouth and pharnyx for evidence of damage (will be sooty).
   * Check for shortness of breath, hoarseness, and difficulty in swallowing.
   * Check for blood-tinged or sooty sputum.
   * Check for cyanosis. (As usual, this is a late sign of damage.)
   * Check for circumferential burns on the chest inhibiting normal chest excursion.
   * Obtain arterial blood gases.
   * Obtain chest x-ray film.

3. Support respiratory function.
   * Keep the airway patent.
   * Suction with extreme care to prevent doing more damage.
   * Administer oxygen therapy as ordered.
   * Entubation and mechanical ventilation may be indicated.

4. Closely monitor vital signs and ECG.
   * Neurological signs should be checked for effects of decreased cardiac output.
   * Pulse and respirations are increased.
   * Blood pressure is decreased and falling (preshock).
   * Notify physician immediately concerning significant findings.

5. Treat shock accordingly if present.

6. Start an IV in a large vein using a large bore needle.
   * Use a peripheral and central line if needed.
   * Administer Ringer's lactate solution as ordered. Several formulas are used to determine composition of fluid and amount. (See Formulas for Estimating Fluid Replacement chart, p 294.)
   * Begin blood transfusions if indicated. (Observe closely for transfusion reactions.)

7. Assess the depth and extent of the burn. (See Table 26-1, Figs. 26-1 and 26-2.)

8. Begin hemodynamic monitoring.
   * Central venous pressure line
   * Pulmonary artery catheter
   * Arterial line

9. Obtain the following laboratory studies:
   * Complete blood cell count
   * Serum electrolytes

- Type and crossmatch (blood)
- Blood urea nitrogen
- Creatinine
- Albumin and total protein
- Arterial blood gases
- Serum glucose
- Urinalysis (glucose, hemoglobin, and myoglobin)
- Bilirubin
- Alkaline phosphatase
- Calcium
- Phosphorus

ONGOING CARE

1. Monitor intake and output strictly.
   - Insert an indwelling urinary catheter.
   - Maintain output with fluid replacement (30–50 ml/hr—adult, 20–30 ml/hr—child over 2 yr; 10–20 ml/hr—infant).
   - Check specific gravity, pH, glucose, and acetone.
   - Infuse large volumes of fluid.
   - Watch patient closely for signs of fluid overload (*e.g.*, pulmonary edema, heart failure)
   - Watch for signs of dehydration. Fluid replacement may not be meeting the specific patient's needs.
   - Weigh patient.
2. Begin ECG monitoring. A 12-lead ECG is indicated in the elderly patient or in the patient with cardiac disease or signs of cardiac complications.
3. Insert a nasogastric tube and attach to low suction to keep the stomach decompressed.
   - Paralytic ileus is not unusual in this situation.
   - An antacid should be instilled every 2 hours or as prescribed to prevent Curling's ulcer (gastrointestinal ulcer), another common complication of severe burns.
   - Fluid should not be given by mouth unless ordered by physician.
     - Electrolyte solutions may be tolerated.
     - Plain tap water may cause water intoxication.
4. Assess for other injuries.
   - The patient should be thoroughly assessed for other injuries and treated accordingly (*e. g.*, fractures, chest injuries, hemorrhage, head injuries, etc.).
5. Administer pain medication as prescribed.
   - Small doses of morphine are usually administered. (Contraindicated in the presence of respiratory depression.)
   - Sedatives may be administered if respiratory depression prevents narcotic administration.
   - Medications should be given IV only in the critically ill patient.
   - Analgesics should be given at least 20 minutes prior to dressing changes.
   - Remember that hypoxia can also cause pain and discomfort.

6. Administer tetanus prophylaxis to prevent disease.
   - Toxoid is administered if the patient was previously immunized.
   - Tetanus immune globulin is administered if the patient was not previously immunized.
7. Administer antibiotics as prescribed.
   - Burn wounds are considered contaminated.
   - Antibiotics are given IV.
8. Place the patient in a flat position until the cardiovascular system is stabilized.
9. Protect the skin from infection.
   - All bedding or clothing in contact with the patient should be sterile.
   - All personnel should wear caps, mask, and sterile gowns and gloves in the vicinity of the patient.
   - Strict aseptic technique should be used with any procedure, including sterile solutions for cleaning the wound.
   - The patient's room should be aseptically clean.
   - Only personnel necessary for assisting in care should be allowed in room.
   - Family members should be required to wear sterile gowns when visiting the patient.

   NOTE. The purpose of the sterile surgical garb should be explained to the patient and family. It may only frighten the patient and make him feel isolated unless adequate explanations are given.

10. Provide emotional support throughout the hospital stay.
    - Explain to the patient what is happening.
    - Organize care to prevent causing undue pain and anxiety.
    - Enlist the patient's and his family's help in his care as much as possible.
    - Spend some time with patient free of painful procedures just to talk and answer any questions he may have.
    - Provide diversional therapy.
11. Meet the patient's nutritional needs.
    - Following the return of bowel sounds, liquids are allowed and the patient advances to a full diet as tolerated (usually by the end of the first week).
    - The diet should be high protein (3 gm of protein/kgm of body weight) and high calorie (3000–6000 calories).
    - Vitamin supplements are administered, especially vitamin C.
    - Electrolytes may be supplemented, depending on lab tests.
    - Nutritional status should be checked by weighing the patient daily.
    - Total parenteral nutrition may be indicated.
12. Properly position the patient throughout his care.
    - If possible, put patient through range of motion exercises (passive initially and active). Check with physician before beginning.
    - Ambulation is started as soon as possible.

- More intense physical therapy may be indicated.
- Circular beds (CircOlectric Bed) or the Stryker frame may be used to assist in position changes for the patient with severe burns.

13. Maintain the proper temperature in the room.
    - The room should be kept at 76°F (24.4°C).
    - If the room is too cold, shivering will occur, using up energy resources.
    - If too warm, increased vasodilation occurs, causing the loss of more fluid by perspiration.
    - Drafts should be prevented because they are painful to the patient.
    - Patient and the room temperature should be checked frequently.

WOUND CARE

1. Clean the wound using strict aseptic technique.
   - Gently remove debris with sterile 4 × 4s and normal saline solution.
   - Commercial cleaners may be indicated for the removal of heavy oil and grease. Do not attempt to scrub these areas. Check with physician.
   - Clean the area according to physician's orders or routine (a mild soap, povidone-iodine, or normal saline may be used).

2. Assist the physician with wound debridement.
   - Escharotomies (incisions made through the dead tissue or eschar) may have to be performed to relieve constriction or compression from circumferential deep burns (full thickness).
   - Hair in and around burn areas should be shaved to lessen the chance of infection.
   - Topical ointment should be applied as ordered.
   - Hands and feet should be splinted and dressed (fingers or toes wrapped separately) in a position of function and elevated to lessen edema.

3. Assist the physician in dressing the wound.
   - Wound may be left open.
   - Immediate grafting may be indicated for extensive burns.
     - Patient should be prepared for emergency surgery.
     - A signed consent form should be obtained.

4. Change dressings as ordered or at least every 24 hours.
   - Pain medication should be administered prior to therapy.

5. Begin hydrotherapy for extensive burns.
   - Dressings should not be forced off.
     - Dressings should be thoroughly soaked so they will lift off with relative ease.
     - Patient may assist in removal (may not be as painful).
   - The temperature of the electrolyte solution should be kept at 37.8°C (100°F) to prevent chilling.
   - Hydrotherapy not only aids in debridement but the patient can also perform range of motion exercises with more comfort.
   - Vital signs should be checked before and after the dressing change utilizing this method.

PREVENTION OF COMPLICATIONS

Complications	**Preventive Actions**
Infection	
Pseudomonas	Administer antibiotics as prescribed.
• Most common	Practice strict aseptic technique.
• Rapid onset (within 36 hours)	Keep environment as clean as possible. Use antiseptic solutions for cleansing. Use wet/dry vacuuming to clean the floor and equipment.
Hemolytic Staphylococcus aureus	
• Insidious onset (up to a week)	
	Use laminar airflow system if available.
	Keep patient isolated.
	Prevent debilitation with proper nutritional status.
Gastrointestinal Problems	
Early complications	
Nausea	Insert and connect nasogastric tube should be to low suction during the acute phase.
Vomiting	
Paralytic ileus	
Gastric distention	
Curling's ulcer (usually seen at end of first week although may occur anytime)	Instill antacids in nasogastric tube every 2 hours.
Pulmonary Problems (may not be evident until day 2 or 3 postburn)	
Respiratory distress syndrome	Perform endotracheal intubation with mechanical ventilation.
• From burn damage to lung tissue	
Pneumonia (resulting from stasis of secretions, inadequate coughing or position changes)	Begin oxygen therapy.
	Remove secretions by suctioning.
	Change patient's position frequently.
	Encourage deep breathing and coughing.
	Assist patient in use of incentive spirometry.

Deformities and Contractures

* Occur during recovery or rehabilitation period or later

Start passive and active range of motion exercises as soon as possible.

Keep the body in normal alignment.

Keep the hands and feet in functional positions. Use handsplints and footboard.

Change position frequently.

Encourage patient to assist with care and movement as possible. Trapeze frame on bed will aid in movement.

VIII

Other Critical Problems

27

Disseminated Intravascular Coagulation

This chapter presents an overview of disseminated intravascular coagulation (DIC). It is a disorder closely associated with shock as either a cause or a result.

Description

It is a coagulation disorder in which, paradoxically an initial hypercoagulable condition (an increased tendency to clot) is followed by a hypocoagulable state (hemorrhage).

Synonyms

Consumption coagulopathy

Defibrination syndrome

Diffuse intravascular clotting

Causes

It is associated with:
Shock due to sepsis or hemorrhage

Pregnancy complications including toxemia, third trimester bleeding, and fetal death

Burns

Multiple trauma

Terminal cancer

Snakebites

Clinical Manifestations

Petechiae and ecchymoses (mucous membranes, skin, or organs)

Hemorrhage (from puncture sites; respiratory, gastrointestinal, and genitourinary tracts; wounds or during childbirth or surgery)

Diagnostic Tests

Platelet count—very low

Prothrombin time—prolonged

Partial thromboplastin time—prolonged

Specific clotting factors

Treatment

Correct the underlying problem (*e.g.*, treat shock).

Stop hemorrhaging.

Administer heparin intravenously to stop clotting.

Treat shock by giving blood transfusions to replace lost blood.

28
Liver Failure

Acute liver failure and associated nursing considerations are discussed in this chapter.

Causes
Parenchymal damage from any of the following causes:
- Circulatory impairment (chronic congestive heart failure)
- Parenchymal disease including hepatitis, nutritional deficiencies, drugs, and metabolic disorders
- Bile flow obstruction
- Direct damage (trauma)

Clinical Manifestations
Anorexia

Weakness

Lethargy

Flapping tremor of hands and feet

Hemorrhage

Fluid and electrolyte imbalance

Change in level of consciousness (from blurring or confusion to unconsciousness)

Muscle twitching

Ascites

Significant blood ammonia elevation

Treatment and Nursing Actions
1. Monitor vital signs and ECG closely.
   - Congestive failure may be an underlying cause.
   - Notify physician of any adverse changes.
2. Support respiratory function.
   - Keep airway patent.

- Suction when necessary.
- Prevent aspiration in the unconscious patient by proper positioning (turn patient from side to side).
- Change position at least every two hours in order to prevent respiratory complications.
- Oxygen therapy and respiratory assistance may be indicated depending on the underlying cause.

3. Start an IV with a large bore needle in a large vein.
   - Administer fluid, blood, and blood byproducts. (Large amounts are ordered.)
   - Provide an emergency drug route.

4. Keep an accurate record of intake and output.
   - An indwelling urinary catheter may be required if the patient is critically ill.
   - Document all measurable intake and output.
   - Record daily weight.
   - Check girth measurements daily.

5. Put the patient on a strict bed rest program.
   - Rest increases the hepatic blood flow which may help healing.
   - It lowers metabolic needs.

6. Administer medications with extreme care.
   - Many medications (*e.g.*, narcotics, sedatives) detoxify in the liver.
   - Closely monitor their effects.

7. If possible, treat and correct the underlying cause.

8. Protect against infections.
   - There is an increased susceptibility to infections.
   - Use strict aseptic techniques for venepuncture, catheter insertion, site care for arterial line, and IV.
   - Instruct the patient to turn, cough, and frequently breathe deeply in order to prevent respiratory infections. If unconscious, frequent change of position is mandatory; respiratory support may be indicated.
   - Notify the physician immediately if infection is detected in the patient.

9. Provide protective measures.
   - Keep side rails up if the patient is not fully alert.

10. Paracentesis may be indicated.

11. Antibiotics such as kanamycin or neomycin may be administered to "sterilize" the bowel and lower the level of blood ammonia.

12. Provide emotional support.
    - The patient may be frightened due to the underlying cause and the clinical manifestation.
    - Complete recovery is a slow process.

13. Be on the alert for signs of complications.
    - Hepatic coma (ammonia intoxication), gastrointestinal hemorrhage, ascites, abnormal bleeding tendencies.
    - Treat accordingly.

29
Hypertensive Crisis

This chapter describes some of the many causes and clinical manifestations associated with hypertensive crisis. Nursing considerations are also discussed.

Causes

Malignant hypertension

Pheochromocytoma

Eclampsia

Encephalopathy (hypertensive)

Dissecting aneurysm (acute)

MAO inhibitor drugs

Acute congestive heart failure

Renal disease (acute and chronic)

Antihypertensive drug therapy that has been stopped abruptly

Severe stress

Clinical Manifestations

Acute blood pressure elevation (diastolic pressure may be 130 mm–140mm Hg or higher)

Severe headache (usually frontal)

Disturbances of vision (blurred, transient blindness)

Nausea

Vomiting

Weakness

Change in level of consciousness (lethargic to stuporous or unconscious)

Abnormal reflexes

Papilledema

Hemiparesis

Numbness in fingers and toes

Renal insufficiency

Nose bleed

NOTE. The patient usually has a history of hypertension.

Treatment and Nursing Actions

1. Monitor vital signs, ECG, and neurologic signs closely.
   - Report adverse changes to physician immediately.
   - Check blood pressure every 5 minutes with antihypertensive drug therapy.
   - Keep emergency drugs and resuscitative equipment readily available.
2. Support respiratory function.
   - Keep the airway patent.
   - Suction as necessary.
   - Respiratory support may be indicated.
3. Start an IV with a large bore needle in a large vein with 5% dextrose in water.
   - Administer all medications IV.
   - Set up IV with keep open rate until therapy can be started.
4. Administer antihypertensive medication as prescribed.
   - Drugs frequently used are diazoxide (Hyperstat), nitroprusside (Nipride) and trimethaphan camsylate (Arfonad) because of their rapid-acting abilities—they work within a few minutes.
   - Drugs such as methyldopa (Aldomet) or hydralazine hydrochloride (Apresoline) take longer to act and are used for long term therapy.
   - Potent diuretics such as furosemide (Lasix) and ethacrynic acid (Edecrin) may be administered as supportive therapy.
5. Monitor urinary output closely.
   - Indwelling urinary catheter may be indicated.
   - Oliguria or anuria should be reported to the physician immediately.
6. Arterial pressure monitoring is indicated.
   - Rapid-acting antihypertensive agents require close monitoring of arterial pressure.
   - The condition itself must be monitored closely.
   - The effectiveness of therapy is indicated by monitoring.
   - Arterial cuff pressures should be monitored closely.
7. Keep the patient on strict bed rest.
   - Elevate the head of the bed 45°.
   - Place the patient in a supine position if hypotension occurs suddenly due to medications.
   - Keep the room quiet and free of unnecessary movement.
8. Obtain routine laboratory studies and tests.
   - 12-lead ECG
   - Chest x-ray film
   - CBC
   - Electrolytes, Urinalysis

9. Do not leave patient unattended.
   - The patient may sense an impending catastrophe and be frightened, which will elevate the vital signs further.
   - The status of this patient is very unstable and requires constant monitoring.
10. Provide protective measures.
   - Keep side rails up if patient is not fully alert.
   - Keep padded tongue blade at bedside for use if convulsions occur.
   - Position on sides if level of consciousness is decreased to prevent aspiration.
   - Keep suction equipment readily available.

30
Acid-Base Imbalances

The causes, clinical manifestations, and treatment of metabolic alkalosis and acidosis, respiratory alkalosis and acidosis, mixed imbalances, and compensated imbalances are discussed in this chapter. Procedures for arterial puncture and for drawing blood from an arterial line are described.

METABOLIC ALKALOSIS

Metabolic alkalosis is an excess of bicarbonate.

Causes

Loss of metabolic acids due to the following:
- Nasogastric suction
- Vomiting
- Decreased serum potassium

Increased bicarbonate level due to excessive intake or retention of alkali
- Excessive ingestion or administration of sodium bicarbonate
- Parenteral administration of solutions without potassium
- Diet low in salt and without supplemental potassium chloride
- Diuretics
- Excessive adrenocortical hormone therapy

Clinical Manifestations

Hypoventilation

Cardiac arrhythmias

Electrolyte imbalances and resulting clinical manifestations—decreased serum potassium and serum calcium (see Electrolyte Imbalances, Chap. 31)

Arterial Blood Gases

CO_2—normal or elevated

pH—elevated

HCO_3—elevated

Treatment
- Treat the underlying cause.
- Correct electrolyte imbalances.
- Administer potassium chloride supplements.

METABOLIC ACIDOSIS

Metabolic acidosis is a deficit of bicarbonate.

Causes

Excessive production or accumulation of metabolic acids due to the following:
- Lactic acidosis (cardiac arrest)
- Diabetic ketoacidosis
- Renal failure
- Elevated serum potassium
- Starvation or other disturbances in food intake
- Hepatitis
- Anesthesia

Excess loss of alkali due to the following:
- Diarrhea
- Excess chloride level
- Conditions of the lower gastrointestinal tract (*e.g.*, fistula)

Clinical Manifestations

Change in level of consciousness (confusion, unconsciousness)

Electrolyte imbalances and resulting clinical manifestations—elevated serum potassium and serum calcium (see Electrolyte Imbalances, Chap. 31)

Hyperventilation

Arterial Blood Gases

pCO_2—normal or decreased

pH—decreased

HCO_3—decreased

Treatment

Treat the underlying cause.

Replace bicarbonates.

Correct electrolyte imbalances.

RESPIRATORY ALKALOSIS

Respiratory alkalosis is a carbonic acid deficit.

Cause

Increased excretion of carbon dioxide due to the following:
- Excessively administered mechanical ventilation

- Lack of oxygen
- Hyperventilation
- Extreme emotion (anxiety, hysteria)
- Pain
- Elevated temperature (due to disease or environment)
- Drug toxicity (*e.g.*, early stage of salicylate intoxication)
- Infections
- Encephalitis

Clinical Manifestations

Change in level of consciousness (light-headedness, unconsciousness)

Convulsions

Electrolyte imbalances and resulting clinical manifestations—decreased serum potassium and serum calcium (see Electrolyte Imbalances, Chap. 31)

Cardiac arrhythmias

Arterial Blood Gases

pCO_2—decreased

pH—elevated

HCO_3—normal or decreased

Treatment

Treat the underlying cause.

Correct electrolyte imbalances.

Utilize methods to increase retention of CO_2 (breathing into a paper bag; decreasing mechanical ventilation).

NOTE. To prevent this condition from occurring, do not overtreat abnormal blood gases with mechanical ventilation. This is especially pertinent for the patient with chronic obstructive pulmonary disease.

RESPIRATORY ACIDOSIS (CARBONIC ACID EXCESS)

Respiratory acidosis is an excess of carbonic acid.

Causes

Retention of carbon dioxide due to the following:
- Depression of the central nervous system due to morphine or barbiturate poisoning
- Improperly administered mechanical ventilation (excessive breathing of carbon dioxide)
- Pulmonary disorder (*e.g.*, emphysema, pneumonia)
- Respiratory complications from neuromuscular disorders (Landry–Guillain–Barré Syndrome)

Clinical Manifestations

Hypoventilation

Acute respiratory failure

Change in level of consciousness (confusion, unconsciousness)

Electrolyte imbalances and resulting clinical manifestations—elevated serum potassium and serum calcium (see Electrolyte Imbalances, Chap. 31)

Arterial Blood Gases

pCO_2—elevated

pH—decreased

HCO_3—normal or elevated

Treatment

Treat the underlying cause.

Replace bicarbonates.

Correct electrolyte imbalances.

Treatment may not be required for compensated chronic obstructive pulmonary disease. In fact, treatment in this situation would cause serious adverse effects.

MIXED IMBALANCE (INADEQUATELY COMPENSATED)

Causes

Two primary imbalances that occur simultaneously

A primary imbalance that is inadequately compensated

Blood Gases

pCO_2—abnormal

pH—abnormal

HCO_3—abnormal

Treatment

Treat the underlying cause.

Correct imbalances.

COMPENSATED IMBALANCE

Cause

The unaffected system attempts to counteract the effects of the abnormal system.

Blood Gases

pCO_2—abnormal

pH—within normal limits

HCO_3—abnormal

Treatment

Treat the underlying cause if possible.

Correct imbalances.

NOTE. Keep in mind that compensation may be chronic (*e.g.*, chronic obstructive pulmonary disease) and requires no treatment.

Compensatory mechanisms may fail.
• Monitor arterial blood gases closely to detect early changes of decompensation.
• Monitor vital signs, ECG, and neurological signs to detect changes of decompensation.

TABLE 30-1. **Guide for Interpreting Arterial Blood Gases**

pH	pCO$_2$	HCO$_3$	Disorder Present	Compensation
Abnormal (acid)	Increased	Normal	Respiratory acidosis	No
Abnormal (alkaline)	Decreased	Normal	Respiratory alkalosis	No
Abnormal (acid)	Normal	Decreased	Metabolic acidosis	No
Abnormal (alkaline)	Normal	Increased	Metabolic alkalosis	No
Normal (acid)	Increased	Increased	Respiratory acidosis	Yes
Normal (alkaline)	Decreased	Decreased	Respiratory alkalosis	Yes
Normal (acid)	Decreased	Decreased	Metabolic acidosis	Yes
Normal (alkaline)	Increased	Increased	Metabolic alkalosis	Yes
Abnormal (acid)	Increased	Increased	Respiratory acidosis	Inadequate
Abnormal (alkaline)	Decreased	Decreased	Respiratory alkalosis	Inadequate
Abnormal (acid)	Decreased	Decreased	Metabolic acidosis	Inadequate
Abnormal (alkaline)	Increased	Increased	Metabolic alkalosis	Inadequate

TABLE 30-2. **Guide for Determining Acid-Base Imbalances—Mixed Disorders**

Disorder	pH	pCO$_2$	HCO$_3$
Respiratory acidosis/ metabolic alkalosis	Slightly abnormal (acid or alkaline)	Increased	Increased
Respiratory alkalosis/ metabolic acidosis	Slightly abnormal (acid or alkaline)	Decreased	Decreased
Respiratory acidosis/ metabolic acidosis	Grossly abnormal (acid)	Increased	Slight increase or decrease
Respiratory alkalosis/ metabolic alkalosis	Grossly abnormal (alkaline)	Decreased	Slight increase or decrease

PROCEDURES FOR OBTAINING ARTERIAL BLOOD

ARTERIAL PUNCTURE

Equipment

10-ml glass or plastic syringe

Sterile 2 × 2s and 4 × 4s

Needles (25-gauge, ½-in; 20-gauge, 1½-in)

Aqueous heparin

Povidone-iodine swabs

Alcohol swabs

Tape

Container with ice

Stopper

Requisition

Preliminary Actions

1. Explain procedure to patient.
2. Prepare equipment.
3. Heparinize syringe. Using the 25-gauge needle, draw 1 ml of heparin into syringe. Pull back the plunger, while gently rotating it at the same time. Push plunger back to hub, leaving at least 0.1 ml of heparin in syringe. Change needles. Push out remainder of heparin.

Procedure

1. Select an artery for puncture.

   The femoral artery is the site of choice during CPR. If the radial artery is chosen, check collateral circulation (ulnar artery) to see if it is sufficient to supply circulation if radial artery occlusion occurs. Use the Allen test, as follows:
   - With patient's wrist resting palm side up on a rolled towel, instruct him to clench his fist.
   - Apply pressure, using index and middle fingers, to both radial and ulnar arteries for a few seconds.
   - While still applying pressure, instruct patient to unclench his fist. (Palm will normally be blanched due to impairment of circulation from pressure.)
   - Release pressure over the ulnar artery. Normally, the hand will flush if collateral circulation is adequate.
   - If collateral circulation is not adequate, check the other wrist.
   - Select another site if collateral circulation is not adequate in the opposite wrist.
2. Prepare the site with povidone-iodine swabs.
3. Insert the needle in the artery (45° angle for radial artery, 90° angle for femoral artery) with bevel up. The syringe will immediately fill with blood when the artery is punctured.

4. Collect the desired amount of blood (usually 3–5 ml but check with laboratory).

5. Apply firm pressure to site with gauze as the needle is withdrawn.

6. Have a second nurse maintain pressure over the artery (approximately 5 min for the radial artery and 10 min for the femoral artery).

7. Remove air bubbles immediately from syringe. Gently rotate the specimen.

8. Put stopper on end of syringe and place in container with ice.

9. Send sample to lab immediately with requisition.

10. Check insertion site for bleeding. Apply sterile pressure dressing. (Check several times following procedure to make sure bleeding has completely stopped.)

DRAWING BLOOD FROM AN ARTERIAL LINE

Equipment

Syringes (5-ml and 10-ml)

Aqueous heparin

Needle (25-gauge)

Stopper

Container with ice

Syringe with heparin flush

Requisition

Procedure

1. Explain procedure to patient.

2. Attach 5-ml syringe to 3-way stopcock of arterial line.

3. Aspirate 4 ml and discard.

4. Attach 10-ml syringe that has been heparinized to line (see Arterial Puncture) and withdraw required amount of blood.

5. Withdraw syringe with specimen, cap and place in container with ice. (Remove any air bubbles.)

6. Attach syringe with heparin flush to 3-way stopcock and immediately flush the catheter to prevent clotting.

7. Remove syringe and cover port on stopcock with sterile cover.

8. Send specimen with requisition to lab immediately.

NOTE. Be sure to turn stopcock to *off* position before attaching or removing syringe.

31

Fluid and Electrolyte Imbalances

The causes, clinical manifestations, and treatment of the various fluid and electrolyte imbalances are covered in this chapter. Deficit and excess in extracellular fluid volume, hypocalcemia, hypercalcemia, hypokalemia, hyperkalemia, hypomagnesemia, and hypermagnesemia are described, and significant laboratory values are listed for each.

DEFICIT IN EXTRACELLULAR FLUID VOLUME

Causes

Decreased water intake

Diarrhea

Vomiting

Drainage from a fistula

Diabetes insipidus

Systemic infection

Renal disease

Adrenal insufficiency

Intestinal obstruction

Gastrointestinal suctioning

Blood loss

Diaphoresis

Burns

Diuretics

Diet low in sodium

Clinical Manifestations

Acute loss of weight

Oliguria or anuria

Dryness of mucous membranes and skin

Longitudinal wrinkling on surface of tongue

Hypotension

Decrease in pulse volume and blood pressure

Narrowed pulse pressure

Change in level of consciousness (confusion, restlessness, delirium, unconsciousness)

Convulsions

Rapid, deep respirations

Significant Laboratory Values

Hematocrit—elevated

Hemoglobin—elevated

Red blood cells—elevated

Serum sodium
- Normal—if deficit is due to severe loss of isotonic fluid (hypovolemia)
- Increased—if deficit is due to severe and greater loss of water than sodium (hypernatremia)
- Decreased—if deficit is due to severe loss of sodium (hyponatremia)

Treatment

Treat the underlying cause.

Replace fluid and electrolytes as follows:
- Hypovolemia—replace fluid and electrolytes using an isotonic solution.
- Hypernatremia—replace fluid with a hypotonic or isotonic solution.
- Hyponatremia—replace sodium with an isotonic or hypertonic solution.

Carefully monitor electrolytes.

Weigh patient daily.

Monitor intake and output closely.

EXCESS IN EXTRACELLULAR FLUID VOLUME

Causes

Congestive heart failure

Hyperaldosteronism

Renal disease

Steroid therapy

Excessive intake of sodium chloride without increased water intake

Excessive intake of water without increased intake of sodium chloride

Excessive administration of isotonic solution of sodium chloride

Excessive administration of sodium bicarbonate

Using water to irrigate nasogastric tubes

Excessive administration of tap-water enemas

Clinical Manifestations

Acute weight gain

Edema

Increase in pulse volume and blood pressure

Increase in urinary output

Rales (moist) in lungs

Change in level of consciousness (confusion, restlessness, unconsciousness)

Headache

Convulsions

Rapid, deep respirations

Shortness of breath

Significant Laboratory Values

Hematocrit—decreased

Hemoglobin—decreased

Red blood cells—decreased

Serum and urinary sodium
• Normal—if excess is due to isotonic fluid overload
• Increased—if excess is due to hypernatremia
• Decreased—if excess is due to hyponatremia

Treatment

Treat the underlying cause.

Remove excess fluid and electrolytes as follows:
• Fluid overload—administer diuretics and salt-poor albumin. Fluid intake should be severely restricted. Dialysis may be indicated.
• Hypernatremia—administer diuretics. Fluid intake should be severely restricted.
• Hyponatremia—administer diuretics and hypotonic intravenous solutions. Fluid intake should be severely restricted.

Carefully monitor electrolytes.

Weigh patient daily.

Take girth measurements daily.

Monitor intake and output closely.

HYPOCALCEMIA

Causes

Diarrhea

Acute pancreatitis

Excessive administration of citrated blood
Massive infection of subcutaneous tissues
Renal failure (diuretic phase)
Generalized peritonitis
Vitamin D deficiency
Burns
Hypoparathyroidism
Intestinal shunt operations

Clinical Manifestations

Muscle cramp
Twitching
Positive Chvostek's sign
Positive Trousseau's sign
Tetany
Hyperactive deep-tendon reflexes
Carpopedal spasms
Abdominal cramps
Nausea
Vomiting
Diarrhea
Irritability
Convulsions
ECG—prolonged QT interval
Laryngeal stridor

Significant Laboratory Tests

Serum calcium—depressed
Sulkowitch urine test—no calcium precipitation
ECG changes (see above)

Treatment

Treat the underlying cause.
Administer calcium supplements.
Take seizure precautions.
Emergency tracheotomy may be necessary.
Closely monitor vital signs and ECG.

HYPERCALCEMIA

Causes

Excessive administration of vitamin D

Hyperparathyroidism

Prolonged immobilization

Excessive calcium intake

Acidosis

Renal failure (oliguria phase)

Malignancy (multiple myeloma)

Tumor of parathyroid glands

Pathologic fractures

Clinical Manifestations

Nausea

Vomiting

Loss of appetite

Hypoactive deep-tendon reflexes

Weight loss

Deep bone pain

Renal calculi

Flank pain

Polydipsia

Polyuria

Dehydration

Constipation

Change in level of consciousness (lethargy, unconsciousness)

Cardiac

Predisposes patient to digitalis toxicity

Bradycardia

Heart blocks

ECG—shortened QT interval

Significant Laboratory Values

Serum calcium—elevated

Sulkowitch urine test—heavy calcium precipitation

ECG changes (see above)

Treatment

Treat the underlying cause.

Administer phosphate (orally or intravenously) as prescribed to increase excretion of excess calcium.

Monitor digitalis blood levels closely. Dosage may be reduced.

Observe ECG closely for signs of digitalis toxicity and hypercalcemia.

Closely monitor vital signs.

Monitor intake and output.

Ensure an adequate intake of fluid.

Strain all urine for calculi.

Protect the patient from trauma.

Monitor patient closely for signs of tetany during treatment. Keep emergency drugs readily available.

HYPOKALEMIA

Causes

Diarrhea

Vomiting

Ulcerative colitis

Draining fistulas

Gastrointestinal drainage

Diuretics

Inadequate dietary intake of potassium

Diabetic acidosis (recovery phase)

Renal failure (diuretic phase)

Steroid therapy

Burns (following third day)

Tumors of the adrenal gland

Severe stress

Diabetes insipidus

Alkalosis

Excessive sweating owing to heat or exercise

Clinical Manifestations

Change in level of consciousness (confusion)

Cardiac

ECG changes—peaked P waves; prolonged PR interval; flattened T waves; prominent U wave

Increased ventricular irritability leading to ventricular fibrillation or asystole

Predisposes patient receiving digitalis to digitalis toxicity

Respiratory
Shortness of breath
Shallow respirations
Respiratory arrest

Gastrointestinal
Vomiting
Nausea
Loss of appetite
Distended abdomen
Paralytic ileus

Skeletal Muscles
Weakness
Fatigue
Hypoactive or absent reflexes
Cramps
Flabby muscles
Paresthesia

Significant Laboratory Tests

Serum potassium—decreased
ECG—as above

Treatment

Treat the underlying cause.

Replace potassium.

Correct the alkalosis.

Remember, transfuse patients in renal failure with fresh blood. Reason: Cells break down in stored blood and release potassium.

Monitor electrolytes.

Watch for ECG changes.

Monitor intake and output closely.

HYPERKALEMIA

Causes

Renal failure (oliguric phase)
Massive crushing injury
Burn (early)
Adrenal insufficiency (Addison's disease)

Excessive parenteral administration of potassium

Excessive intake of potassium

Rapid administration of stored bank blood (contains high concentration of potassium)

Acidosis

Clinical Manifestations

Cardiac

ECG changes

- Early changes—high, peaked T waves; ST-segment depression; prolonged PR interval; prolonged duration of QRS complex; height of R wave decreased
- Late changes—no P waves; QRS complex widens and amplitude decreases; rate slows; arrhythmias (including ventricular fibrillation or asystole)

Skeletal Muscles

Cramps

Twitching

Hyperactive reflexes

Paresthesia

Paralysis

Abdominal

Cramps

Abdominal distention

Nausea

Diarrhea

Ileus

Significant Laboratory Values

Serum potassium—elevated

ECG—as above

Treatment

Treat the underlying cause.

Correct the acidosis.

Remove excess potassium:
- Infusion of insulin and dextrose
- Ion exchange resins (Kayexalate)
- Dialysis (may be indicated)

Limit intake of potassium.

Closely monitor vital signs and ECG.

Monitor electrolytes.

Monitor intake and output closely.

HYPOMAGNESEMIA

Causes

Vomiting

Diarrhea

Nasogastric suctioning

Impaired gastrointestinal absorption in the surgical patient and the medical patient (hyperaldosteronism; hyperparathyroidism; renal failure—diuretic phase; malnutrition)

Chronic alcoholism

Enterostomy drainage

Prolonged intravenous therapy with magnesium-free solution

Clinical Manifestations

Tetany

Hyperactive deep reflexes

Muscle cramps

Twitching

Convulsions

Tremors

Mental changes—disorientation, confusion, hallucinations, delusions, combativeness

Positive Chvostek's sign

Significant Laboratory Test

Serum magnesium—decreased

Treatment

Treat the underlying cause.

Administer magnesium supplements.

Promote the intake of foods rich in magnesium.

Monitor the patient closely for signs of hypermagnesemia during treatment.

HYPERMAGNESEMIA

Causes

Excessive parenteral administration of magnesium

Renal insufficiency (retention of magnesium)

Excessive administration of enemas containing magnesium sulfate

Severe dehydration

Oliguria

Clinical Manifestations

Loss of deep-tendon reflexes

Paralysis of skeletal muscles

Extreme sedative effects, including deep unconsciousness

Respiratory arrest

Cardiac

ECG changes—prolonged PR interval

Prolonged QRS complex

Elevated T wave

Tachycardia, eventually resulting in bradycardia

Hypotension

Cardiac arrest (resulting from cardiac arrhythmias)

Significant Laboratory Test

Serum magnesium—elevated

Treatment

Treat the underlying cause.

Administer calcium gluconate immediately.

Stop parenteral administration of magnesium immediately.

Treat the symptoms appropriately. Have emergency drugs and equipment readily available, including mechanical ventilation.

Closely monitor vital signs and ECG.

Dialysis may be indicated.

Decrease the intake of foods containing excessive amounts of magnesium.

Avoid use of antacids containing magnesium in the patient with renal insufficiency.

32

Fetal Distress—Monitoring the Fetal Heart Rate

A general overview of the methods of monitoring the fetal heart rate and the basic terminology are presented in this chapter. The normal and abnormal fetal heart rates are discussed, as well as nursing intervention for the abnormal rates.

TYPES OF MONITORING

External monitors
* Fetoscope
* Doppler ultrasound
* Fetal monitors
  * Phonotransducer—microphone is placed directly on the mother's abdomen over the approximate position of the fetal heart.
  * Abdominal electrodes—electrodes are attached directly to the mother's abdomen; two abdominal electrodes are attached above the position of the head and back, and a suction electrode is attached over the position of the buttocks of the fetus. It provides a maternal-fetal ECG in addition to monitoring the fetal heart rate.

NOTE. In the maternal-fetal ECG, the maternal complexes are tall and the fetal complexes are very small in comparison.

Internal monitors
* Electrode is attached directly to the presenting part, except if the presenting part is the face or the genital area. The cervix must be partially dilated and the membranes ruptured.

FETAL HEART RATE

Normal fetal heart rate is 120 to 160 beats/min (Fig. 32–1).

Baseline of fetal heart rate is normally irregular (Fig. 32–2).

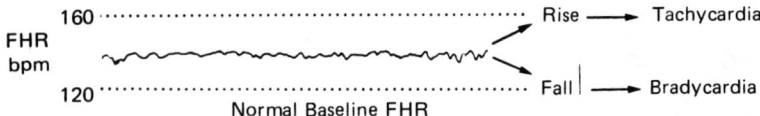

FIG. 32-1. *Normal fetal heart rate.* (From Hon EH: An Atlas of Fetal Heart Rate Patterns. New Haven, Harty Press, 1968)

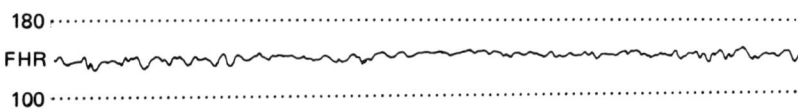

FIG. 32-2. *Average irregularity of normal fetal heart rate baseline.* (From Hon EH: An Atlas of Fetal Heart Rate Patterns. New Haven, Harty Press, 1968)

NOTE. Baseline is defined as the fetal heart rate in the absence of labor or contractions, or the period of time between changes in the fetal heart rate.

Changes in fetal heart rate are referred to as fluctuations and are further classified as either acceleration or deceleration.

SUMMARY OF ABNORMAL FETAL HEART RATE CHANGES

Rate changes
- Bradycardia—fetal heart rate is below 120 beats/min and varies from moderate to severe.
- Tachycardia—fetal heart rate is above 160 beats/min and varies from moderate to severe.

Baseline variability
- Minimal variability—baseline varies under 6 beats/min.
- Increased variability—baseline varies more than 10 beats/min.
- No variability—baseline does not vary (smooth line).

Periodic fetal heart rate patterns (Fig. 32-3)
- Early deceleration—there is a uniform appearance; fetal heart rate does not fall below 100, with lowest level occurring at the peak of the contraction; it has mirror image of uterine activity; fetal acid-base status is usually unchanged; this pattern is benign.
- Late deceleration—there is a uniform appearance; effects on fetal heart rate begin at peak of contraction; irregularities in fetal heart rate may be noted; meconium may be passed; fetal acid-base status is affected (associated with progressive fetal acidosis and hypoxia).
- Variable deceleration—there is an irregular appearance; decreased fetal heart rate occurs at any time without any relationship to uterine activity; fetal heart rate falls below 100; acceleration may precede and follow deceleration.

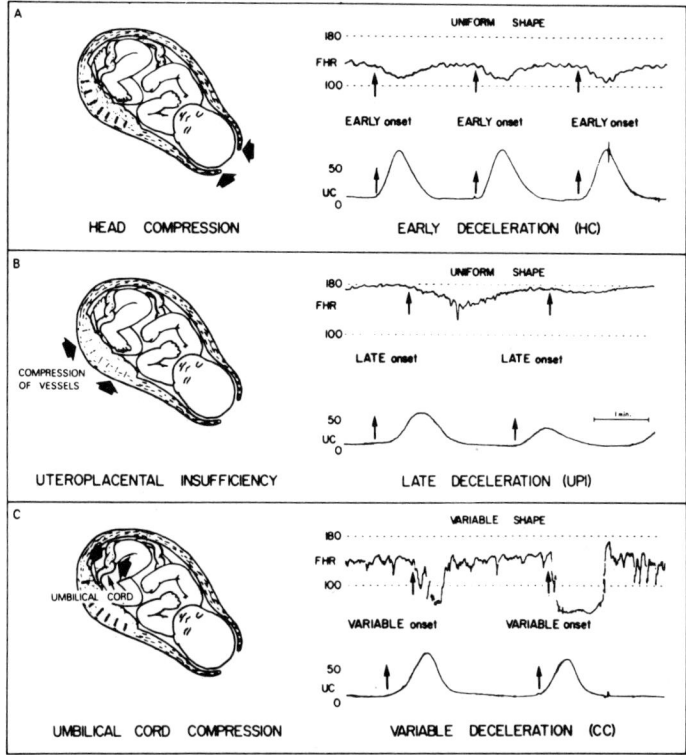

FIG. 32-3. *Periodic FHR patterns.* (From Hon EH: An Atlas of Fetal Heart Rate Patterns. New Haven, Harty Press, 1968)

NURSING INTERVENTION FOR PERIODIC CHANGES IN FETAL HEART RATE

EARLY DECELERATION

- Usually no treatment is required because this change is considered benign.
- Continue to monitor the fetal heart rate (FHR) closely.

LATE DECELERATION (DEPENDS ON UNDERLYING CAUSE)

Uterine hyperactivity
- Discontinue oxytocin.
- Administer oxygen.

Maternal hypotension
- Turn mother to left side.
- Elevate legs.
- Administer oxygen.

Uteroplacental insufficiency
- Administer oxygen.
- Increase rate of IV fluid.

- Prepare the patient for delivery if the pattern becomes ominous.
- Obtain a fetal blood sample to assess the degree of fetal hypoxia. Fetal compromise is indicated by the following:
  - pH decrease (normal 7.30–7.40)
  - pCO_2 increase
  - pO_2 decrease[1]

VARIABLE DECELERATION

- Change position of mother to relieve compression on umbilical cord.
- Administer oxygen.
- Prepare the patient for delivery.
- Discontinue oxytocin.

REFERENCE

1. Brunner LS, Suddarth DS: The Lippincott Manual of Nursing Practice, 2nd ed. Philadelphia, JB Lippincott, 1978

IX

Interpretation of Vital Signs

33
Quick Reference for Critical Vital Signs

The normal and abnormal vital signs for all age groups and the significance of abnormal findings are presented in this chapter. Temperature, patterns of respiration, breath sounds, adventitious sounds, voice sounds, pulse rates, heart sounds, and blood pressure are included.

TEMPERATURE

Normal
Adult
- Oral—37°C (98.6°)
- Axillary—usually 1° lower than oral
- Rectal—usually 1° higher than oral

Temperatures are usually lower early in the morning.

Child
- Oral—36.4°C to 37.4°C (97.6°F–99.3°F)
- Axillary—35.9°C to 36.7°C (96.6°F–98°F)
- Rectal—36.2°C to 37.8°C (97°F–100°F)[1]

Hyperthermia
Temperature above normal

Significance—head injury, following neurosurgery; infection; environmental temperatures (excessively hot)

Hypothermia
Temperature below normal

Significance—induced hypothermia for medical reasons; environmental temperatures (excessively cold)

RESPIRATORY SIGNS

PATTERNS OF RESPIRATION—NORMAL AND ABNORMAL

Eupnea—Normal Respirations

Adult
- 14 respirations/minute to 20 respirations/minute

Child
- Newborn: 30 respirations/minute to 50 respirations/minute
- 11 months: 26 respirations/minute to 40 respirations/minute
- 2 to 4 years: 20 respirations/minute to 30 respirations/minute
- 6 years: 20 respirations/minute to 26 respirations/minute
- 8 to 10 years: 18 respirations/minute to 24 respirations/minute
- Adolescence: 12 respirations/minute to 20 respirations/minute[1]

Bradypnea

Slower than normal; regular

Significance—sleep pattern; morphine; alcohol; increase an intracranial pressure; diabetic coma

Tachypnea

Faster than normal; regular

Significance—fever; pain; exertion; respiratory distress; pneumothorax; abdominal distention; overweight

Apnea

Cessation of breathing that may be periodic

Significance—deep sleep; hyperventilation; coma; central nervous system injury; cardiac disease

Hyperpnea

Increase in respiratory rate and depth

Significance—exertion; pain; fever; fear; cardiac disease; respiratory disease

Kussmaul's Respiration (Air Hunger)

Respirations are deep and gasping or sighing; regular

Significance—diabetic acidosis; uremia; acute hemorrhage

Cheyne–Stokes Respiration

Gradual increase in rate and amplitude until a climax is reached, followed by a gradual decrease and then a period of apnea (may last from 5 seconds–50 seconds)

Cycle begins again following the period of apnea

Significance—increased intracranial pressure; cardiac failure; head injury; narcotics

Biot's Respiration

Periods of apnea alternate irregularly with periods of hyperpnea.

Breaths are equal in length, end abruptly, and are followed by period of apnea.

Significance—meningitis

Apneustic Respiration
Prolonged inspiratory phase

Expiratory phase is shortened and inefficient

Significance—damage or lesions in the respiratory center of the brain

Paradoxical Respiration
Affected area of chest rises on exhalation and falls on inspiration

Significance—flail chest; paralysis of diaphragm

BREATH SOUNDS: CHARACTERISTICS

TYPE	*LOCATION*	*CHARACTERISTICS*
Vesicular	Most of lung surface	Soft, whishing sound; normal breathing Inspiratory phase is long and expiratory phase is very short
Bronchovesicular	Above the sternum and in the upper interscapular region	Sound is between vesicular and bronchial sounds or medium in pitch Duration of inspiration and expiratory phases are about equal Abnormal if heard in any other area of the lung
Bronchial (tubular)	Over the trachea	Sound is loud and high-pitched Inspiratory phase is short and expiratory phase is long Abnormal sound; does not normally occur Result of lung consolidation
Tracheal	Above the sternal notch and over the sixth and seventh cervical vertebrae	Sound is loud and high-pitched (compared to blowing air through a hollow tube), but has more of a harsh and hollow quality than bronchial breathing Normal sound

ADVENTITIOUS SOUNDS

Definition
Abnormal breath sounds

Rales
Also referred to as crackles

Occurrence—noncontinuous

Description—bubbling or crackling sound (resembles sound obtained by rubbing strands of hair together or the crackle of crumbling tissue paper)

Significance—pulmonary edema, pneumonia, tuberculosis

Classifications—fine, medium, coarse
* Fine—secretions in alveoli; crackling sound
* Medium—secretions in bronchioles; sound of air passing through secretions
* Coarse—secretions in bronchi and trachea; sound of air passing through secretions (loud and gurgling)

Rhonchi
Occurrence—continuous; louder during expiration

Description—wheezing (sibilant) or snoring sound

Significance—obstructed airway; chronic obstructive pulmonary disease; asthma

Classifications—wheezing, sonorous
* Wheezing—high-pitched rhonchi
* Sonorous—low-pitched rhonchi

Pleural Friction Rub
Occurrence—on inspiration and expiration; may not be constant

Description—the sound of rubbing leather together or a grating (resembles the sound produced by rubbing the thumb and the forefinger together)

Significance—inflammation of pleural surface

Decreased or Absent Breath Sounds
Significance—pneumothorax; pleural effusion; emphysema, atelectasis

VOICE SOUNDS
Normally, whispered or spoken words are heard indistinctly and faintly over the peripheral lung.

TYPE	DESCRIPTION	SIGNIFICANCE
Whispered pectoriloquy	Whispered words are heard distinctly	Pulmonary consolidation
Bronchophony	Spoken words are heard distinctly and clearly	Pulmonary consolidation

(Continued)

TYPE	*DESCRIPTION*	*SIGNIFICANCE*
Egophony	Spoken words have a nasal quality (compared to the bleat of a goat)	Pleural effusion

CARDIOVASCULAR SIGNS

PULSE RATES

Normal

Regular in rate and rhythm

Adult:
- 60 beats/minute to 80 beats/minute

Child:
- Newborn—70 beats/minute to 170 beats/minute
- 11 months—80 beats/minute to 160 beats/minute
- 2 years—80 beats/minute to 130 beats/minute
- 4 years—80 beats/minute to 120 beats/minute
- 6 years—75 beats/minute to 115 beats/minute
- 8 to 10 years—70 beats/minute to 110 beats/minute
- Adolescence—60 beats/minute to 110 beats/minute[1]

Dicrotic Pulse

Double pulsation, the latter being weaker than the former

NOTE. When counting the pulse rate, count only the stronger beat.

Significance—fever; toxic conditions

Waterhammer Pulse (Corrigan's; Bounding)

Rapid and strong pulsation is followed by sudden collapse

Significance aortic regurgitation; thyrotoxicosis

Pulsus Paradoxus

Pulse decreases in strength on inspiration

Significance—cardiac tamponade; pericardial effusion; pericarditis (constrictive)

Pulsus Alternans

Alternating strong and weak beats

Regular rhythm

Significance—weakness of the myocardium

Pulsus Bigeminus-(Bigeminy)

Two beats separated by a short pause occurring close together (coupled), followed by a longer pause

Significance—premature ventricular contractions

HEART SOUNDS

First Heart Sound (S_1)

"Lubb"

Caused by closure of the tricuspid and mitral valves

Normal

Second Heart Sound (S_2)

"Dubb"

Caused by closure of the semilunar valves (aortic and pulmonary)

Normal

Location of areas of heart valves:
- Aortic valve area—second intercostal space to right of sternum
- Pulmonic valve area—second intercostal space to left of sternum
- Tricuspid valve area—fifth intercostal space to left of sternum
- Mitral valve area—apex of heart

Variations in Heart Sounds

According to area of heart valves:
- Aortic valve area—S_2 is louder than S_1
- Pulmonic valve area—S_2 is louder than S_1
- Tricuspid valve area—S_1 and S_2 are almost of the same intensity
- Mitral valve area—S_1 is slightly louder than S_2

Components of Heart Sounds

S_1: mitral closure (M_1) and tricuspid closure (T_1)
- The first heart sound is slightly longer in duration than the second heart sound as a result of the slight asynchronous closure of the components.

S_2: aortic closure (A_2) and pulmonic closure (P_2)
- Normally, the aortic valve closes before the pulmonary valve, producing an interval (splitting) between the two components that may be detected on inspiration. (On expiration, the interval is smaller and may not be detectable.)

Third and Fourth Heart Sounds

Usually not detectable

Third heart sound (S_3)
- Caused by rapid filling of ventricles during diastole (early)
- May be heard in children and young adults and is considered normal
- Occurs after the second heart sound

Fourth heart sound (S_4)
- Caused by atrial contraction and resulting ventricular distention
- Occurs immediately before the first heart sound

Murmur

Caused by vibrations from movement of blood within the heart and great vessels

Abnormal (Blood flow is normally silent.)

Duration is longer than that of heart sounds

May not be significant

Described according to time of occurence (systole or diastole), intensity, duration, pitch, quality and location

SUMMARY OF ABNORMAL HEART SOUNDS

First Heart Sound

Accentuated
- *Significance*—mitral stenosis; tachycardia (from fever, anemia, exercise, hyperthyroidism, etc.)

Diminished
- *Significance*—first-degree heart block; calcification of mitral valve (from acute rheumatic fever) causing severe restriction in movement; thickened chest wall (from obesity, emphysema, etc.)

Variation
- *Significance*—atrial fibrillation; atrial flutter with varying block; complete heart block; ventricular tachycardia

Splitting
- *Significance*—may be normal; right bundle branch block

Second Heart Sound

Aortic component
- Accentuated
  - *Significance*—arterial hypertension; coarctation of the aorta; aortic regurgitation
- Diminished
  - *Significance*—aortic stenosis

Pulmonic component
- Accentuated
  - *Significance*—pulmonary hypertension
- Diminished
  - *Significance*—pulmonic stenosis

Pathological splitting, wide
- *Significance*—pulmonic stenosis; right bundle branch block; delayed closure of pulmonic valve; early closure of aortic valve (mitral regurgitation)

Paradoxical
- Obvious on expiration, absent on inspiration
- *Significance*—left bundle branch block; aortic stenosis

Fixed
- Unaffected by respiration
- *Significance*—right ventricular failure; atrial septal defect

Third Heart Sound

Ventricular gallop

Significance—failure of the myocardium
- Right ventricular gallop—right-sided heart failure
- Left ventricular gallop—left-sided heart failure

(This sound resembles a galloping horse or the word Kentucky in rhythm.)

Fourth Heart Sound

Atrial gallop

Significance—hypertensive cardiovascular disease; aortic stenosis; myocardiopathy; may in normal in some cases

BLOOD PRESSURE

Normal

Adult
- Systolic: 95 mm Hg to 140 mm Hg
- Diastolic: 60 mm Hg to 90 mm Hg

Child
- See Table 33-1.

TABLE 33-1. **NORMAL BLOOD PRESSURE VALUES AT VARIOUS AGES***

Age in Years	Mean Systolic	Range in 95% of Normal Children	Mean Diastolic	Range in 95% of Normal Children
½–1 year	90	± 25	61	± 19
1–2 years	96	± 27	65	± 27
2–3 years	95	± 24	61	± 24
3–4 years	99	± 23	65	± 19
4–5 years	99	± 21	65	± 15
5 years	94	± 14	55	± 9
6 years	100	± 15	56	± 8
7 years	102	± 15	56	± 8
8 years	105	± 16	57	± 9
9 years	107	± 16	57	± 9
10 years	109	± 16	58	± 10
11 years	111	± 17	59	± 10
12 years	113	± 18	59	± 10
13 years	115	± 19	60	± 10
14 years	118	± 19	61	± 10
15 years	121	± 19	61	± 10

*From Johns Hopkins Hospital: The Harriet Lane Handbook, 7th ed. Copyright 1975 by Year Book Medical Publishers, Inc., Chicago, p 265.

Data for ½–5 years from Allen–Williams GM: Pulse-rate and blood pressure in infancy and early childhood. *Arch Dis Child* 20:125, 1945.

Data for 5–15 years from Graham AW, Hines EA JR, Gage RP: Blood pressure in children between the ages of five and sixteen years. Am J Child 69:203, 1945.

NOTE. Formula for determining mean arterial blood pressure: ⅓ systolic pressure + ⅔ diastolic pressure = mean arterial pressure

Hypertension

Blood pressure elevated above normal limits

Significance—eclampsia; cerebrovascular accidents; renal disease; cardiac disease; of unknown cause

Hypotension

Blood pressure decreased below the patient's normal limit or general normal limits

Significance—shock; myocardial infarction; cardiac tamponade

Postural Hypotension (Orthostatic)

Although normal in the recumbent position, the blood pressure falls significantly upon arising, which may cause the patient to faint

Significance—antihypertensive agents (ganglionic blocking agents); prolonged bed rest; varicosities of the lower extremities

Narrowed Pulse Pressure

Difference between systolic and diastolic pressures is reduced below 30 mm Hg

Significance—pericarditis (constrictive); pericardial effusion; tachycardia

Widened Pulse Pressure

Difference between systolic and diastolic pressures is greater than 40 mm Hg

Significance—coarctation of the aorta; patent ductus arteriosus; hypertension; emotional states

REFERENCE

1. Brunner LS, Suddarth DS: The Lippincott Manual of Nursing Practice, 2nd ed. Philadelphia, JB Lippincott, 1978

X

Emergency Drug Therapy

34

Alphabetical Guide to Commonly Used Emergency Drugs

Emergency drugs most commonly used in the critical care unit are presented in this chapter. Dosages for the different age groups are included as well.

NOTE. It is imperative that the nurse checks current drug literature prior to administering any drug and that medications are administered under the direction of a physician.

ARAMINE (METARAMINOL BITARTRATE)

Dosage

Adult
- Prevention of hypotension—2 mgm to 10 mgm (0.2–1.0 ml) administered IM or SC
- Direct IV injection for severe shock—0.5 mgm to 5 mgm (0.05–0.5 ml) pushed over 5 minutes; IV infusion of 15 mgm to 100 mgm (1.5–10 ml) in 500 ml of sodium chloride or 5% dextrose should follow

NOTE. Administration by IV push should be used in extreme emergencies only.

- Treatment of hypotension—15 mgm to 100 mgm (1.5–10 ml) in 500 ml of sodium chloride or 5% dextrose; rate should be adjusted to maintain blood pressure at desired level

Child
- IV—0.01 mgm/kgm slow IV push; follow with IV infusion 1 mgm/25 ml 5% dextrose in water (titrate)
- IM injection—0.1 mgm/kgm

Side-effects

Hypertension

Cardiac arrest

Nervousness

Arrhythmias (*e.g.*, sinus bradycardia and tachycardia, ventricular tachycardia, AV dissociation)

Dizziness

Headache

Convulsions

Incompatibilities

Dilantin

Levophed

Heparin sodium

Ampicillin

Morphine

Whole blood

Keflin

Solu-Cortef

Ringer's solution

Lactated Ringer's solution

Sodium bicarbonate

Contraindications

Hypersensitivity

Use with halothane or cyclopropane

Comments

Blood pressure should be checked every 5 minutes until stable and then every 15 minutes during therapy.

Continuous ECG monitoring is indicated

Extravasation may result in tissue sloughing and necrosis.

ATROPINE SULFATE

Dosage

Adult

- 0.5 mgm IV push over 2 minutes and repeat in 5 min intervals if necessary (the total amount not to exceed 2 mgm)

Child

- IV push
- 0.01 mgm/kgm to 0.02 mgm/kgm

NOTE. Atropine sulfate may be administered undiluted or diluted in 10 ml of sterile water.

Maternity
• Safety not established

Side-effects

Dryness of mouth
Postural hypotension
Bradycardia (temporary)
Blurred vision
Headache
Urinary retention
Delirium
Flushing
Tachycardia
Pupil dilation
Skin rash
Temperature elevation (in children)
Disorientation
Coma

Contraindications

Glaucoma
Asthma
Adhesions between iris and lens of eye

Incompatibilities

Sodium bicarbonate
Adrenalin
Heparin
Aramine
Staphcillin
Chloromycetin
Nembutal

Comments

Do not add atropine sulfate to IV solution bottle.

Use it with caution in the following situations: prostatic hypertrophy, pediatric patients, urinary retention.

BRETYLOL (BRETYLIUM TOSYLATE)

Dosage

Adult
- Ventricular fibrillation or other life-threatening ventricular rhythms—IV rapid injection 5 mgm/kgm (undiluted); may increase to 10 mgm/kgm and repeat every 15 to 30 minutes, the total amount not to exceed 30 mgm/kgm
- Other ventricular arrhythmias—one 10 ml ampule of Bretylol (500 mgm) diluted to 50 ml (minimum) with normal saline or 5% dextrose; administer 5 mgm/kgm to 10 mgm/kgm over a period greater than 8 minutes; may repeat in 1 to 2 hours
- IM injection—5 mgm/kgm to 10 mgm/kgm (undiluted); may repeat in 1 to 2 hours; administer same dosage every 6 to 8 hours for maintenance
- IV maintenance
  - Constant—1 mgm/min to 2 mgm/min of diluted solution
  - Intermittent—5 mgm/kgm to 10 mgm/kgm of diluted solution over a period greater than 8 minutes; repeat every 6 hours

Child
- Not recommended

Maternity
- Not recommended (Use must be weighed against nonuse.)

Side-effects

Severe nausea and vomiting with rapid infusion

Hypotension

Postural hypotension

Incompatibilities

None known

Contraindications

None

Comments

Continuous ECG monitoring is required.

Other resuscitative measures are necessary.

Ventricular fibrillation is generally suppressed within minutes following administration.

Ventricular tachycardia (or other arrhythmias of ventricular origin) is generally suppressed within 20 minutes to 2 hours.

Bretylol should be used with caution in patients with fixed cardiac output (*i.e.*, severe pulmonary hypertension).

Bretylol should not be used in the digitalized patient because it aggravates digitalis toxicity; however, it may be used for a life-threatening arrhythmia that is not caused by digitalis toxicity and when other antiarrhythmic drugs are ineffective.

CALCIUM CHLORIDE

Dosage
Adult
- 5 ml to 10 ml of 10% solution IV bolus; slow push over 5 minutes to 10 minutes

Children
- 1 ml to 4 ml of 10% solution IV bolus; slow push over 5 minutes to 10 minutes

NOTE. Calcium chloride may be given intracardiac but this route should be avoided if possible.

Side-effects
Bradycardia

Arrhythmias

Cardiac Arrest

Tingling sensation

Hypercalcemia

Incompatibilities
Adrenalin

Terramycin

Tetracycline

Staphcillin

Keflin

Contraindications
Digitalis toxicity

Ventricular fibrillation

Hypercalcemia

Comments
Calcium chloride is more potent (three times) than calcium gluconate.

It is a very sclerosing agent. Infiltration will cause tissue sloughing and necrosis.

Continuous ECG monitoring is required.

Calcium chloride increases digitalis toxicity.

DILANTIN (PHENYTOIN)

Dosage

Adult
- Antiarrhythmic—50 mgm to 100 mgm slow IV push every 5 minutes to 10 minutes as indicated (total dosage not to exceed 1 gm)
- Anticonvulsant—150 mgm to 250 mgm administered slow IV push initially; 100 mgm to 150 mgm may be administered slow IV push 30 minutes later if necessary

Child
- 2 mgm/kgm to 5 mgm/kgm slow IV push over a period of 5 minutes

NOTE. Do not administer more than 50 mgm of phenytoin per minute intravenously.

NOTE. Oral administration is the preferred method (100 mgm to 300 mgm PO 4 times a day).

Side-effects

Heart block
Respiratory arrest
Seizures (tonic)
Nervousness
Tremors
Bradycardia
Cardiac arrest
Ventricular fibrillation
Confusion
Severe hypotension
Skin eruptions

Incompatibilities

Any drug in syringe or solution
Aminophyllin
Insulin
Levophed
Aramine
Demerol
Morphine sulfate
Benadryl

Contraindications

Hypersensitivity

Second-degree heart block

Complete heart block

Sinus bradycardia

SA block

Adams–Stokes syndrome

Comments

Extravasation will cause tissue sloughing.

Normal saline is used to flush IV line before and after administration.

The solution should be clear and free of precipitate.

Action is more potent when used with other drugs, including anticoagulants, valium, amphetamines, analeptics, sulfonamides, and myocardial depressants.

Dilantin cannot be used with digitalis.

DOPAMINE HYDROCHLORIDE (INTROPIN)

Dosage

Adult

- Use microdrip to administer 2 mcgm/kgm/min to 5 mcgm/kgm/min diluted in IV infusion
- Increase dosage gradually by 5 mcgm/kgm/min until desired response (up to 20 mcgm/kgm/min to 50 mcgm/kgm/min)
- If doses higher than 50 mcgm/kgm/min are used, urine output must be closely watched.

NOTE. See dilution methods under comments.

Pregnancy
- Use with extreme caution and only if the benefits outweigh the risks

Child
- Safety not established

Side-effects

Anginal pain

Ectopic beats

Vomiting

Hypotension or hypertension

Vasoconstriction

Aberrant conduction

Azotemia

Bradycardia

Nausea

Headache

Widened QRS complex

Piloerection

Incompatibilities

Sodium bicarbonate

Alkaline solutions

Contraindications

Pheochromocytoma

Uncorrected tachyarrhythmias

Ventricular fibrillation

Comments

Dilute dopamine hydrochloride in a 250-ml or 500-ml bottle in one of the following sterile solutions: normal saline, 5% dextrose in water, 5% dextrose in normal saline (0.9% or 0.45%), sodium lactate (one-sixth molar solution), or lactated Ringer's solution.

NOTE. If a 5-ml (200-mgm) ampule is diluted in 250 ml of solution, each milliliter contains 800 mcgm of dopamine. If a 5-ml (200 mgm) ampule is diluted in 500 ml of solution, each milliliter contains 400 mcgm of dopamine.

Check arterial blood pressure (A-line and cuff) every 3 to 5 minutes initially and closely throughout therapy.

Monitor ECG continuously.

If a disproportionate rise in the diastolic pressure is noted (pulse pressure is markedly narrowed), slow down the infusion and notify the physician immediately.

Monitor urine output closely. If it decreases, slow down the infusion and notify the physician immediately.

Discard discolored solutions and those that are over 24 hours old.

Infuse dopamine hydrochloride in a large vein. Tissue sloughing and necrosis may follow extravasation.

Do not add other medications to the solution.

Use it with caution in patients taking MAO inhibitors (require 1/10 of normal dose) and with patients with occlusive vascular disease. It may cause severe hypertension in patient receiving oxytocin or ergonovine.

EPINEPHRINE (ADRENALIN)

Dosage

Bronchodilator or Allergic Reactions

Adult

• 0.2 ml to 1 ml of 1:1000 solution SC

Child
• 0.05 mgm to 0.3 mgm of 1:1000 solution SC

Cardiac Arrest

Adult
• 0.5 mgm to 1 mgm (5–10 ml of a 1:10,000 dilution) may be administered IV or intracardiac; repeat every 5 minutes

Child
• 0.03 mgm to 0.2 mgm (0.3–2 ml of 1:10,000 dilution) may be administered IV or intracardiac; repeat every 5 minutes

Newborn
• 0.1 mgm to 0.2 mgm (1–2 ml of 1:10,000 dilution) may be administered intracardiac

NOTE. 1:10,000 solution is obtained by diluting 1 ml of a 1:1000 solution of aqueous epinephrine in 10 ml of normal saline.

IV Infusion

Adult
• 1 mgm epinephrine added to 250 ml of 5% dextrose in water; start with 1 mcgm/kgm/min

Child
• Start with 0.1 mcgm/kgm/min

NOTE. Only aqueous epinephrine may be given intravenously or intracardiac.

Side-effects

Pulmonary edema

Hypertension

Hypotension

Palpitations

Restlessness

Pupillary dilation

Headache

Tachycardia

Anginal pain if coronary insufficiency present

Death

Contraindications

Glaucoma (narrow-angle)

Digitalized patient

Hyperthyroidism

Hypertension

During labor

Shock (except anaphylactic)

Anesthesia with cyclopropane or halogenated hydrocarbons

Organic brain damage

Coronary insufficiency

Incompatibilities

Alkaline solutions

Calcium chloride

Calcium gluconate

Pronestyl

Aminophylline

Thorazine

Compazine

Valium

NOTE. Do not mix epinephrine with any other drug. If administering **IV** push following alkaline solutions, flush the line before injecting.

Comments

Epinephrine cannot be administered concurrently with other cardiac stimulants (Isuprel, calcium chloride).

Acidosis must be corrected prior to epinephrine administration.

It deteriorates rapidly. Protect from heat and light, and referigerate if possible.

Epinephrine should be clear. Discard it if sediment is noted or if it is brown in color.

Administration of epinephrine with MAO inhibitors may result in a hypertensive crisis.

Continuous ECG monitoring is indicated.

Blood pressure should be checked frequently (every 5 min during therapy).

Effects of epinephrine are immediate.

Epinephrine must be administered with caution in the following situations: pregnancy, hypertension, diabetes, and in the elderly patient.

HYPERSTAT IV (DIAZOXIDE)

Dosage

Adult

• Rapid IV push (30 sec or less)—1 mgm/kgm to 3 mgm/kgm maximum

dose being 150 mgm; repeat at 5 minute to 15 minute intervals until
desired reduction in blood pressure is achieved

Child
* 5 mgm/kgm rapid IV push

Maternity
* Safety not established

Side-effects

Sodium and water retention

Hypotension (severe)

Palpitations

Supraventricular tachycardia

Angina

Seizures

Coma

Congestive heart failure

Dizziness

Flushing

Headache

Hyperglycemia

Incompatibilities

Do not mix with any other drug

Contraindications

Compensatory hypertension (aortic coarctation or AV shunt)

Hypersensitivity to Hyperstat or other thiazides

Pregnancy

Children

NOTE. Diazoxide is not effective in lowering blood pressure if it is caused
by pheochromocytoma.

Comments

Patient should remain supine during therapy and immediately afterward
(approximately 30 minutes).

Potent diuretic (Lasix or Edecrin) should be administered during therapy.

Continuous ECG monitoring is indicated.

Blood pressure should be monitored closely during therapy (blood pressure will generally decrease in 5 min or less following administration),
following administration until stabilized, and then hourly.

INDERAL (PROPRANOLOL HYDROCHLORIDE)

Dosage

Adult
- 1 mgm to 3 mgm (diluted in 50 ml of 5% dextrose in water or undiluted) IV push administered 1 mgm/min; may be repeated once if necessary in 2 minutes; further administration should not be attempted any sooner than 4 hours
- Intravenous administration for extreme emergencies only

NOTE. Oral administration is the route of choice. This method should be employed as soon as possible. Dosage is highly individualized.

Child
- Data not available

Maternity
- Safety not established

Side-effects

Bradycardia

Hypotension

Congestive heart failure

AV block

Cardiac arrest

Respiratory distress

Agranulocytosis

Light-headedness

Weakness

Fatigue

Emotional lability

Memory loss (short term)

Hallucinations

Nausea

Vomiting

Diarrhea

Abdominal cramps

Incompatibilites

Any other drug in solution or syringe

Contraindications

Cardiogenic shock

Sinus bradycardia

Heart block greater than first degree

Right ventricular failure occurring secondary to pulmonary hypertension

Bronchial asthma

Allergic rhinitis

Antidepressants (including MAO inhibitors)

Comments

Monitor ECG continuously.

Monitor blood pressure closely.

Discontinue the medication slowly.

Be aware that propranolol hydrochloride may mask the warning symptoms of acute hypoglycemia.

Discontinue the drug 48 hours prior to surgery, with the exception of surgery for pheochromocytoma. If this is not possible, it can be reversed by the administration of Levophed or Isuprel. The anesthesiologist *must* be informed that the patient was receiving Inderal, even if the effects have been reversed (severe complications may follow reversal, including severe, prolonged hypotension).

Notify physician immediately if significant side-effects occur.

Keep emergency drugs and equipment readily available.

ISUPREL (ISOPROTERENOL)

Dosage

Adult

- Use microdrip to administer IV infusion—1 mcgm to 4 mcgm/min of a 1:250,000 solution
- IV push (over 1 min)—initially, 0.02 mgm to 0.06 mgm (1–3ml of a 1:50,000 solution)
- Intracardiac—0.02 mgm (0.1 ml of 1:5000 solution undiluted)
- Titrate

NOTE. To obtain 1:50,000 solution, 1 ml of solution 1:5000 (0.2 mgm) is diluted with 10 ml of sodium chloride or 5% dextrose. To obtain 1:250,000 solution, 10 ml of solution 1:5000 (2 mg) is diluted in 500 ml of 5% dextrose.

Child

- 1 mgm to 4 mgm diluted at rate of 0.1 mcgm/kgm/min to 0.5 mcgm/kgm/min (titrated)
- Use microdrip

Side-effects

Anginal pain

Palpitation

Nausea

Sweating

Headache

Flushing of face

Nervousness

Incompatibilities

Inderal

MAO inhibitors

Valium

Contraindications

Tachycardia caused by digitalis toxicity

Precautions

Do not administer isoproterenol concurrently with other cardiac stimulants (*e.g.*, epinephrine).

Administer with extreme caution in patients with coronary insufficiency, hyperthyroidism, diabetes, or sensitivity to sympathomimetic amines.

Comments

Adjust infusion speed based on heart rate, blood pressure, central venous pressure, and urinary output.

Decrease infusion if heart rate exceeds 110 beat/min. Notify physician.

Monitor ECG continuously.

LANOXIN (DIGOXIN)

Dosage

Parenteral (IM or IV) Administration

Adults and children over 10 years of age

- Digitalizing dose—0.5 mgm to 1 mgm
- Initial dose—0.25 mgm to 0.5 mgm
- Additional doses may have to be administered every 4 to 6 hours. (additional doses—0.25 mgm)
- Digitalization may not occur until a total of 1 mgm has been administered.
- Maintenance dose—0.125 mgm to 0.5 mgm (usually 0.25 mgm) usually through oral administration; parenteral administration will be used if lesions of the GI tract are present or the patient cannot tolerate PO medication (administered as one dose or divided doses)

Parenteral (IM or IV) Administration
Infants and children under 10 years of age
• Digitalization is highly individualized.
• Digitalizing dose (total amount given in divided doses) is as follows:
    • Ages 2 to 10 years—25 mcgm/kgm of body weight to 40 mcgm/kgm of body weight
    • Infant (from 2 wk) to 2 years—35 mcgm/kgm of body weight to 50 mcgm/kgm of body weight.
    • Premature and infants under 2 weeks old—25 mcgm/kgm of body weight to 40 mcgm/kgm of body weight
• Initial dose—one fourth to one half of total dose
• Subsequent doses—one fourth of total dose is administered every six hours until patient is digitalized
• Maintenance dose—20% to 30% of total digitalizing dose (administered as one dose or divided doses)

NOTE. Administer digoxin slow IV push 0.25 mgm over 1 minute. IV administration is the preferred route.

Side-effects
Signs of toxicity

Adult
GI symptoms (most common early signs of toxicity)
• Nausea
• Vomiting
• Loss of appetite
• Diarrhea
Headache
Weakness
Disturbances in vision (yellow vision, blurred vision)
Almost any type of arrhythmia
• Premature ventricular contractions (most common)
• PAT
• Nodal rhythms (paroxysmal and nonparoxysmal)
• AV dissociation
• Conduction disturbances (heart block of increasing degree may progress to complete block)
ECG changes (prolonged PR interval, sagging of ST segment, bigeminy may be present)

Child
Cardiac arrhythmias (most frequent sign of toxicity in this age group)
• Atrial arrhythmias

- PAT with block
- Atrial ectopic rhythms
- Nodal systole

Premature ventricular contractions (rarely seen)
Ventricular arrhythmias (rarely seen)

Newborn
SA arrest
Prolonged PR interval
Undue slowing of sinus rate

NOTE. Neurological changes, vision disturbances, and GI symptoms occur only rarely as initial signs of toxicity.

Incompatibilities
Calcium preparations
Protein hydrolysate (Amigen)
Acid solutions
Alkali solutions

Contraindications
Ventricular fibrillation
Toxic effects caused by a digitalis preparation
Sensitivity reaction

Comments
Give digoxin undiluted through 3-way stopcock directly IV.

Do not add it to IV solution.

Avoid IM administration because it is very painful.
- If administration is ordered IM, use deep IM technique.
- Massage the injection site immediately.
- Do not administer more than 0.5 mgm/site to lessen discomfort.

Monitor ECG continuously.

Monitor electrolytes closely.
- Hypokalemia predisposes the patient towards digitalis toxicity.
- Abnormalities should be corrected.

Take an apical-radial pulse for a full minute. Significant abnormalities should be reported to the physician immediately.

Administer with caution in the patient with advanced heart failure, acute myocardial infarction, and severe pulmonary disease.

Withhold drug for at least 2 days prior to cardioversion.

Administer lower digitalizing and maintenance doses to patients with renal failure.

Take the apical pulse for a full minute prior to administration. If pulse is below 60 or grossly irregular, withhold digoxin administration and notify the physician.

Check blood levels frequently.

LEVOPHED OR NOREPINEPHRINE (LEVARTERENOL BITARTRATE)

Dosage
Adult
- 2 mcgm to 4 mcgm (0.5–1 ml) min diluted solution (titrate)

Child
- 0.1 mcgm/kgm/min to 1 mcgm/kgm/min diluted solution (titrate)

NOTE. For diluted solution add 4 ml of Levophed to 1000 ml of either 5% dextrose in water or 5% dextrose in saline, providing a concentration of 4 mcgm/ml.

Side-effects
Bradycardia

Headache (may indicate overdosage)

Chest pain

Incompatibilities
Valium

Aramine

Dilantin

Heparin solution

Oxytocin

Staphcillin

Keflin

Sodium bicarbonate

Pentothal

Diuril

Contraindications
Hypotension due to blood loss

Use with cyclopropane and halothane anesthesia

Mesenteric or peripheral vascular thrombosis

Comments
Extravasation causes tissue sloughing and necrosis.

If extravasation occurs, infiltrate the area with Regitine (5–10 mgm diluted in 10–15 ml of saline solution) as soon as possible. Regitine may be added to IV solution (5–10 mgm).

Blood pressure should be checked every 2 minutes during initial therapy and then every 5 minutes thereafter. Arterial pressure readings and cuff pressures are recommended.

Infusion should be through a catheter located in a large vein.

Patient should not be left alone during therapy.

Constant ECG is indicated.

Levaterenol bitartrate should be discontinued gradually.

LIDOCAINE HYDROCHLORIDE (Xylocaine)

Dosage

Adult
- Bolus—50 mgm to 100 mgm (1 mgm/kgm body weight) administered
- 25 mgm/min to 50 mgm/min; repeat every 3 minutes to 5 minutes, total amount not exceeding 200 mgm to 300 mgm in 1 hour
- IV infusion—1 mgm/min to 4 mgm/min (Add 1 gram Lidocaine to 1000 ml 5% dextrose.)

Child
- Bolus—1 mgm/kgm body weight, slow push
- IV infusion—1 mgm/kgm every hour

Side-effects

Convulsions

Coma

Slurred speech

Blurred or double vision

Respiratory depression and arrest

Hypotension

Bradycardia

Cardiovascular collapse and arrest

Confusion

Restlessness

Tinnitus

Twitching

Incompatibilities

Should not be mixed with other drugs due to the rate adjustments that have to be made

Contraindications

Hypersensitivity

Adam–Stokes syndrome

Severe heart block (of SA, AV or intraventricular origin)

Comments

Monitor ECG continuously.

Stop infusion immediately if signs of excessive cardiac conductivity depression (prolonged PR interval and QRS complex) or arrhythmias (either sudden appearance or increase of preexisting ones) occur.

Use lidocaine hydrochloride with caution in hepatic failure, congestive failure, and elderly patients. These patients require 50% of the normal loading dose and a reduced maintenance dose.

MAGNESIUM SULFATE

Dosage

Adult
- 4 gm in 250 ml of 5% dextrose in water IV
- 4 gm to 5 gm deep IM

Child
- 0.2 ml/kgm of a 50% solution IM every 4 hours to 6 hours as necessary or 100 mgm/kgm of a 10% solution IV very slowly (titrate)

NOTE. Do not infuse more than 150 mgm/min of magnesium sulfate.

Side-effects

Drowsiness

Depressed reflexes (knee jerk reflex is absent)

Flushing

Circulatory collapse

Cardiac arrest

Heart block

Respiratory depression

Respiratory failure

Hypocalcemic tetany

Incompatibilities

Calcium gluconate

Sodium bicarbonate

Aquamephyton

Thorazine

Contraindications

Heart block

Myocardial damage

Renal failure

Respiratory depression

During labor

Comments

Check respirations for a full minute before each dose. There should be approximately 16 breaths/min. If respirations are depressed, notify physician before administering magnesium sulfate.

Monitor ECG continuously.

NOTE. Watch for heart block.

Check vital signs frequently (every 15 min) during therapy.

Monitor urinary output closely. Notify physician immediately if oliguria develops.

Keep an IV preparation of calcium gluconate at the bedside at all times in case magnesium intoxication develops.

Check serum magnesium levels during therapy.

If side-effects occur, withhold medication and notify physician immediately.

NIPRIDE (SODIUM NITROPRUSSIDE)

Dosage

Adult and Child

• Use microdrip to administer 3 mcgm/kgm/min of diluted solution (normal range from 0.5-10mcg/kgm/min); titrate

NOTE. Diluted solution is obtained by the following method. Mix 50 mgm (one vial) of Nipride with 2 ml to 3 ml of dextrose in water. This stock solution should then be diluted in 250 ml to 1000 ml of 5% dextrose in water.

• 50 mgm (1 vial) Nipride in 250 ml 5% dextrose in water will yield a concentration of 200 mcgm/ml.
• 50 mgm (1 vial) Nipride in 500 ml 5% dextrose in water will yield a concentration of 100 mcgm/ml.
• 50 mgm (1 vial) Nipride in 1000 ml 5% dextrose in water will yield a concentration of 50 mcgm/ml.

NOTE. Sodium nitroprusside must be diluted.

Maternity

• Safety not established

Side-effects

Muscle twitching

Diaphoresis

Restlessness

Headache

Apprehension

Nausea

Abdominal pain

Palpitations

Retrosternal discomfort

Dizziness

Cyanide toxicity

Retching

Incompatibilities

Do not add any other drug to this solution.

Contraindications

Compensatory hypertension (coarctation of the aorta or arteriovenous shunt)

Comments

Wrap infusion bag or bottle and tubing in foil to protect from light.

Monitor ECG continuously.

Check blood pressure every minute until the desired level is reached, and then every 5 minutes to 15 minutes according to the patient's status.

Do not leave patient unattended during therapy.

Effects are almost immediate following infusion with the diastolic pressure being lowered and maintained at 30 to 40% below the pretreatment level.

The blood pressure will usually return to pretreatment levels within 1 minute to 10 minutes after the infusion is slowed or stopped.

Use sodium nitroprusside with extreme caution with the elderly. They require lower dosages.

Discard the prepared solution after 4 hours.

The solution normally has a very faint brownish tint.

Reduce the dosage of other antihypertensive agents being administered concurrently.

Check thiocyanate levels of patients receiving long-term therapy or high doses (greater than 10 mcgm/kgm/min).

Blood pressure should be reduced gradually.

Take precautions to prevent extravasation. Watch patient closely.

Administer solium nitroprusside with caution in the presence of hypothyroidism, severe renal impairment, or hepatic insufficiency.

POTASSIUM CHLORIDE

Dosage

Adult
- IV infusion—usually no more than 10 mEq/hour of a diluted solution, not to exceed a total daily dose of 150 mEq

NOTE. In an extreme emergency (*e.g.*, serum potassium under 2 mEq/liter), 40 mEq/hr may be administered with extreme caution.

Child
- IV infusion—total dose for 24 hours should not exceed 3 mEq/kgm of body weight

NOTE. To make diluted solution add 20 mEq to 40 mEq in 500 ml to 1000 ml 5% dextrose in water.

Side-effects

ECG changes (shortened QT interval, widened QRS complex, prolonged PR interval, P wave diminished in size or absent, peaked T wave, ST segment depression)

Bradycardia

Heart block

Ventricular fibrillation

Ventricular asystole

Cardiac arrest

Weakness

Voluntary muscle paralysis

Mental confusion

Paresthesia of the extremities

Incompatibilities

Protein hydrolysate (Amigen)

Amphotericin B (Fungizone)

Contraindications

Oliguria

Kidney failure

Shock with hemolytic reactions

Dehydration

Hyperkalemia

Adrenal cortex insufficiency

Comments

Parenteral administration should be slow IV only. Never give IM or IV push.

Potassium chloride must be diluted.

Potassium blood levels should be monitored closely.

Continuous ECG monitoring is indicated.

Potassium chloride should be administered with extreme caution in the cardiac patient.

PRONESTYL (PROCAINAMIDE)

Dosage

Adult (The following two approaches may be used in extreme emergency:)

• Administer 100 mgm diluted in 10 ml of 5% dextrose in water, slow IV push (do not exceed 50 mgm/min) every 5 minutes until the arrhythmia ceases, side-effects occur, or a total of 1 gm has been administered; follow by IV infusion of 2 mgm/minute to 6 mgm/minute for maintenance therapy.

• Infuse 500 mgm to 600 mgm diluted in 5% dextrose in water (do not exceed 25 mgm–50 mgm) over 25 minutes to 30 minutes; follow by IV infusion of 2 mgm/minute to 6 mgm/minute for maintenance therapy

NOTE. Prepare IV infusion by adding 1 gm of Pronestyl to 500 ml of 5% dextrose in water (concentration is 2 mgm Pronestyl/ml). Titrate.

NOTE. The preferred parenteral route is IM (0.5 mgm–1 gm every 6 hr until medication can be administered orally). Intravenous administration should be used for extreme emergencies only.

Side-effects

Severe hypotension (with IV administration)

Ventricular asystole (with IV administration)

Ventricular fibrillation (with IV administration)

Ventricular tachycardia (with IV administration)

Lupus erythematuslike syndrome

ECG changes (prolonged PR interval, widening QRS complex, prolonged QT interval)

Nausea

Vomiting

Elevated temperature

Chills

Diarrhea

Weakness

Giddiness

Mental depression

Hallucinations

Elevated SGOT

Incompatibilities

Dilantin

Should not be mixed with other drugs due to rate adjustments that are necessary

Contraindications

Hypersensitivity

Myasthenia gravis

Complete heart block

High-degree AV block (unless pacemaker has been inserted)

Comments

Monitor ECG constantly.

Monitor blood pressure constantly.

Keep patient in the supine position during IV therapy.

Use procainamide with extreme caution in the following situations: acute MI, hepatic insufficiency, renal insufficiency, digitalis intoxication, AV block, and bundle branch block.

Keep in mind that small emboli may dislodge after atrial fibrillation has been corrected.

Do not leave patient unattended during IV therapy.

Watch closely for significant side-effects and notify physician immediately if any develop.

NOTE. If ECG changes are noted, withhold the medication and notify the physician immediately. Document changes with rhythm strip.

Keep emergency drugs and equipment readily available.

Use an infusion pump to administer procainamide. Dosage must be precise.

SODIUM BICARBONATE

Dosage

Adult

• 1 to 2 ampules IV push initially, followed by 1 ampule every 10 minutes

Child

• 1 mEq/kgm IV push every 5 minutes to 10 minutes.

NOTE. Approximately one half of the initial dose is repeated every 10 minutes according to arterial blood gas reports.

Maternity
• Monitor closely for symptoms of fluid and sodium retention

Side-effects
Alkalosis

Hypernatremia

Incompatibilities
Atropine

Calcium chloride

Calcium gluconate

Lactated Ringer's solutions

Ringer's solution

Antibiotics (*e.g.*, tetracycline, Staphcillin, streptomycin)

Levophed

Codeine

Demerol

Morphine

Magnesium sulfate

Comments
Arterial blood gases must be monitored closely and the dosage adjusted accordingly.

METHODS OF CALCULATING PEDIATRIC DOSAGE

$$\frac{\text{Adult dose} \times \text{age of child}}{\text{Age of child} + 12} = \text{Pediatric dose}$$

Clark's Rule

$$\frac{\text{Child's weight in pounds}}{150} \times \text{Adult dose} = \text{Pediatric dose}$$

$$\frac{\text{Body surface area in square meters}}{1.75} \times \text{Adult dose} = \text{Pediatric dose}$$

BIBLIOGRAPHY

Abels Linda F: Mosby's Manual of Critical Care. St. Louis, CV Mosby, 1979
Andreoli Kathleen, Fowkes Virginia Hunn, Zipes Douglas P et al: Comprehensive Cardiac Care, 4th ed. St Louis, CV Mosby, 1979
Assessing Vital Functions Accurately. Nursing Skillbook. Horsham, PA, Intermed Communications, Inc., 1977
Barry Jeanie. Emergency Nursing. New York, McGraw–Hill, 1978
Bates Barbara: A Guide To Physical Examination, 2nd ed. Philadelphia, JB Lippincott, 1979
Beeson Paul B, McDermott Walsh, Wyngarrden, James B: Cecil Textbook of Medicine, 15th ed., Vol 1. Philadelphia: WB Saunders, 1979
Blowers Margaret G, Smith Roberta J. How to Read An ECG. Oradell, NJ, Medical Economics, 1977
Brunner Lillian S, Suddarth Doris S: Textbook of Medical–Surgical Nursing 4th ed. Philadelphia, JB Lippincott, 1980
Brunner Lillian S, Suddarth Doris S: The Lippincott Manual of Nursing Practice, 2nd ed. Philadelphia, JB Lippincott, 1978
Combating Cardiovascular Diseases Skillfully. Nursing Skillbook. Horsham, PA, Intermed Communications, Inc., 1978
Cosgriff James H: An Atlas of Diagnostic and Therapeutic Procedures for Emergency Personnel. Philadelphia, JB Lippincott, 1978
Cosgriff James H, Anderson Diann L: The Practice of Emergency Nursing. Philadelphia, JB Lippincott, 1975
Dealing with Emergencies. Nursing Photobook. Horsham, PA, Intermed Communications, Inc., 1980
Dubin D: Rapid Interpretation of EKG's, 3rd ed. Tampa, Cover Publishing, 1979
Gahart Betty L: Intravenous Medications, 2nd ed. St. Louis, CV Mosby, 1977
Giving Emergency Care Competently. Nursing Skillbook. Horsham, PA, Intermed Communications, 1978
Hamilton Ardith J: Selected Subjects for Critical Care Nurses. Missoula, Mountain Press Publishing, 1975
Holloway Nancy M: Nursing the Critically Ill Adult. Reading, MA, Addison–Wesley Publishing Co, 1979
Hudak Carolyn M: Critical Care Nursing, 2nd ed. Philadelphia, JB Lippincott, 1977
Meltzer Lawrence E, Pinneo, Rose, Kitchell J. Roderick: Intensive Coronary Care, 3rd ed. Bowie, MD, The Charles Press Publishers, 1977
Reading EKGs Correctly. Nursing Skillbook. Horsham, PA, Intermed Communications, Inc., 1977
Millar Sally (ed): Methods in Critical Care—The A.A.C.N. Manual. Philadelphia, WB Saunders, 1980
Nursing Critically Ill Patients Confidently. Nursing Skillbook. Horsham, PA, Intermed Communications, Inc., 1979
Physicians Desk Reference. Oradell, NJ, The Medical Economics Company, 1981
Providing Respiratory Care. Nursing Photobook Series. Horsham, PA, Intermed Communications, Inc., 1979

Standards and Guidelines for Cardiopulmonary Resuscitation (CPR) and Emergency Cardiac Care (ECC). JAMA 244, 5:453–509, 1980

Schroeder John S, Daily Elaine K: Techniques in Bedside Hemodynamic Monitoring. St. Louis, CV Mosby, 1976

Swift Nancy, Mabel Robert M: Manual of Neurological Nursing. Boston, Little, Brown & Co, 1978

Using Monitors. Nursing Photobook Series. Horsham, PA, Intermed Communications, Inc., 1979

Vinsant Marielle Ortiz, Spence Martha I, Hagen Dianne Chapell: A Commonsense Approach to Coronary Care: A Program, 2nd ed. St. Louis, CV Mosby, 1975

Appendix

NOMOGRAM FOR ESTIMATING SURFACE AREA OF INFANTS AND YOUNG CHILDREN

Height		Surface Area	Weight	
Feet	*Centimeters*	*In Square Meters*	*Pounds*	*Kilograms*

To determine the surface area of the patient draw a straight line between the point representing his height on the left vertical scale to the point representing his weight on the right vertical scale. The point at which this line intersects the middle vertical scale represents the patient's surface area in square meters. (Courtesy, Abbott Laboratories.) **379**

NOMOGRAM FOR ESTIMATING SURFACE AREA OF OLDER CHILDREN AND ADULTS

Height		Surface Area	Weight	
Feet	*Centimeters*	*In Square Meters*	*Pounds*	*Kilograms*

Height (Feet / Centimeters):
7′ — 220, 215, 210
10″ — 205
8″ — 200
6″ — 195, 190
4″ —
2″ — 185
6′ — 180
10″ — 175
8″ — 170
6″ — 165
4″ — 160
2″ — 155
5′ — 150
10″ — 145
8″ — 140
6″ — 135
4″ — 130
2″ — 125
4′ — 120
10″ — 115
8″ — 110
6″ — 105
4″ — 100
2″ — 95
3′ — 90
10″ — 85
8″ — 80
6″ — 75

Surface Area (In Square Meters):
3.00, 2.90, 2.80, 2.70, 2.60, 2.50, 2.40, 2.30, 2.20, 2.10, 2.00, 1.95, 1.90, 1.85, 1.80, 1.75, 1.70, 1.65, 1.60, 1.55, 1.50, 1.45, 1.40, 1.35, 1.30, 1.25, 1.20, 1.15, 1.10, 1.05, 1.00, .95, .90, .85, .80, .75, .70, .65, .60

Weight (Pounds):
440, 420, 400, 380, 360, 340, 320, 300, 290, 280, 270, 260, 250, 240, 230, 220, 210, 200, 190, 180, 170, 160, 150, 140, 130, 120, 110, 100, 90, 80, 70, 60, 50

Weight (Kilograms):
200, 190, 180, 170, 160, 150, 140, 130, 120, 110, 100, 95, 90, 85, 80, 75, 70, 65, 60, 55, 50, 45, 40, 35, 30, 25, 20

(Courtesy, Abbott Laboratories.)

Table for Calculating the Heart Rate by Measuring the Number of Large Squares

Number of Large Squares	Rate
1	300
2	150
3	100
4	75
5	60
6	50
7	43
8	38
9	33
10	30

Table for Calculating the Heart Rate if the Second R Wave Falls Between Two Heavy Black Lines

Heavy Black Lines	Interval	Value of Each Small Line Between Interval
1	300–150	250
		214
		187
		167
2	150–100	136
		125
		115
		107
3	100–75	94
		88
		83
		79
4	75–60	71
		68
		65
		62
5	60–50	58
		55
		54
		52

Table for Calculating the Heart Rate by Measuring the Number of Small Squares or Time Interval

Number of Small Squares	Time (Measured in Sec)	Rate
3	0.12	500
4	0.16	375
5	0.2	300
6	0.24	250
7	0.28	214
8	0.32	188
9	0.36	167
10	0.4	150
11	0.44	136
12	0.48	125
13	0.52	115
14	0.56	107
15	0.6	100
16	0.64	94
17	0.68	88
18	0.72	83
19	0.76	79
20	0.8	75
21	0.84	71
22	0.88	68
23	0.92	65
24	0.96	63
25	1	60
26	1.04	58

(Continued)

**Table for Calculating the Heart Rate by Measuring the Number of Small Squares
or Time Interval** *(Continued)*

Number of Small Squares	Time (Measured in Sec)	Rate
27	1.08	56
28	1.12	54
29	1.16	52
30	1.2	50
31	1.24	48
32	1.28	47
33	1.32	46
34	1.36	44
35	1.40	43
36	1.44	42
37	1.48	41
38	1.52	40
39	1.56	39
40	1.6	38
41	1.64	37
42	1.68	36
43	1.72	35
44	1.76	34
45	1.8	33
46	1.84	(32.6) = 33
47	1.88	32
48	1.92	31
49	1.96	(30.6) = 31
50	2	30

LABORATORY VALUES

Normal Arterial Blood Gases

Arterial Blood Gases	Normal Value
pH	7.35–7.45
pCO_2	35 mm Hg–45 mm Hg
pO_2	80 mm Hg–100 mm Hg
O_2 saturation	95%–100%
HCO_3^-	22 mEq/liter–26 mEq/liter
H_2CO_3	1.05 mEq/liter–1.35 mEq/liter
Base excess	−2 to +2

Acid-Base Status Vigorous Term Infants*

Determination	Vaginal Delivery	Birth	First Hour	Third Hour	24 Hours	Two Days	Three Days
pH	Umbilical artery	7.26					
	Umbilical vein	7.29					
pCO_2 mm Hg	Arterial	54.5	38.8	38.3	33.6	34	35
	venous	42.8					
O_2 sat.	Arterial	19.8	93.8	94.7	93.2		
	venous	47.6					
pH	Left atrial		7.30	7.34	7.41	7.39 (temp. artery)	7.38 (temp. artery)
CO_2 content mEq/liter			20.6	21.9	21.4		

Premature Infants

	Capillary			7.36	7.35	7.35
pH	Below 1250 gm			7.36	7.35	7.35
pCO_2 mm Hg				38	44	37
pH	Above 1250 gm			7.39	7.39	7.38
pCO_2 mm Hg				38	39	38

*(Avery GB: Neonatology. Philadelphia, Lippincott, 1975. Data of Weisbort LM et al: J Pediatr 52:395, 1958; and Bucci E et al: Biol Neonate, 8:81, 1965)

Blood Chemistry for an Adult

Determination	Normal Value*
Ammonia (plasma)	5 mcgm/dl†–70 mcgm/dl
Bilirubin	Total—0.1 mgm/dl–1 mgm/dl Direct—0.1 mgm/dl–0.2 mgm/dl Indirect—0.1 mgm/dl–0.8 mgm/dl
Calcium	8.5 mgm/dl–10.5 mgm/dl
Chloride	95 mEq/liter–105 mEq/liter
Creatinine	0.7 mgm/dl–1.4 mgm/dl
Glucose	Fasting—60 mgm/dl–110 mgm/dl Postprandial (2 hr)—65 mgm/dl–140 mgm/dl
Magnesium	1.8 mEq/liter–2.2 mEq/liter
Osmolality	280 milliosmoles/kgm–300 milliosmoles/kgm
Potassium	3.5mEq/liter–5.0 mEq/liter
Sodium	135 mEq/liter–145 mEq/liter
Urea nitrogen (BUN)	10 mgm/dl–20 mgm/dl

*Normal values vary according to different hospitals' laboratory practices
†dl equals 100 ml.

Blood Chemistry for a Child

Determination	Normal Value
Ammonia	below 150 mcgm % (Seligson blood ammonia)

*Bilirubin	Cord—up to 1.8 mgm %
	2–4 days—mean peak 7 mgm %
	      range 2 mgm %–12 mgm %
	After newborn period—less than 0.8 mgm %
	    total

*Calcium	9.0 mgm %–11.5 mgm %
*Chloride	94 mEq/liter–106 mEq/liter
*Creatinine	0.7 mgm %–1.5 mgm %
*Glucose (fasting)	55 mgm %–100 mgm %
*Potassium	0–10 days—up to 7 mEq/liter Thereafter—3.5mEq/liter–5.0 mEq/liter
*Sodium	136 mEq/liter–145 mEq/liter
*Urea nitrogen (Nonpro- tein nitrogen)	6 mgm %–23 mgm %

*These determinations are done by the Johns Hopkins Hospital routine laboratory on serum, and the values quoted apply to their methods. Values for other determinations are taken from the literature and may not be valid for a given laboratory.

(Johns Hopkins Hospital. The Harriet Lane Handbook. 7th ed. Chicago, Year Book Medical Publishers, Inc., 1975)

Hematology for an Adult

Determination	Normal Value
Erythrocyte count (Red blood cell)	Males—4,600,000–6,200,00 Females—4,200,000–5,400,000
Erythrocyte sedimentation rate	Males—0 mm/hr–9 mm/hr Females—0 mm/hr–20 mm/hr
Hematocrit	Males—42%–50% Females—40%–48%
Hemoglobin	Males—13 gm/dl–16 gm/dl Females—12 gm/dl–14 gm/dl
Leukocyte count (WBC)	Total—5,000 cu/mm–10,000/cu mm
Neutrophils	60%–70%
Eosinophils	1%–4%
Basophils	0%–0.5%
Lymphocytes	20%–30%
Monocytes	2%–6%
Partial thromboplastin time (activated)	20 sec–45 sec
Platelets	200,000/cu mm—350,000/cu mm
Prothrombin time	70%–100% of control

Hematology for a Child

	Gm Hgb	% Hct	WBC/cu mm	% Polys	% Retics
1 day	16–22*	53–73*	18,000 (7,000–35,000)	45–85	2.5–6.5
1 wk	13–20*	43–66*	10,000 (4,000–20,000)	30–50	0.1–4.5
1 mo	16	53	10,000 (6,000–18,000)	30–50	0.1–1.0
3 mo	11.5	38	10,000 (6,000–17,000)	30–50	0.7–3.0
6 mo	12	40	10,000 (6,000–16,000)	30–50	0.7–2.3
1 yr	12	40	10,000 (6,000–15,000)	30–50	0.6–1.7
2–6 yr	13	43	9,000 (7,000–13,000)	35–55	0.5–1.0
7–12 yr	14	46	8,500 (5,000–12,000)	40–60	0.5–1.0

Absolute eosinophil count—100/cu min–600/cu mm, average 250

*Under the age of 1 month capillary Hgb and Hct exceed venous as follows:
1 hour: 3.6 gm average difference
5 days: 2.2 gm average difference
3 weeks: 1.1 gm average difference
(Johns Hopkins Hospital. The Harriet Lane Handbook, 7th ed. Chicago, Year Book Medical Publishers, Inc., 1975)

Urinalysis—Ranges from Newborn/Infant to Adult

Determination	Age/Sex	Normal Value		
Addis count				
Leukocytes		below 10		
Erythrocytes		below 5		
Casts		occasional hyaline		
Colony count,				
colonies/ml.				*Suprapubic*
urine (fresh	*Clean catch,*			*Bladder*
specimen)·	*Midstream*	*Catheterization*		*Puncture*
Infant/child	below 1,000	100		0
Thereafter	below 10,000	100		0
Microscopic				
Leukocytes		0 per high-power field– 4 per high-power field		
Erythrocytes		Rare per high-power field		
Casts		Rare per high-power field		
Osmolarity	Premature/ newborn	50 mOsm/liter–600 mOsm/liter		
	Thereafter	50 mOsm/liter–1400 mOsm/liter		
	Thereafter	Above 850 mOsm/liter (after fluid restriction)		
*p*H	Newborn/ neonate	5.0–7.0		
	Thereafter	4.8–7.8		
Protein				
Qualitative		Negative		
Quantitative		10 mgm/day–100 mg/day (higher after strenuous exercise)		
Specific gravity	Newborn/infant	1.001–1.020		
(random)	Thereafter	1.001–1.030		
	Thereafter	Above 1.025 (after fluid restriction)		
Sugar, qualitative (including glucose)		Negative		
Volume	Newborn/neonate	50 ml/day–300 ml/day		
	Infant	350 ml/day–550 ml/day		
	Child	500 ml/day–1000 ml/day		
	Adolescent	700 ml/day–1400 ml/day		
	Thereafter—male	800 ml/day–2000 ml/day		
	female	800 ml/day–1600 ml/day		

*Pure cultures with colony counts >100,000 are considered diagnostic in adults, whereas colony counts of >10,000 are usually considered diagnostic in children. Intermediate counts must be interpreted relative to the clinical situation. For females, the physician must be aware of the cleanliness and care used in collecting the specimen. Urine obtained by means of a plastic collection device or by voiding into a container without prior preparation of the patient is usually contaminated and has limited usefulness in evaluating the possibility of urinary tract infections.

(Vaughn VC, McKay RJ, Behrman RE: Nelson's Textbook of Pediatrics, 11th ed. Philadelphia, WB Saunders, 1979)

Cerebrospinal Fluid for an Adult

Determination	Normal Value
Cell count	0 mononuclear cells/cu mm– 5 mononuclear cells/cu mm
Chloride	100 mEq/liter–130 mEq/liter
Colloidal gold	0000000000
Glucose	50 mgm/dl–75 mgm/dl
Protein	
Lumbar	15 mgm/dl–45 mgm/dl
Cisternal	15 mgm/dl–25 mgm/dl
Ventricular	5 mgm/dl–15 mgm/dl

Cerebrospinal Fluid for a Child

Determination	Normal Value
Amount (obtainable by LP)	
Newborn	up to 5 ml
Adult	100 ml–150 ml
Initial pressure	
Newborn	50 mm CSF–90 mm CSF
Infant	40 mm CSF–150 mm CSF
Child	70 mm CSF–200 mm CSF
Specific gravity	1.005–1.009
pH at 38°C	7.33–7.42
Calcium	4.5 mm %–5.5 mm % (approximate ionized serum Ca)
Cell count	
Newborn	up to 25 WBC (average of 8) and up to 650 RBC/ cu mm
After first month	up to 7 lymphocytes
Glucose	40 mgm %–80 mgm % (at least half of blood sugar)
Pandy test (mainly globulin)	0 (may be positive in newborn)
Protein (80% albumin)	
Ventricular	5 mgm %–15 mgm %
Cisternal	5 mgm %–25 mgm %
Lumbar	5 mgm %–40 mgm % up to 150 mgm % in newborn*
G-O transaminase	4 U–14 U, often about half of SGOT

*Because of insufficient available data on newborn CSF, it is not possible to define normal limits or to make fine diagnostic distinctions.

(Johns Hopkins Hospital: The Harriet Lane Handbook, 7th ed. Chicago, Year Book Medical Publishers, Inc., 1975)

CONVERSION TABLES

System of Weights

Metric System	Apothecaries System
0.3 mgm	1/200 gr
0.4 mgm	1/150 gr
0.6 mgm	1/100 gr
1000 mcgm (1 mgm)	1/60 gr
(2 mgm)	1/30 gr
(4 mgm)	1/16 gr
(8 mgm)	1/8 gr
(15 mgm or 16 mgm)	1/4 gr
(30 mgm)	1/2 gr
(60 mgm)	1.0 gr
1 gm (1000 mgm)	15 gr
2 gm (2000 mgm)	30 gr (1/2 dr)
4 gm (4000 mgm)	60 gr (1 dr)
15 gm	4 dr
30 gm	1 oz
1000 gm (1 kgm)	2.2 lb

Conversion Formulas

Use the following equation to convert milligrams to grains:
$$mgm \times 0.0154 = gr$$

Use the following equation to convert grams to grains:
$$gm \times 15 = gr$$

Use the following equation to convert grams to drams:
$$gm \times 0.257 = dr$$

Use the following equation to convert grams to ounces:
$$gm \times 0.0311 = oz$$

Use the following equation to convert ounces to grams:
$$oz \times 30 = gm$$

Use the following equation to convert grains to grams:
$$gr \div 15 = gm$$

Use the following equation to convert drams to grams:
$$dr \times 4 = gm$$

Use the following equation to convert grains to milligrams:
$$gr \times 60 = mgm$$

Temperature Equivalents

Centigrade	Fahrenheit
36	96.8
36.5	97.7
37	98.6
37.5	99.5
38	100.4
38.5	101.3
39	102.2
39.5	103.1
40	104
40.5	104.9
41	105.8
41.5	106.7
42	107.6

Conversion Formulas

Use the following equation to convert degrees F to degrees C:

$$(F° - 32) \times \frac{5}{9} = C°$$

Use the following equation to convert degrees C to degrees F:

$$(C° \times \frac{9}{5}) + 32 = F°$$

Equivalent Units of Length

Measurement	Centimeters	Inches
1 mm	.100	0.039
1 cm	1	0.394
1 in	2.54	1
1 ft	30.48	12
1 y	91.4	36
1 m	100	39.4

Length

Inches	Centimeters
1	2.5
2	5.1
4	10.2
6	15.2
8	20.3
12 (1 ft)	30.5
18 (1½ ft)	46
24 (2 ft)	61
30 (2½ ft)	76
36 (3 ft)	91
42 (3½ ft)	107
48 (4 ft)	122
54 (4½ ft)	137
60 (5 ft)	152
66 (5½ ft)	168
72 (6 ft)	183
78 (6½ ft)	198

Equivalent Liquid Measures

Metric System	Apothecaries System
0.065 ml*	1 min
1 ml	15 min
4 ml	1 fl dr
30 ml	1 fl oz
500 ml	1 pt
1000 ml (1 liter)	1 qt
4000 ml	1 gal

Conversion formulas

Use the following equation to convert minims to milliliters:
$$\text{Number of minims} \div 15 = \text{milliliters}$$

Use the following equation to convert fluid ounces to milliliters:
$$\text{Number of fluid ounces} \times 30 = \text{milliliters}$$

*A cubic centimeter (cc) is approximately equivalent to a milliliter (ml); therefore, the two terms are used interchangeably.

Household Equivalents

Household	Apothecaries	Metric
1 tsp or 60 drops	1 fl dr	4 ml–5 ml
1 dessertspoonful	2 fl dr	8 ml–10 ml
3 tsp	1 T or ½ fl oz	15 ml
2 T	1 fl oz	30 ml
4 T	¼ c or 2 fl oz	60 ml
8 T	½ c, 4 fl oz, or 1 teacupful	120 ml
16 T	1 c or 8 fl oz	240 ml
1 pt	16 fl oz	500 ml
1 qt	32 fl oz	1000 ml
1 gal	64 fl oz	4000 ml

Weight Equivalents

Pounds	Kilograms	Pounds	Kilograms
1	0.5	140	63.6
2	0.9	150	68.1
3	1.4	160	72.6
4	1.8	170	77.2
5	2.3	180	81.7
6	2.7	190	86.3
7	3.2	200	90.8
8	3.6	210	95.3
9	4.1	220	100
10	4.5	230	104.4
20	9.1	240	109
30	13.6	250	113.5
40	18.2	260	118
50	22.7	270	122.6
60	27.2	280	127.1
70	31.8	290	131.7
80	36.3	300	136.2
90	40.9	310	140.7
100	45.4	320	149.8
110	50	330	150
120	54.5	340	154.4
130	59	350	158.9

WEIGHT RANGES

Conversion formulas

Use the following equations to convert pounds to kilograms:

$$\text{Pounds} \times 0.454 = \text{kilograms; or,}$$
$$\text{Pounds} \div 2.2 = \text{kilograms}$$

Use the following equation to convert kilograms to pounds:

$$\text{Kilograms} \times 2.2 = \text{pounds}$$

NOTE. 1 lb = 0.454 kgm; 1 kgm = 2.2 lb

100 mmHg ≈ 13.3 kPa.

Index

The letter *t* following a page number indicates tabular material.

Infant
  CPR for, 97–98
  premature, acid-base values for, 384
  surface area estimation in, 379
  term, acid-base values for, 384
Intestine, obstructed, 260–262
Intoxication, 197
Intra-aortic balloon pump, 233
Intracranial pressure
  increased, 195–196
  monitoring of, 213–215
  normal value of, 213
Intracranial pressure waves, 215–218, *215*
Intraventricular pressure monitoring, 214
Intropin (dopamine HCl), 357–358
Intubation, 148–165
  cuff inflation in, 150–151
  endotracheal, 148–150
Isoenzyme studies, 6
Isoproterenol (Isuprel), 363–364
Isuprel (isoproterenol), 363–364

Junctional beats
  nonparoxysmal tachycardia, 47–48
  paroxysmal tachycardia, 48–49
  premature, 46–47
Junctional rhythm, 45–46

Kidney failure, 181–186
  acute, 182–186
  chronic, 181–182
Kussmaul's respiration, 340

Laboratory values, normal, 384–388
Lactic dehydrogenase, 6
Lanoxin (digoxin), 364–367
Larynx, fractured, 117–118
Lavage
  gastric, 269
  peritoneal, 272–274
Length equivalents, 390–391
Levarterenol bitartrate (Levophed or
  Norepinephrine), 367–368
Levin tube, 274–276
Levophed (levarterenol bitartrate), 367–368
Lidocaine HCl (Xylocaine), 368–369
Liquid measure equivalents, 391
Liver
  failure of, 311–312
  injury to, 257
Lown-Ganong-Levine syndrome, 68
Lumbar puncture, 209–211
Lung. See also Respiratory failure.
  edema of, 109–112
  embolus of, 107–109
  manual hyperinflation of, 140

Mafenide acetate (Sulfamylon cream), 298
Magnesium sulfate, 369–370
Mediastinal shift, 116–117
Metabolic acidosis, 317
Metabolic alkalosis, 316–317
Metaraminol bitartrate (Aramine), 351–352
Metric weights, 389
Military anti-shock trousers, 231
Miller-Abbott tube, 278–279
Monitoring
  central venous pressure, 238–242, 241t
  fetal heart, 333–336, *335*
  hemodynamic, 234–253
Murmur, heart, 345
Myocardial contusion, 70–71
Myocardial infarction, 3–12
  cardiac rest in, 9
  CCU transfer in, 12
  clinical manifestations in, 3–4
  comfort in, 8
  complications related to, 13–21
  diagnostic tests in, 4–7
  ECG changes in, 4–5
  emergencies in, 11–12
  emotional support in, 10–11
  history in, 11
  isoenzymes in, 6
  monitoring in, 7–8
  nutrition and elimination in, 10
  oxygen therapy in, 11
  recurrent, 20
  serum enzymes in, 5–6
  treatment and nursing actions in, 7–12

Neurogenic shock, 221, 228–229
Neurological disorders, 195–201
  agitation or restlessness in, 205–206
  eye care in, 207
  general treatment and nursing
    considerations in, 202–208
  intake and output in, 206
  mechanical hyperventilation in, 204
  medications in, 204–205
  neurological status in, 203–204
  nutrition and fluid in, 206
  patient positioning in, 207
  postural abnormalities in, 204
  respiratory function in, 202–203
  seizures in, 208
  special procedures in, 209–218. See also
    individual procedure.
  spinal fluid leakage in, 207
  ventriculostomy tubes in, 208
Nipride (sodium nitroprusside), 370–372
Nomogram for surface area estimation   s
  infants and children, 379
  older children and adults, 380
Norepinephrine (levarterenol bitartrate),
  367–368
Nutrition, total parenteral, 281–285